Public Health: Ethics and Drug Resistance

Public Health: Ethics and Drug Resistance

Edited by Ezekiel Wilson

STATES
ACADEMIC PRESS
www.statesacademicpress.com

States Academic Press,
109 South 5th Street,
Brooklyn, NY 11249, USA

Visit us on the World Wide Web at:
www.statesacademicpress.com

ISBN: 978-1-63989-452-9

Cataloging-in-Publication Data

Public health : ethics and drug resistance / edited by Ezekiel Wilson.
p. cm.
Includes bibliographical references and index.
ISBN 978-1-63989-452-9
1. Public health. 2. Public health--Moral and ethical aspects. 3. Drug resistance.
4. Medical ethics. 5. Bioethics. I. Wilson, Ezekiel.
RA427.25 .P83 2022
362.1--dc23

Table of Contents

Preface

This book has been an outcome of determined endeavour from a group of educationists in the field. The primary objective was to involve a broad spectrum of professionals from diverse cultural background involved in the field for developing new researches. The book not only targets students but also scholars pursuing higher research for further enhancement of the theoretical and practical applications of the subject.

The decrease in the effectiveness of a drug, while treating a disease, is termed as drug resistance. The resistance to antibiotics is generally observed in cases where the medication focuses on a specific bacteria molecule. The specificity of the drug can result in it becoming ineffective if there is any mutation in the molecule of the bacteria. This issue is compounded if the antibiotics are used indiscriminately in livestock. The antibiotics in livestock can result in super-resistant bacteria. The resistance to antibiotics by the bacteria can be either through the bacteria altering the targeted enzyme or using the enzyme to neutralize the antibiotic itself. This book covers in detail some existent theories and innovative concepts revolving around ethics and drug resistance. Different approaches, evaluations, methodologies and advanced studies on public health have been included herein. The book is appropriate for students seeking detailed information in this area as well as for experts.

It was an honour to edit such a profound book and also a challenging task to compile and examine all the relevant data for accuracy and originality. I wish to acknowledge the efforts of the contributors for submitting such brilliant and diverse chapters in the field and for endlessly working for the completion of the book. Last, but not the least; I thank my family for being a constant source of support in all my research endeavours.

Editor

1

Surveillance and Control of Asymptomatic Carriers of Drug-Resistant Bacteria

Euzebiusz Jamrozik and Michael J. Selgelid

Abstract Drug-resistant bacterial infections constitute a major threat to global public health. Several key bacteria that are becoming increasingly resistant are among those that are ubiquitously carried by human beings and usually cause no symptoms (i.e. individuals are asymptomatic carriers) until a precipitating event leads to symptomatic infection (and thus disease). Carriers of drug-resistant bacteria can also transmit resistant pathogens to others, thus putting the latter at risk of infections that may be difficult or impossible to treat with currently available antibiotics. Accumulating evidence suggests that such transmission occurs not only in hospital settings but also in the general community, although much more data are needed to assess the extent of this problem. Asymptomatic carriage of drug-resistant bacteria raises important ethical questions regarding the appropriate public health response, including the degree to which it would be justified to impose burdens and costs on asymptomatic carriers (and others) in order to prevent transmission. In this paper, we (i) summarize current evidence regarding the carriage of key drug-resistant bacteria, noting important knowledge gaps and (ii) explore the implications of existing public health ethics frameworks for decision- and policy-making regarding asymptomatic carriers. *Inter alia*, we argue that the relative burdens imposed by public health measures on healthy carriers (as opposed to sick individuals) warrant careful consideration and should be proportionate to the expected public health benefits in terms of risks averted. We conclude that more surveillance and research regarding community transmission (and the effectiveness of available interventions) will be needed in order to clarify relevant risks and design proportionate policies, although extensive community surveillance itself would also require careful ethical consideration.

E. Jamrozik (✉)
Monash Bioethics Centre, Monash University, Clayton, VIC, Australia

Royal Melbourne Hospital Department of Medicine, University of Melbourne, Parkville, VIC, Australia

Wellcome Centre for Ethics and the Humanities and The Ethox Centre, Nuffield Department of Population Health, University of Oxford, Oxford, UK
e-mail: zeb.jamrozik@gmail.com

M. J. Selgelid
Monash Bioethics Centre, Monash University, Melbourne, VIC, Australia

Keywords Antimicrobial resistance · Drug resistance · Asymptomatic infection · Drug-resistant infection · Ethics · Public health ethics

Introduction

The human body contains more bacterial cells than human cells. We all, thus, "carry" bacteria--especially in our digestive, respiratory, and urogenital tracts – and on our skin (Sender et al. 2016). Bacteria travel with and between human beings, following the daily flux of commuters in cities and crossing the world with international travellers. These 'fellow travellers' are often unsuspected since most of these bacteria cause no overt symptoms (i.e. the human carriers are mostly 'asymptomatic'), and some even have symbiotic benefits for humans.[1] Yet, under certain circumstances (e.g., skin breakdown, bowel surgery, or the use of immunosuppression), some ubiquitous species of bacteria cause 'invasive' disease that may require antibiotic treatment and be life threatening if such treatments are ineffective or unavailable. With increasing use (and overuse) of antibiotics in recent decades, such ubiquitously carried bacteria have in many cases become increasingly resistant to first line (and, in some cases, second line and/or 'reserve') treatments (See Table 12.1). Some have become effectively untreatable with standard antibiotics, and those who develop invasive disease are at high risk of death and/or permanent morbidity (Klein et al. 2007; Tischendorf et al. 2016).

Asymptomatic carriers of resistant ubiquitous bacteria vastly outnumber symptomatic cases (Tischendorf et al. 2016; Smith et al. 2004; Safdar and Bradley 2008) and may carry them unknowingly for months or years (Smith et al. 2004; Carlet 2012; Zimmerman et al. 2013; Marchaim et al. 2007; Kennedy and Collignon 2010), creating risks of disease for carriers as well as risks of transmission to others

Table 12.1 Pathogens frequently carried by healthy individuals

Pathogen	Examples of resistant form(s) of public health importance[b]	Site of carriage
Enterobacteriaceae[a]	CRE (carbapenem resistant enterobacteriaciae)	Digestive tract
Enterococcus faecium	VRE (vancomycin-resistant enterococci	Digestive tract
Clostridium difficile	Vancomycin resistant strains	Digestive tract
Staphylococcus aureus	MRSA (methicillin-resistant *S. aureus*)	Skin, nose
Streptococcus pneumonia	Penicillin resistant strains	Respiratory tract
Haemophilus influenzae	Penicillin / macrolide resistant strains	Respiratory tract

[a]Enterobacteriaciae include: *Klebsiella pneumoniae, Escherichia coli, Enterobacter spp., Serratia spp., Proteus spp.,* and *Providencia spp, Morganella spp.* [b]Adapted from WHO List of Priority Resistant Pathogens

[1] Others can lead to indirect benefits because their presence in the ecological niche of asymptomatic carriage excludes and/or inhibits other more harmful organisms.

(Klein et al. 2007; Tischendorf et al. 2016; Safdar and Bradley 2008; Carlet 2012; Giske et al. 2008). In light of the potential transmission of resistant bacteria from asymptomatic carriers to others, asymptomatic carriage (otherwise referred to as asymptomatic infection, colonization, commensalism, persistence, the carrier state, etc. (Casadevall 2000)) has underexplored ethical implications for public health programs aimed at controlling the spread of drug resistant bacteria.

Though infection control policies often focus on symptomatic cases, in some cases they also apply to apparently healthy individuals (for example, quarantine involves those suspected, but not known, to be infected (Morgan et al. 2017; Kass 2001; Selgelid 2009; Millar 2009)). As more knowledge is gained regarding *community* (as opposed to in-hospital) transmission of drug-resistant bacteria, policymakers will need to determine appropriate responses to this relatively new set of public health problems in the general community. Policy options could include screening and other kinds of interference with the lives of apparently healthy individuals. When potentially transmissible (resistant) asymptomatic carriage is diagnosed, there may sometimes be an ethical rationale for public health interventions to prevent transmission, and these measures (as well as screening itself) may entail significant burdens[2] for carriers (and others) as well as public health benefits. Beyond screening, interventions could include reporting the diagnosis of asymptomatic carriage to authorities, notification of third parties, monitoring of carriers, restrictions on freedom of movement (e.g. quarantine, isolation, travel bans), exclusion of carriers from working in certain occupations, and/or possibly even requirements for treatment of carriers in certain circumstances (See Table 12.1). Where the rate of carriage of highly resistant (i.e. effectively untreatable) bacteria is increasing and/or where community transmission poses significant risks, such public health interventions could have wide-ranging effects on social norms and the everyday lives of healthy individuals (as was the case for tuberculosis and HIV prior to the availability of effective treatments (Fitzgerald 2007)) resulting in stigma and/or social exclusion, in addition to the direct burdens of complying with public health interventions.

A key ethical question concerns whether or not, or the extent to which, public health decision makers should be especially reluctant to impose public health measures that infringe upon the lives of those who are healthy (as opposed to those who are sick). In this chapter, we summarize current knowledge regarding asymptomatic carriage and community transmission, and argue that (i) beliefs that only those with symptoms pose risks to others (and related views, such as 'microbial determinism' – i.e. the idea that all those who acquire a pathogen will develop symptoms) should be discarded, (ii) policymakers should consider the risks posed by asymptomatic carriers of resistant organisms, and (iii) policy formation should be guided public health ethics frameworks such that the burdens imposed on carriers (and others) are minimized (and/or offset) and proportionate to the public health benefits in terms of risks averted; and (iv) designing proportionate interventions will require, *inter alia*, careful assessments of the risks related to asymptomatic carriage, including through expanded, ethically designed, public health surveillance programs.

[2] In this chapter we use the term 'burden' to refer to compromises of people's (especially carriers') liberties and/or wellbeing.

History

In the late nineteenth and early twentieth centuries, pioneering microbiologists such as Robert Koch significantly improved scientific understanding of the microbial agents of infectious disease. In 1890, Koch laid out criteria for inferring causal links between pathogens and disease states, including a requirement that every person with the microbe must show signs of the relevant disease. Only 3 years later Koch realized that this was an error since many people carry pathogenic microbes and can transmit them to others, without themselves showing signs of disease. This insight went against common wisdom at the time and was illustrated in famous cases such as that of 'Typhoid Mary' in New York in 1907: despite being asymptomatic, Mary Mallon transmitted typhoid to many other people through her work as a cook, resulting in several deaths (Soper 1939).

Against Microbial Determinism

Despite this, people might be tempted to think that such cases (of asymptomatic carriage) are exceptions and that the acquisition of potentially pathogenic microbes by a human being (or other animal) will always (or almost always) lead to symptomatic infection (i.e. disease). In some ways, the false view that one's infectious disease status is determined by the pathogens in one's body (which we call 'microbial determinism') is akin to an erroneous view in genetics ('genetic determinism'), according to which phenotype is determined by genotype (de Melo-Martín 2005). Just as particular genetic polymorphisms do not always give rise to particular phenotypes (because many environmental factors as well as cellular and other causal processes are required), acquiring particular pathogens does not always lead to the relevant infectious diseases. Upon acquisition of a pathogen, a complex set of host-pathogen interactions (involving immunological and other causal processes) can lead to a variety of outcomes – e.g. the microbe being eliminated without symptoms, short- or long-term asymptomatic carriage, or symptomatic infection/disease (with rapid or delayed onset)(Casadevall 2000).

Key Drug-Resistant Pathogens

This chapter focuses on the ethical implications associated with a subset of WHO Priority Resistant Pathogens (World Health Organisation 2017a): among those with resistance profiles of public health concern, we concentrate on pathogens that are ubiquitous organisms in the bacterial flora of the human body in healthy individuals (Table 12.1) where – in the majority of carriers, whether the bacteria are resistant or not – they usually cause no symptoms[3] until a precipitating event leads to invasive disease (Tischendorf et al. 2016; Safdar and Bradley 2008; Carlet 2012). Such invasive disease can occur in otherwise completely healthy carriers, although it is more common in those with comorbidities, especially those associated with reduced immune function (e.g. diabetes, HIV etc.). We are also particularly concerned with community as opposed to in-hospital transmission, as the latter has received more analysis elsewhere (Millar 2012), including in this volume.

Many of our arguments may be relevant to other increasingly resistant bacteria, including (i) gastro-intestinal and sexually transmitted pathogens that are associated with a high rate of symptomatic infection when a person is first exposed (e.g. *Campylobacter, Salmonella* (including typhoid), *Shigella,* and *Gonorrhea*) following which only some people will become chronic asymptomatic carriers, and (ii) *Helicobacter pylori*, a less ubiquitous pathogen for which carrier status is associated with a range of clinical severity from no symptoms to mild indigestion to overt peptic ulcer disease and/or stomach cancer.

The Public Health Problem

With widespread use (and overuse) of antibiotics, the number of asymptomatic carriers of resistant bacteria (henceforth 'asymptomatic carriers') is increasing. It is difficult to characterize the overall carriage rates of the many different types of clinically significant resistant organisms, since the rate of carriage (and the rate of invasive infection) of each varies considerably between populations, and quoted rates will depend on the quality and extent of public health surveillance in different settings (Laxminarayan et al. 2016; Bryce et al. 2016; Bernabé et al. 2017; Nordmann et al. 2011; Schwaber and Carmeli 2013). In any case, *symptomatic* resistant bacterial infections already cause hundreds of thousands of deaths globally per year (although few estimates of the total burden are available) (Laxminarayan et al. 2016; O'Neill 2015) and increase healthcare costs by billions of dollars (Klein et al. 2007; Giske et al. 2008; O'Neill 2015). The true population prevalence of *asymptomatic* carriage of resistant bacteria is often unknown, because not enough community surveillance data are available. Most data come from hospital settings and are biased by the inclusion of a disproportionate number of symptomatic cases and a focus on patients who have contact with healthcare institution(s) as opposed to the wider community (World Health Organization 2014).

Globally, the rate of carriage and/or disease from resistant organisms tracks disadvantage, with higher rates in many low- and middle-income countries (LMICs) (Bernabé et al. 2017). For example, a recent study in a Malaysian hospital found that around 50% of patients screened on arrival to hospital were carrying

[3] Emerging microbiome research programs are, however, seeking links between strains of colonization and a wide range of 'subclinical' physical and mental health outcomes.

carbapenem resistant Enterobacteriaciae (CRE)[4] in their digestive tract (Zaidah et al. 2017) – of whom perhaps up to 1 in 6 can be expected to develop invasive disease, with overall mortality among carriers reportedly around 10% (Tischendorf et al. 2016). In general, there is a much higher rate of mortality from resistant infections in poor communities, including among infants – some of whom acquire resistant infections from mothers and/or family members (and/or, for infants admitted to hospital, from staff or other patients) who are asymptomatic carriers (Chan et al. 2013). One 2016 estimate suggested that of the 680,000 annual neonatal deaths due to bacterial infection, the vast majority of which occur in LMICs, around 31% (214,500) were due to resistant infections (Laxminarayan et al. 2016).

Yet the problem is by no means confined to developing regions. A 2016 systematic review of *E. coli*[5] urinary infections among children (with the usual source of such infections being asymptomatic carriage of *E. coli* in the child's digestive tract) found that the highest rates of resistance to first-line penicillin antibiotics occurred in (lower income) non-OECD countries (79.8%), but rates in (higher income) OECD countries were still relatively high (53.4%) (Bryce et al. 2016).

More epidemiological research is urgently needed to quantify the rates of carriage of key pathogens in different populations, as well as the rates of disease among carriers and the rates of transmission from (symptomatic and asymptomatic) carriers to others in different contexts. Novel, less expensive, genomic screening techniques are expected to facilitate such investigations (Kwong et al. 2017).

Antibiotic Use and Drug Resistance

The use of antibiotics that kill sensitive bacteria in the human microbiome inevitably leads to the evolutionary selection of drug resistant bacteria. Despite concerns regarding underuse, the vast majority of drug resistant bacteria in humans arise due to antibiotic overuse and 'appropriate' use (Llewelyn et al. 2017).[6] Importantly, when antibiotics are prescribed/taken to treat one type of (suspected or confirmed) infection, many other bacteria carried in the body are exposed to the same antibiotics, which select for resistant strains by killing sensitive ones. It is mainly these 'off-target' effects that lead to asymptomatic carriage of resistant forms of ubiquitous bacteria (Llewelyn et al. 2017). This means that whether a given prescription for antibiotics is 'appropriate' (e.g. because the patient actually has a symptomatic infection with the pathogen for which she is being treated) or not, each additional dose of antibiotics potentially adds to the burden of resistant bacteria carried in the

---

[4] i.e. highly resistant bacteria predominantly found in the digestive tract, a group considered "critical" (i.e. of highest importance) on the WHO Priority list.

[5] *E. coli* is an important species in the family of *Enterobacteriaciae*, carried primarily in the digestive tract (see Table 12.1 and footnote above).

[6] In this paper we focus on human use, although animal and agricultural use is an important contributor to drug-resistant human infection.

body (Carlet 2012). Furthermore, at the population level, it is otherwise relatively healthy occasional users of antibiotics (taken together) who contribute the most to the prevalence of (asymptomatic carriage of) drug-resistant bacteria, rather than the relatively few, relatively sick individuals whose antibiotic use is more frequent and/or intensive (Olesen et al. 2018). In any case, although reducing the use of antibiotics is one important policy to reduce carriage of drug-resistant bacteria, this chapter focuses on other potential community interventions that have received less ethical analysis in this context (Bryce et al. 2016; Barbosa and Levy 2000; Bronzwaer et al. 2002).

Transmission

Even those who never use antibiotics can acquire resistant pathogens through (direct or indirect) contact with carriers (Zimmerman et al. 2013; Schwaber and Carmeli 2013; Waters et al. 2004; Paterson 2006). Living in close contact with carriers (Eveillard et al. 2004; Granoff and Daum 1980), hospitalization(Eveillard et al. 2004; Cronin et al. 2017), working in healthcare (Eveillard et al. 2004; Albrich and Harbarth 2008), and travel to countries with high rates of resistant organisms (Kennedy and Collignon 2010) are all risk factors for the acquisition of resistant pathogens via transmission. Increasingly, outbreak investigations have demonstrated transmission networks that connect symptomatic and asymptomatic individuals both within hospitals and in the wider community (Smith et al. 2004; Kwong et al. 2017). Community transmission of some pathogens is relatively well understood; for example, colonization with methicillin resistant *S. aureus* (MRSA) is associated with transmission within families (Eveillard et al. 2004; Fritz et al. 2014; Manian 2003), while the transmission of many other resistant pathogens has been primarily studied in the hospital setting (if at all).

Duration of Carriage

Once an individual becomes a carrier of resistant bacteria, the duration of carriage depends on complex local factors at the site of carriage including competition from other strains or other species of bacteria, as well as the carrier's immune response, and whether (more) antibiotics are used (Andersson and Hughes 2010). Few studies have estimated the average duration of carriage of key resistant bacteria in the general population; studies in returned travellers have suggested a decrease in carriage over months, with most individuals carrying detectable levels of resistant strains for a few months and a minority (around 10%) developing long-term carriage of 6 months or more (Kennedy and Collignon 2010).

Potential Public Health Responses

Strategies for preventing the transmission of drug-resistant bacteria from asymptomatic carriers include a wide range of potential interventions (Table 12.2). Each of these interventions could involve burdens for carriers (and others, for example family members) – to a greater or lesser degree, depending on the chosen policy and its implementation. Such burdens may include reduced well-being, infringements on privacy,[7] restrictions of other freedoms (including freedom of movement and freedom to decide on the medical interventions to which one will be subjected (Table 12.2)[8]) (Inness 1996), and significant financial costs.[9] Interventions can be more or less coercive ranging from being offered, recommended, or self-enforced to strictly coerced and/or backed by legal sanctions including fines and/or prison terms.

Thus, the design and implementation of infection control policy will inevitably involve ethical tradeoffs (Millar 2009; Millar 2012). The focus of most drug-resistant infection policy regarding asymptomatic carriers has been on healthcare contexts (primarily hospitals), yet – with few exceptions (Millar 2009; Millar 2012) – there has been little explicitly ethical analysis of such policies. There has

Table 12.2 Infection control interventions and potential burdens

Public health interventions that could lead to reduced well-being, privacy infringements, and reductions in other freedoms (e.g. freedom of movement, freedom to decide on medical interventions)	
Intervention Types	**Description/examples**
Screening	Testing apparently healthy individuals for carriage
Informing carriers of their status	Communicating and explaining the diagnosis of a carrier state
Notifying public health authorities	Requirements for health workers to report the diagnosis of carrier status
Monitoring	Serial (re)testing to assess carrier status
Treatment or decolonization	Skin/nasal decolonization of MRSA; faecal transplant for CRE
Limitations on freedom of movement	Isolation, quarantine, travel bans
Limitations on social practices	Change of occupation, altered norms of social interaction

[7] We consider privacy to be a freedom; see, for example, Inness (1996).

[8] This paper focuses on burdensome interventions for carriers; there are of course a range of other interventions including nudging or minimally-burdensome behavioral interventions (we thank an anonymous reviewer for pointing this out) and interventions to change healthcare worker behaviors such as antibiotic prescribing (which have received some discussion elsewhere).

[9] Costs arise both for the individuals directly affected and, where public health measures are financed through taxation, for the whole community.

been even less ethical analysis of public health infection control interventions to prevent the transmission of drug resistant bacteria in the general community (i.e. outside healthcare settings).

Surveillance, Notification, and Monitoring

Screening is routinely used to detect asymptomatic carriage of resistant bacteria among hospital patients (Morgan et al. 2017; Perencevich et al. 2004; Cooper et al. 2004). In many jurisdictions, hospitals are required to notify or report the diagnosis of asymptomatic carriage to local infectious diseases departments and/or central agencies, resulting in exceptions to the usual right to privacy over one's own health information (Morgan et al. 2017; Inness 1996; World Health Organisation 2017b). In order to form a more accurate estimate of the reservoir of asymptomatic infection in the community, and accurately assess the transmissibility and invasiveness (i.e. propensity to cause symptomatic disease) of a given pathogen, surveillance would ideally go beyond (hospital) patients and include members of the general community such as (but not necessarily limited to) the close contacts of those known to be carriers. Yet this raises questions regarding how policy should address potential scenarios in which large numbers of asymptomatic carriers of highly resistant pathogens are identified. Furthermore, the accuracy of tests used in surveillance has ethical implications especially where, for example, a false positive test result leads to significant burdens for someone who is not actually a carrier of resistant microbes (or where a false negative result provides false reassurance).

Restrictions of Freedom of Movement (Isolation, Quarantine, Travel Bans)

Although isolation and quarantine of asymptomatic carriers and/or their contacts have sometimes been successful in hospitals, whether such measures would be feasible and/or successful in the general community (e.g. where community members are identified as carriers by public health surveillance) remains uncertain. Restricting the freedom of movement of healthy carriers (or those suspected to be carriers) in the general community would plausibly involve significant infringements on individual liberty, and such restrictions might often lead to greater burdens for healthy carriers than for those suffering with the symptoms of the relevant disease (or, for example, confined to hospital for other reasons), as discussed below (See Sect. 12.4.2).

Treatment and Decolonization

Many asymptomatic bacterial infections in certain populations – for example, asymptomatic bacteriuria in most females – do not require treatment because they lead to a low rate of disease in the carrier (Nicolle et al. 2005). In other cases, either because of risks to the carrier or to others, treatment may lead to a net benefit (although not necessarily to the carrier herself). Treatment of asymptomatic *resistant* bacteria is often more difficult and sometimes referred to as decolonization. Decolonization strategies have been used for MRSA, primarily carried on the skin and in the nose – which allows for topical (i.e. non-invasive) bactericidal treatment[10] (Coates et al. 2009). Although decolonization has primarily been used in carriers with recurrent symptomatic infection in order to benefit the carrier herself, they have also been used in family members (and pets) of at-risk patients and healthcare workers in order to prevent harm to others (Albrich and Harbarth 2008; Guardabassi et al. 2004).

Decolonization for organisms carried in the digestive tract is sometimes more invasive than decolonization of the skin. For example, an effective, last-line treatment for resistant *C difficile*[11] is faecal transplantation (i.e. decolonization (Morgan et al. 2015)), whereby the bowel microbiome of the patient is replaced by feces from a healthy donor (Van Nood et al. 2013). There have been recent reports of the successful use of fecal transplantation to clear (symptomatic or asymptomatic) carriage of ubiquitous bowel organisms that have become highly resistant (e.g. CRE), Freedman and Eppes 2014; Manges et al. 2016; Crum-Cianflone et al. 2015). At present, the use of such procedures has been largely confined to unwell patients, including in intensive care units (Carlet 2012). Yet if such strategies prove to be safe, effective and reliable, they could be more widely implemented to address the carriage and transmission of resistant bowel organisms.

Ethical Issues

Asymptomatic infection raises a number of important ethical issues. In this chapter we focus on ethical considerations related to policy responses to the problem of asymptomatic carriage of resistant strains of ubiquitous bacteria because, as described earlier (i) asymptomatic carriers of such pathogens vastly outnumber symptomatic cases, (ii) carriers are at risk of severe and difficult to treat invasive disease, (iii) carriage of resistant pathogens places others in the community at risk,

---

[10] One limitation of *S. aureus* decolonization is that it uses bactericidal products (albeit with different formulations to other relevant antibiotics) to which the organism can also become resistant.

[11] *C. difficile*: a species of bacteria that is commonly (but not ubiquitously) carried asymptomatically in the bowel and most frequently causes disease in individuals already treated with antibiotics for other conditions.

and (iv) public health interventions to prevent the transmission of resistant bacteria are potentially associated with significant burdens for carriers (and others). Determining the appropriate responses will thus require scientific data regarding the risks involved (e.g. for a given pathogen or resistance mechanism in a given population) as well as moral judgments about the degree to which burdensome interventions to prevent these risks would be justified. An initial question relates to the extent to which the ethical permissibility of a burdensome infection control measure depends on whether contagious carriers are symptomatic as opposed to asymptomatic (i.e. 'healthy'). We begin by arguing for a useful way of applying existing public health ethics frameworks to policy questions, and then give an account of how the principles in such frameworks should be used to inform policy related to asymptomatic carriers.

Applying Public Health Ethics Frameworks

Existing public health ethics frameworks are applicable to the problem of the carriage and community transmission of resistant bacteria by asymptomatic carriers. The principles in different frameworks overlap considerably; Table 12.3 provides a list of relevant principles and examples of how they might be interpreted (based on previous work (Selgelid 2009)). These principles are usually framed as necessary conditions for determining when a given intervention would be justifiable. However, were this to be so, it might seem that certain principles would be difficult to satisfy

Table 12.3 Principles from public health ethics Frameworks

Public Health Ethics Principle	Interpretation/Example
Need for evidence	Evidence of efficacy is needed to justify imposition of potentially burdensome public health interventions.
Least restrictive alternative	Where two interventions are expected to be equally effective, the intervention that involves the least restrictions of liberty should be selected.
Proportionality	The burdens involved in an intervention should be outweighed by public health benefits achieved.
Equity	The intervention should be implemented (and burdens imposed) in an equitable, non-discrimintory manner.
Least harmful alternative	Where two interventions are expected to be equally effective, the intervention that involves the least harms should be selected.
Reciprocity	Those who benefit from public health policies/interventions have a reciprocal duty to assist and/or compensate those on whom burdens are imposed.
Due legal process	Appropriate legal procedures should be followed and individuals should have the right of appeal.
Transparency	Policymaking should be transparent and democratic.

(as necessary conditions) in the context of asymptomatic carriage of drug-resistant bacteria (and/or in many other public health contexts). If the existence of evidence of an intervention's effectiveness is conceived as a necessary condition, for example, then some might think that the current lack of evidence (e.g. of the risks of community transmission of resistant bacteria) precludes the implementation of relevant public health interventions. Such an approach would likely reduce the scope of legitimate public health interventions to a very narrow set (for example, those for which we have very substantial evidence regarding the effectiveness of relevant interventions, and where the attendant burdens are well characterized, etc.). For this and other reasons it is arguably more useful to conceive of such principles as pointing to ethically relevant desiderata the are achieved to a greater or lesser degree (i.e. on a scale) rather than as necessary conditions that are either satisfied or unsatisfied depending on whether some threshold has been crossed (Selgelid 2016).[12] For example, there can be more or less (reliable) evidence regarding the expected public health benefits associated with a given intervention—and a relative lack of evidence (such as the current gaps regarding our knowledge of community transmission of drug-resistant pathogens) might suggest that an intervention should first be instituted as (public health) research (rather than suggesting that it would be ethically unacceptable to implement it at all), and re-evaluated as more evidence comes to light. Furthermore, since there is not likely to be widespread agreement among public health practitioners on any threshold that could be used to characterize a sufficient amount of evidence to justify the implementation of a given intervention (in public health practice, rather than in research), policymakers should consider both evidence and ethical acceptability as matters of degree existing on a scale—the idea being that the more (reliable) evidence one has that an intervention is likely to create a net public health benefit, the more ethically acceptable it would be to implement it in policy, other things being equal.

Likewise the harms of potential interventions should be considered to exist on a spectrum from least to most harmful, liberty infringements on a spectrum from least (e.g., minor and/or short-term) to most restrictive (e.g. major and/or longer duration),[13] and transparency of policy making on a spectrum from least to most

[12]For illustration of how such an approach might work in the context of public health policy regarding gain-of-function research see Selgelid (2016).

[13]Although the Least Restrictive Alternative and Least Harmful Alternative principles are usually framed as necessary conditions, there are often cases where policymakers will be uncertain whether one intervention is more effective and/or less restrictive or harmful than another. In such cases of uncertainty, a scalar framing of the principles might run as follows: "The more confidence policymakers have that two interventions are associated with similar expected public health benefits and significantly different restrictions, the more moral considerations would support selecting the less restrictive alternative, other things being equal. The more confidence policymakers have that two interventions are associated with similar expected public health benefits and significantly different burdens, the more moral considerations would support selecting the less harmful/burdensome alternative, other things being equal." However, in a restricted set of cases where policymakers are very certain that one intervention is equally (or more) effective and less restrictive or harmful, interpreting the principles as necessary conditions will yield similar guidance, other

transparent, and so on—the idea being that the ethical acceptability of interventions will be a matter of degree, and a function of the extent to which they are harmful, restrictive, transparent, etc., other things being equal (Allen and Selgelid 2017). There might often be reasonable disagreement about exactly how the estimated degrees of evidence, harmfulness, restrictiveness, transparency, etc. can/should determine what ultimately ought to be done; but, as a starting point, policymakers should consider how well, or poorly, each available intervention fares with respect to the values/concerns highlighted by each principle before making *judgements* regarding what policies/interventions should be implemented. We consider this to be a practical approach to ethically sensitive public health policymaking; in the next section we illustrate such an approach in the context of asymptomatic carriage of drug resistance.

Public Health Intervention for Healthy Carriers

One might think that public health agencies should be more reluctant to interfere with the lives of healthy asymptomatic carriers as opposed to sick individuals who carry, and/or are suffering from clinical infection due to, the same (resistant) pathogens. The proportionality principle may help to explain such intuitions. Firstly, one way in which it may make a difference, ethically speaking, whether a carrier is symptomatic or not when imposing potentially burdensome public health interventions is that asymptomatic carriers are more likely to be living active lives in general society; whereas the more symptomatic one is, the more likely it is that they will be bedbound and/or admitted to a healthcare facility. In the latter kind of case, one's liberty and well-being are in a sense already impaired by illness, and so some restrictions (to prevent transmission of drug-resistant bacteria) may impose few, if any, additional burdens.[14] For example, public health measures limiting the freedom of movement of carriers (See Table 12.2) would be a more significant burden for healthy carriers whereas the isolation of sick individuals is a relatively minor additional burden, since such individuals are more likely to be restricted in their movement (e.g. confined to a healthcare facility) due to illness.[15] Thus, if the risk of transmission from a healthy individual is similar to, or less than, the risk from a sick

things being equal. We thank an anonymous reviewer for pressing us on this point. For more on this kind of approach to public health ethics frameworks, see Allen and Selgelid (2017).

[14] Those who are ill may also be more likely to understand and comply with burdensome restrictions because they can more easily perceive that they are infected and a risk to others; in some such cases restrictive measures may even be unnecessary since voluntary measures suffice. We thank an anonymous reviewer for suggesting this point.

[15] Some might worry that the systematic imposition of additional burdens on those who are already (in one sense) badly off due to illness would be inequitable; arguably, this would be particularly worrisome if these burdens were disproportionate (see following discussion of proportionality) to the risks averted which is less likely in cases where (i) the additional burden is small and/or (b) the risk of transmission from sick individual carriers is at least as high as, or higher than, the risk from healthy carriers (i.e. most cases).

individual, the burdens would be higher when imposing a given intervention on healthy carriers. Secondly, there may be cases in which healthy carriers and sick carriers impose different risks of transmission to others. Sick carriers may impose higher risks of transmission because (i) in at least some cases, the degree of symptoms (e.g. related to the resistant bacterial infection in question) is correlated with the risk of transmission[16] (Lerner et al. 2015) or because (ii) hospitalisation for illness places one in (direct or indirect) contact with other patients who are at particularly high risk of acquiring and suffering from (resistant) infection due to medical comorbidities and/or contamination of the shared hospital environment. In cases where such conditions hold, not only would the burdens of certain interventions be lower among sick carriers (as discussed above), but the risks (to others) averted would be greater, meaning that imposing similarly restrictive interventions on healthy carriers would be comparatively less proportionate (because more significant burdens would be imposed to avert lower risks). On the other hand, there might be cases in which healthy carriers impose higher risks on others. For example, healthcare workers or food handlers who carry resistant pathogens might impose increased risks on others because of the nature of their work. In such cases, it may be more justifiable to impose burdensome restrictions on such individuals, because these would be more proportionate to the risks involved (c.f. vaccination of healthcare workers (van Delden et al. 2008)).

Burdens of Interventions and Support for Carriers

As noted previously, public health interventions to control the spread of resistant bacteria in the general community could potentially burden carriers to a greater or lesser degree. They may also involve burdens for family members and contacts of known carriers, as well as direct financial costs for those involved and funding costs of relevant public health policy options (which are borne by the wider community and/or lead to forgoing other opportunities to improve public health)[17]. While the threat of drug-resistant infections as an urgent public health problem might prompt some to consider or propose particularly far-reaching and/or coercive interventions, several other public health ethics principles (in addition to the proportionality principle) can provide useful guidance regarding the ethical reasons to ensure that the burdens (and costs) of an intervention are not only proportionate to the public health benefits but also as low as possible (i.e. without unduly compromising the goals of a policy to reduce risks and thereby lead to public health benefits).

[16] for example, urinary frequency and incontinence related to urinary tract infection (e.g. with *E.* coli), diarrhea (e.g. from resistant *Clostridium difficile*), etc. potentially increase the risk of transmission to others.

[17] We thank anonymous reviewers for emphasizing the implications for family members and for pointing out the opportunity cost of public health policies.

First, the least harmful alternative principle holds that interventions must be no more harmful to carriers than necessary (i.e. minimally harmful) – because compromising individuals' well-being requires justification. If two alternative policies/ interventions are expected to be equally beneficial interms of public health protection, then the alternative that is less harmful to carriers should be preferred, other things being equal – See Table 12.3. Second, the reciprocity principle entails that policymakers should consider obligations to assist and support carriers as part of policy implementation so as to reduce or offset the 'net burdens' for those affected. This could include preferential/non-discriminatory access to healthcare, psychological support, assistance with finances or finding other employment, etc.

More broadly, public health agencies should aim to reduce burdens related to stigma through public education campaigns and through informing carriers about important aspects of carriage (for example, that carriage of resistant organisms is frequently not permanent) at the time of diagnosis. Overly burdensome interventions may also lead to perverse incentives for (potential) carriers to avoid diagnosis and/or contact with health authorities, which could lead to greater risks for the carrier and others, undermining the purported public health benefits of a given policy (meaning that the need for evidence includes evidence regarding how well a policy actually works in practice).[18]

The Need for More Surveillance and Research

Practical ethical deliberations guided by the above principles should always be informed by the best available empirical data on the relevant risks related to carriage of a given pathogen and the expected benefits of an intervention. An initial challenge is that, for many infections transmitted by asymptomatic carriers, the risks are not yet well understood because few data are available. There is thus an ethical imperative for increased public health surveillance and research on such infections, including programs aimed at collecting and analyzing long-term data (i.e. involving monitoring) related to asymptomatic carriage in the general community. This again requires careful ethical consideration, since ethically appropriate surveillance also requires striking a balance between public health goals and individual interests; here, too, public health ethics principles and analysis should help to guide policy formation (World Health Organisation 2017b). Likewise, there is an urgent need for more research regarding the relative effectiveness of different potential public health interventions, as well as qualitative research aimed at better characterizing the burdens experienced by carriers. Being able to draw on such empirical data will only serve to improve public health ethics analysis and, ultimately, public health policy.

[18] We thank the participants at the 2018 Brocher workshop "Invisible epidemics: ethics and interventions for asymptomatic carriers of infectious diseases.", in particular Niels Nijsingh and Christian Munthe for helpful discussions of this point.

Conclusions

All human beings are asymptomatic carriers of bacteria, meaning that 'microbial determinism' is false. The increasing prevalence of carriage of *resistant* strains of ubiquitous bacteria is an urgent public health issue, and many apparently healthy individuals are at risk of resistant infections and risk transmitting such pathogens to others. Deliberations regarding the design and implementation of public health policy should be guided not only by empirical data regarding the health risks of a given resistant strain and the public health benefits of a given intervention (and much more data are needed to clarify these risks and benefits), but also by ethical analysis regarding the justification of burdens imposed on carriers. Principles of existing public health ethics frameworks should help policymakers identify important considerations that have particular implications for the design and implementation of infection control policies regarding asymptomatic carriers. The proportionality principle in particular provides reasons for being wary about imposing potentially burdensome interventions on otherwise healthy carriers of drug resistant pathogens—which is not to say that such interventions would never be ethically appropriate.

Acknowledgement Reprinted with permission of John Wiley and Sons (Licence 4890151079850); original citation: Jamrozik, E., & Selgelid, M. J. (2019). Surveillance and control of asymptomatic carriers of drug-resistant bacteria. *Bioethics*, 33(7), 766–775.

References

Albrich, W.C., and S. Harbarth. 2008. Health-care workers: Source, vector, or victim of MRSA? *The Lancet Infectious Diseases* 8 (5): 289–301.

Allen, T., and M.J. Selgelid. 2017. Necessity and least infringement conditions in public health ethics. *Medicine, Health Care and Philosophy* 20 (4): 525–535.

Andersson, D.I., and D. Hughes. 2010. Antibiotic resistance and its cost: Is it possible to reverse resistance? *Nature Reviews Microbiology* 8 (4): 260–271.

Barbosa, T.M., and S.B. Levy. 2000. The impact of antibiotic use on resistance development and persistence. *Drug Resistance Updates* 3 (5): 303–311.

Bernabé, K.J., C. Langendorf, N. Ford, J.-B. Ronat, and R.A. Murphy. 2017. Antimicrobial resistance in West Africa: A systematic review and meta-analysis. *International Journal of Antimicrobial Agents*.

Bronzwaer, S.L.A.M., O. Cars, U. Buchholz, et al. 2002. The relationship between antimicrobial use and antimicrobial resistance in Europe. *Emerging Infectious Diseases* 8 (3): 278.

Bryce, A., A.D. Hay, I.F. Lane, H.V. Thornton, M. Wootton, and C. Costelloe. 2016. Global prevalence of antibiotic resistance in paediatric urinary tract infections caused by Escherichia coli and association with routine use of antibiotics in primary care: systematic review and meta-analysis. *BMJ* 352: i939.

Carlet, J. 2012. The gut is the epicentre of antibiotic resistance. *Antimicrobial Resistance and Infection Control* 1 (1): 39.

Casadevall, A. 2000. Pirofski L-a. Host-pathogen interactions: Basic concepts of microbial commensalism, colonization, infection, and disease. *Infection and Immunity* 68 (12): 6511–6518.

Chan, G.J., A.C.C. Lee, A.H. Baqui, J. Tan, and R.E. Black. 2013. Risk of early-onset neonatal infection with maternal infection or colonization: A global systematic review and meta-analysis. *PLoS Medicine* 10 (8): e1001502.

Coates, T., R. Bax, and A. Coates. 2009. Nasal decolonization of Staphylococcus aureus with mupirocin: Strengths, weaknesses and future prospects. *Journal of Antimicrobial Chemotherapy* 64 (1): 9–15.

Cooper, B.S., S.P. Stone, C.C. Kibbler, et al. 2004. Isolation measures in the hospital management of methicillin resistant Staphylococcus aureus (MRSA): Systematic review of the literature. *BMJ* 329 (7465): 533.

Cronin, K.M., Y.S.P. Lorenzo, M.E. Olenski, et al. 2017. Risk factors for KPC-producing Enterobacteriaceae acquisition and infection in a healthcare setting with possible local transmission: A case–control study. *Journal of Hospital Infection* 96 (2): 111–115.

Crum-Cianflone, N.F., E. Sullivan, and G. Ballon-Landa. 2015. Fecal microbiota transplantation and successful resolution of multidrug-resistant-organism colonization. *Journal of Clinical Microbiology* 53 (6): 1986–1989.

de Melo-Martín, I. 2005. Firing up the nature/nurture controversy: Bioethics and genetic determinism. *Journal of Medical Ethics* 31 (9): 526–530.

Eveillard, M., Y. Martin, N. Hidri, Y. Boussougant, and M.-L. Joly-Guillou. 2004. Carriage of methicillin-resistant Staphylococcus aureus among hospital employees: Prevalence, duration, and transmission to households. *Infection Control & Hospital Epidemiology* 25 (2): 114–120.

Fitzgerald, C. 2007. Kissing can be dangerous. The public health campaigns to prevent and control tuberculosis in Western Australia, 1900–1960. *Australian Journal of Social Issues Subscriptions* 42 (2): 273.

Freedman, A., and S. Eppes. 2014. Use of stool transplant to clear Fecal Colonization with Carbapenem-Resistant Enterobacteraciae (CRE): Proof of concept. *Open Forum Infectious Diseases* (1):S65. Oxford University Press.

Fritz, S.A., P.G. Hogan, L.N. Singh, et al. 2014. Contamination of environmental surfaces with Staphylococcus aureus in households with children infected with methicillin-resistant S aureus. *JAMA Pediatrics* 168 (11): 1030–1038.

Giske, C.G., D.L. Monnet, O. Cars, and Y. Carmeli. 2008. Clinical and economic impact of common multidrug-resistant gram-negative bacilli. *Antimicrobial Agents and Chemotherapy* 52 (3): 813–821.

Granoff, D.M., and R.S. Daum. 1980. Spread of Haemophilus influenzae type b: Recent epidemiologic and therapeutic considerations. *The Journal of pediatrics* 97 (5): 854–860.

Guardabassi, L., S. Schwarz, and D.H. Lloyd. 2004. Pet animals as reservoirs of antimicrobial-resistant bacteria Review. *Journal of Antimicrobial Chemotherapy* 54 (2): 321–332.

Inness J.C. 1996. *Privacy, intimacy, and isolation*: Oxford University Press on Demand.

Kass, N.E. 2001. An ethics framework for public health. *American Journal of Public Health* 91 (11): 1776–1782.

Kennedy, K., and P. Collignon. 2010. Colonisation with Escherichia coli resistant to "critically important" antibiotics: A high risk for international travellers. *European Journal of Clinical Microbiology & Infectious Diseases* 29 (12): 1501–1506.

Klein, E., D.L. Smith, and R. Laxminarayan. 2007. Hospitalizations and deaths caused by methicillin-resistant Staphylococcus aureus, United States, 1999–2005. *Emerging Infectious Diseases* 13 (12): 1840.

Kwong, J.C., C. Lane, F. Romanes, et al. 2017. *bioRxiv* 175950.

Laxminarayan, R., P. Matsoso, S. Pant, et al. 2016. Access to effective antimicrobials: A worldwide challenge. *The Lancet* 387 (10014): 168–175.

Lerner, A., A. Adler, J. Abu-Hanna, S.C. Percia, M.K. Matalon, and Y. Carmeli. 2015, 21. Spread of KPC-producing carbapenem-resistant Enterobacteriaceae: the importance of super-spreaders and rectal KPC concentration. *Clinical Microbiology and Infection* (5): 470. e1–70. e7.

Llewelyn, M.J., J.M. Fitzpatrick, E. Darwin, et al. 2017. The antibiotic course has had its day. *BMJ* 358: j3418.

Manges, A.R., T.S. Steiner, and A.J. Wright. 2016. Fecal microbiota transplantation for the intestinal decolonization of extensively antimicrobial-resistant opportunistic pathogens: A review. *Infectious Diseases* 48 (8): 587–592.

Manian, F.A. 2003. Asymptomatic nasal carriage of mupirocin-resistant, methicillin-resistant Staphylococcus aureus (MRSA) in a pet dog associated with MRSA infection in household contacts. *Clinical Infectious Diseases* 36 (2): e26–e28.

Marchaim, D., S. Navon-Venezia, D. Schwartz, et al. 2007. Surveillance cultures and duration of carriage of multidrug-resistant Acinetobacter baumannii. *Journal of Clinical Microbiology* 45 (5): 1551–1555.

Millar, M. 2009. Do we need an ethical framework for hospital infection control? *Journal of Hospital Infection* 73 (3): 232–238.

———. 2012. 'Zero tolerance'of avoidable infection in the English National Health Service: Avoiding the redistribution of burdens. *Public Health Ethics* 6 (1): 50–59.

Morgan, D.J., S. Leekha, L. Croft, et al. 2015. The importance of colonization with Clostridium difficile on infection and transmission. *Current Infectious Disease Reports* 17 (9): 43.

Morgan, D.J., R.P. Wenzel, and G. Bearman. 2017. Contact precautions for endemic MRSA and VRE: Time to retire legal mandates. *JAMA* 318 (4): 329–330.

Nicolle, L.E., S. Bradley, R. Colgan, J.C. Rice, A. Schaeffer, and T.M. Hooton. 2005. Infectious Diseases Society of America guidelines for the diagnosis and treatment of asymptomatic bacteriuria in adults. *Clinical Infectious Diseases*: 643–654.

Nordmann, P., T. Naas, and L. Poirel. 2011. Global spread of carbapenemase-producing Enterobacteriaceae. *Emerging Infectious Diseases* 17 (10): 1791.

Olesen, S.W., M.L. Barnett, D.R. MacFadden, et al. 2018. The distribution of antibiotic use and its association with antibiotic resistance. *bioRxiv* 473769.

O'Neill, J. 2015. Antimicrobial resistance: Tackling a crisis for the health and wealth of nations. The Review on Antimicrobial Resistance. Chaired by Jim O'Neill. December 2014.

Paterson, D.L. 2006. The epidemiological profile of infections with multidrug-resistant Pseudomonas aeruginosa and Acinetobacter species. *Clinical Infectious Diseases* 43 (Supplement_2): S43–S48.

Perencevich, E.N., D.N. Fisman, M. Lipsitch, A.D. Harris, J.G. Morris Jr., and D.L. Smith. 2004. Projected benefits of active surveillance for vancomycin-resistant enterococci in intensive care units. *Clinical Infectious Diseases* 38 (8): 1108–1115.

Safdar, N., and E.A. Bradley. 2008. The risk of infection after nasal colonization with Staphylococcus aureus. *The American Journal of Medicine* 121 (4): 310–315.

Schwaber, M.J., and Y. Carmeli. 2013. An ongoing national intervention to contain the spread of carbapenem-resistant Enterobacteriaceae. *Clinical Infectious Diseases* 58 (5): 697–703.

Selgelid, M.J. 2009. A moderate pluralist approach to public health policy and ethics. *Public Health Ethics* 2 (2): 195–205.

———. 2016. Gain-of-function research: Ethical analysis. *Science and Engineering Ethics* 22 (4): 923–964.

Sender, R., S. Fuchs, and R. Milo. 2016. Revised estimates for the number of human and bacteria cells in the body. *PLoS Biology* 14 (8): e1002533.

Smith, D.L., J. Dushoff, E.N. Perencevich, A.D. Harris, and S.A. Levin. 2004. Persistent colonization and the spread of antibiotic resistance in nosocomial pathogens: resistance is a regional problem. *Proceedings of the National Academy of Sciences of the United States of America* 101 (10): 3709–3714.

Soper, G.A. 1939. The curious career of Typhoid Mary. *Bulletin of the New York Academy of Medicine* 15 (10): 698.

Tischendorf, J., R.A. de Avila, and N. Safdar. 2016. Risk of infection following colonization with carbapenem-resistant Enterobactericeae: A systematic review. *American Journal of Infection Control* 44 (5): 539–543.

van Delden, J.J.M., R. Ashcroft, A. Dawson, G. Marckmann, R. Upshur, and M.F. Verweij. 2008. The ethics of mandatory vaccination against influenza for health care workers. *Vaccine* 26 (44): 5562–5566.

Van Nood, E., A. Vrieze, M. Nieuwdorp, et al. 2013. Duodenal infusion of donor feces for recurrent Clostridium difficile. *New England Journal of Medicine* 368 (5): 407–415.

Waters, V., E. Larson, F. Wu, et al. 2004. Molecular epidemiology of gram-negative bacilli from infected neonates and health care workers' hands in neonatal intensive care units. *Clinical Infectious Diseases* 38 (12): 1682–1687.

World Health Organisation. 2017a. *WHO guidelines on use of medically important antimicrobials in food-producing animals*. Geneva: WHO.

———. 2017b. *WHO guidelines on ethical issues in public health surveillance*. Geneva.

World Health Organization. 2014. *Antimicrobial resistance: global report on surveillance*: World Health Organization.

Zaidah, A.R., N.I. Mohammad, S. Suraiya, and A. Harun. 2017. High burden of Carbapenem-resistant Enterobacteriaceae (CRE) fecal carriage at a teaching hospital: Cost-effectiveness of screening in low-resource setting. *Antimicrobial Resistance & Infection Control* 6 (1): 42.

Zimmerman, F.S., M.V. Assous, T. Bdolah-Abram, T. Lachish, A.M. Yinnon, and Y. Wiener-Well. 2013. Duration of carriage of carbapenem-resistant Enterobacteriaceae following hospital discharge. *American Journal of Infection Control* 41 (3): 190–194.

2

Providing Universal Access While Avoiding Antiretroviral Resistance: Ethical Tensions in HIV Treatment

Bridget Haire

Abstract The provision of effective antiretroviral therapy is an ethical imperative, and global access to antiretroviral drugs is an important aspect of this. The other less recognised aspect of effective HIV management is in ensuring that HIV does not become resistant to the drugs used in treatment (and increasingly also in prevention), as multi-drug resistant HIV poses a major threat to the sustainability of current responses to HIV control. In resource-constrained environments, the rapid scale up of access to life-saving anti-HIV treatment was achieved using a public health approach that standardised antiretroviral regimens, minimised laboratory monitoring, and devolved responsibilities from clinicians where necessary. In recent years demand for antiretroviral treatment has increased due to new understandings of the clinical importance of early treatment, but global investment has declined. Exponential growth of the population using antiretrovirals without careful monitoring increases the risk of significant antiretroviral drug resistance. In this chapter, I consider the example of single-drug interventions to prevent parent-to-child HIV transmission, and how the implementation of that strategy increased health risks for mothers. I argue that while global antiretroviral scale up must continue, laboratory monitoring at individual and national levels needs to improve to maintain treatment effectiveness, and protocols for moving people from failing regimens need to be strengthened.

Keywords Ethics · Public health · Infectious diseases

B. Haire (✉)
Kirby Institute, University of NSW, Sydney, Australia
e-mail: b.haire@unsw.edu.au

Introduction

With an estimated 36.9 million people living with HIV worldwide (WHO 2018), the provision of effective antiretroviral therapy (ART) is an ethical imperative. Ensuring that people with HIV can access ART is an important part of this, but another less recognised aspect is ensuring that the HIV does not become resistant to the drugs used in the treatment, as multi-drug resistant HIV poses a major threat to the sustainability of current responses to HIV control. There are, however, ethical tensions about striking the right balance between maximising ART access and minimising the risk of the emergence of drug resistant HIV. In resource-constrained environments these tensions are concerned with relative investment in drugs as compared with laboratory monitoring, and sometimes 'blaming' discourses regarding non-adherent people with HIV.

In 1996 it was established that antiretroviral drugs used in combination could control HIV replication ('viral load') in individuals and thus prevent HIV from destroying the CD4 cells that protect against infection (Arts and Hazuda 2012). Over time, the control of viral replication was shown to prevent people with HIV from becoming immune suppressed and developing the opportunistic infections associated with acquired immune deficiency syndrome (AIDS) (Moore and Chaisson 1999). ART could also reverse immune damage, to some extent (Kaufmann et al. 2005). Thus, combination ART could prevent AIDS and prolong, and perhaps save, the lives of people with HIV. Initial drug regimens however were often highly complex. The drugs were associated with serious side effects and were prohibitively expensive, as were the laboratory tests used to monitor both the impact of the drugs on viral load (viral load tests) and the degree of immune functionality (measured by CD4 cell tests). Hence there were significant barriers to access to these regimens for the majority of people living with HIV.

The stark injustice of life saving medication being inaccessible to the majority of those living with HIV, concentrated predominantly in low and middle income countries (LMIC) and especially in sub-Saharan Africa, was the catalyst for a worldwide treatment access movement that put pressure on governments, drug companies and non-government organisations to find solutions to make ART access more equitable. In response to the treatment access movement the World Health Organization launched its first 'public health' program for HIV treatment, an approach that aimed for universal access, starting with the initial goal of getting 3 million people onto ART by 2005, the '3 by 5 Programme' (WHO 2003a, b). This approach was supported and facilitated by the creation of two major donor organisations – The Global Fund for HIV, TB and Malaria (the Global Fund), and the (US) President's Emergency Program for AIDS Relief (PEPFAR) – that supplied drugs to LMIC (Smart 2006). Even with these donors, it was not feasible to mimic the highly individualised approach to ART prescription in affluent countries that relied heavily on expensive and resource-intensive laboratory monitoring. Accordingly, the program standardised both ART regimens (the drugs) and monitoring (including tests that measure the effect of the drugs on viral load and those that measured the impact of

HIV on the immune system). In some LMIC, nurse-practitioners performed roles usually reserved for doctors. Thus, the 'public health' approach was designed to facilitate ART delivery in resource-poor settings with limited health infrastructure, simplifying, standardising and devolving responsibilities as required (WHO 2003a, b). (Note, while the '3 by 5 Programme' was the initial iteration of this approach, the WHO has continued to champion universal access programmatically using a public health approach. For simplicity's sake, in this chapter I will treat the WHO universal access/public health approach as a strategy that started with '3 by 5' and has continued to this day, albeit with various adjustments and shifts in nomenclature.)

This chapter will first describe the mechanism for the development of HIV drug resistance and detail elements of the 'public health' approach to ART. It will then discuss how and why the 'public health' approach to ART in lower income countries was a reasonable trade-off that enabled widespread access to HIV treatment, despite increasing the likelihood of the development of drug resistance. In the medium to long term, however, strategies to avoid, contain and diagnose drug resistance will be critical to the sustained management of the epidemic, and to reaching the global goal of virtual elimination of new HIV infections. The tensions between a public health approach that focuses on access and an increasing emphasis on effective use of resources will be explored, using the history of mother-to-child prevention programs as a case study. The increasing use of ART-based prevention strategies for sexual transmission will also be considered. Finally consideration will be given to issues likely to impact on responses to drug resistant HIV in a context where guidelines recommend universal treatment, but access to uninterrupted drug supplies and high quality monitoring standards are limited.

Drug Resistant HIV

HIV is a highly mutable virus, meaning that as it replicates it makes errors and hence changes and evolves over time within the human host. These changes are random, though the principles of natural selection mean that over time and in the absence of treatment, changes that make the virus more replication competent will crowd out those that make it less fit.

Drug resistant HIV develops when a person is taking ART that is insufficient to fully suppress viral replication. This creates the conditions of selective pressure, so that viral copies that are less sensitive to the drugs have a competitive advantage over other viral copies, and begin to push the evolution of HIV in the particular body to become increasingly resistant. If the ART regimen is sufficient to fully suppress replication, this will not occur and hence resistance will not develop. Standard ART regimens will fully suppress viral replication if adherence is good, if no biological event disrupts individual drug absorption and metabolism, and unless the person was infected with a strain of HIV that had already evolved to be resistant to some or all of the drugs in the particular ART regimen.

In terms of the potential development of ART resistance, all ART drugs are not equal – the strength of antiretroviral action can differ, and some drugs are more vulnerable to the development of resistance. ART drugs work by targeting and blocking selected enzymes or proteins of HIV that enable it to replicate and infect cells. Changes to particular HIV regions that the ART drugs target make the drugs less effective. Some regions of HIV are more prone to mutation than others, and some drugs lose their effectiveness in the face of HIV evolution faster than others. For example, a single mutation reduces susceptibility to the drug nevirapine (this is called having a low genetic barrier to resistance) (Luber 2005). Drug resistance is also not a black and while phenomenon, in that a particular mutation or set of mutations may diminish susceptibility to particular drugs, but not completely stop working in terms of controlling HIV replication. For example, a person taking ART who has a detectable but low viral load may have some drug resistance, but may also be receiving clinical benefit from the drugs.

ART drugs are classified into classes that are determined by where and how they target HIV replication. While ART drugs within the designated classes work in slightly different ways, developing resistance to one drug in a class can also confer either resistance (or at least reduced sensitivity) to other drugs in the class. Accordingly, if a person has to change from one ART regimen to another, the second regimen needs to comprise drugs to which there is no likely pre-existing cross resistance to maximise the likely success. Further, in high income countries like Australia, when a person is first diagnosed with HIV, genetic resistance testing determines whether the person has been infected with a resistant strain of HIV that is less likely to respond optimally to standard treatment (if resistance is found, different regimens are used).

In summary, there are four main causes of drug resistance: acquiring a drug resistant strain; being prescribed a regimen that is incompletely suppressive (usually single or dual therapy combinations, or a triple combination that is too weak); non-adherence (failing to take pills as prescribed and on time); and taking drugs intermittently (where fluctuating blood levels of medication allow HIV replication under selective pressure).

A Word on HIV Monitoring

There are two highly significant tests used to monitor HIV disease progression and the effectiveness of ART in an individual: Tests that count CD4 cells per cubic ml of blood, and viral load tests. CD4 cells are immune cells that are targeted by HIV. A healthy person would have a CD4 cell count in excess of 500. Once a person's CD4 cell count drops to 200 or below s/he is at serious, imminent risk of HIV-related opportunistic infections. A person with HIV who has a CD4 cell count above 200 but below 500 is showing some HIV-related damage. There is a strong relationship between declines in CD4 cell count and disease progression, and in CD4 cell recovery and effective ART treatment (Mellors et al. 1997). CD4 counts are thus a useful tool in the management of HIV disease.

Viral load tests measure viral RNA in the peripheral blood. The higher the viral RNA number is, the greater the level of viral replication, and the greater the risk of disease progression (Mellors et al. 1996). 'Undetectable viral load' means that viral replication is suppressed below the level of detection on the test used (tests have become much more sensitive since they were first available). An undetectable viral load is the individual goal of ART treatment. At the strategic level, having 90% of people who know their HIV status on ART, and 90% of those with an undetectable viral load is a current global goal (UNAIDS 2017).

Key Elements of the 'Public Health' Approach to HIV

To maximise access to life-saving ART, WHO prioritised getting ART drugs into the bodies of people with HIV, and maximising the capacity to deliver ART by processes of standardisation, simplification and, where necessary, syndromic management rather than laboratory monitoring. The core underlying principles were identified as urgency, equity and sustainability (Macklin 2004).

Standardised first line and second line ART regimens were a critical aspect of the approach. In determining the drugs used in these regimens, a balance had to be struck between user-friendliness (pill burden, dosing routine, side effect profile), effectiveness (probability of viral load suppression), and cost (WHO 2003a). Further, the second line regimen had to be effective against the ART resistance likely to develop (for whatever reason) to the drugs in the first line regimen. (Third line regimens are also detailed in guidelines.) These standardised regimens were presented as algorithms that were flexible enough to allow for the different availability of certain drugs in particular countries due to purchasing arrangements, and to allow some substitutions for people who had different health needs, such as those who were pregnant, had other infections like TB or viral hepatitis. The standard algorithms for first and second line treatment have changed since the first iteration of the WHO universal access program, as further information about drug efficacy emerged (for example, a first line regimen recommended in 2003 was found to be insufficient of suppress very high viral loads found in people initiating treatment in advanced disease), and alternative drugs became available to replace ART associated with significant toxicities (Gulick et al. 2004). Both inadequate viral suppression and high levels of side effects are significant for the development of resistance – incomplete suppression create the conditions for the emergence of resistance, and ART toxicities can reduce adherence, also potentially resulting in incomplete suppression.

The issue of how to prioritise people for treatment access was another critical element of the approach. Utility, equity and concern for the worst-off (the principle of maximin) were key considerations (Macklin 2004). Initial WHO guidance for resource constrained settings recommended that ART should be commenced in those at high and proximate risk of clinical disease progression and/or death (those diagnosed with Stage IV HIV disease regardless of CD4 cell count; those with CD4 cell counts below 200 regardless of disease staging; those with stage III HIV disease and CD4 counts below 35) (WHO 2003a). Targeting ART at those at experiencing or at imminent risk of serious HIV disease was acceptable in a moral sense as it prioritised treatment for those with greatest clinical need, and it also greatly reduced the pool of people eligible for treatment, as only a fraction of those living with HIV would require treatment under such guidance. The downside to this approach was that many people tested and found HIV positive would not be eligible for treatment, increasing the potential of significant loss to follow-up (Rosen and Fox 2011). It is important to note that while WHO guidelines play an important normative role in shaping standards, they are in no sense binding, and the expectation of their use is that countries draw from them and adapt them according to relevant contextual factors (WHOF 2006).

Laboratory monitoring was simplified in WHO guidance documents, with CD4 cell tests recommended but not mandatory both at baseline and for subsequent monitoring of treatment efficacy at 6–12 month intervals. Haemoglobin testing would occur depending on the drug regimen (it was required if AZT was included.) Other blood work such as white blood cell and liver function tests were to be ordered as determined by clinical symptoms, and viral load testing – the gold standard for measuring ART response – not even mentioned. Developing guidelines for the surveillance of drug resistance was however one of the itemised strategic actions of the initial '3 by 5 Programme' (WHO 2003a, b). The low level of laboratory monitoring was contentious, given that the longer a person stays on a failing regimen, the greater the opportunity both for the development of resistance and the loss of clinical benefit. Accordingly, a randomised control trial (RCT) investigated whether (and to what extent) ART could be delivered safely without laboratory monitoring (the DART study). This study, first reported in 2009 and published in 2010, found that differences in outcomes occurred after the second year of treatment. Investigators argued that this justified only introducing CD4 cell tests at 24 months, and prioritising spending on ART drugs rather than resource-intensive monitoring (DART Trial Team 2010). Of note, this study only looked at clinical outcomes, in people who already had advanced HIV disease, not at the drug resistance outcomes.

Changes in Eligibility for ART

At the inception of the global universal access program, there was no clear scientific evidence as to the best time to commence ART, except that it clearly prolonged life for those who commenced with low CD4 counts (below 200). From the mid 1990s, many argued on the basis of modelling from other infectious diseases that HIV replication should be suppressed as early and as completely as possible. 'Hit hard, hit early', was the catch cry (Ho 1995). Mitigating against this was the fact that serious HIV disease did not usually occur until 6–10 years after infection, and the problem that ART regimens in the mid to late 1990s were hard to take (with high pill burdens, specific food and or fasting requirements for dosing particular drugs, and high rates of side effects). Of course the rapacious cost of ART was also significant – for example in 1997, 6 months use of the drug AZT was costed at $US 800 – it is now an estimated $US 237 (Pharmacychecker 2017).

From the late 90s, a series of RCTs clarified issues pertaining to treatment commencement, indicating that better outcomes were achieved with earlier treatment initiation. These included CIPRA-HT001, a study in Haiti that showed that people who started ART with CD4 counts higher than 200 had a significantly reduced risk of death (Severe et al. 2010). This result was underscored by findings from the SMART Study, which was designed to test whether structured ART treatment interruptions were safe (people with HIV took treatment interruptions or 'holidays' for a variety of reasons, including relief from side effects). The SMART Study found that not only did treatment interruptions increase the risk of disease progression at any CD4 level, but that the greater time spent with a CD4 count below 350, the greater the risk of HIV disease progression and death (Strategies for Management of Antiretroviral Therapy Study Group 2008). These findings together were the catalyst for a revision of WHO guidelines for resource-constrained environments to recommend ART commencement at the higher CD4 level of 350 (WHO 2009). Two further studies have been critical in pushing WHO ART guidelines toward recommending treatment at higher levels – the HPTN 052 Study, which showed that early ART treatment reduced onward HIV transmission to sexual partners by 96 % (Cohen et al. 2011), and then the START Study, reported in 2015, which showed a clear clinical benefit from early treatment initiation (at CD4 levels of 500 and above), with people who initiated treatment immediately showing significant benefit compared with those who did not initiate ART until their CD4 counts had dropped to 350 or below (The Insight START Study Group 2015). This finding resulted in a revision of WHO guidelines, such that immediate ART therapy is now recommended for any person diagnosed with HIV, regardless of CD4 cell count.

This change to WHO ART guidelines is based in robust evidence about the beneficial impact of immediate ART on health, and where taken up in national guidelines, may reduce the numbers of people diagnosed with HIV who get lost to follow -up due to being deemed ineligible for immediate ART. It also has some problematic implications. Firstly, it increases exponentially the estimates of people living with HIV who require ART, which may increase the likelihood of rationing taking place where supplies are inadequate. Secondly, notwithstanding the fact that some resource-poor countries may continue to align their national guidelines to earlier iterations of the WHO guidance, the expansion of eligibility for ART puts greater demand on ART stocks, and increases the risks of stock-outs, which could have an impact on the development of drug resistance. Even if drug supplies were perfect, human adherence will not be, so the logical result of millions more people taking lifelong ART over many decades must be an increase in drug resistance. Thirdly, increasing the number of people eligible for treatment may increase pressure at country level to continue to prioritise wider access to ART drugs at the expense of improving monitoring, exponentially expanding the risk that large scale poorly monitored ART use poses with regard to development and transmission of drug resistant ART (at higher CD4 cell counts, the risk of death is far more remote that at lower one, so the risks of drug resistance are not so obviously balanced by the overwhelming benefit of prevention of illness and death). Fourthly, there is a major paradigm shift in terms of health communication in shifting ART treatment from something required for people with ill or declining health status to treating people who are well, and requiring this treatment to be maintained over a lifespan. Thus, well-targeted health promotion, innovative and effective adherence support, improved monitoring to detect signs of resistance early, and affordable, tolerable second, third and fourth line (or rescue) regimens all need to be integrated into this ambitious expansion of ART eligibility.

ART in Pregnancy in LMIC: A Case Study

"*Once started, antiretroviral therapy is for life....*" states the introduction to the '3 by 5 Programme' (WHO 2003a, b). The reason that ART treatment, once started, is to be continued for life is to maximise health by maintaining a supressed HIV viral load, and preventing the development of drug resistance that could occur if ART is started and stopped (as the various drugs in combination ART regimens have different half-lives, it is complex to stop a regimen in a way that ensures that there is no lingering, suboptimal antiviral activity that could provide the conditions for drug resistance to develop). A brief look at the history of interventions aimed at preventing vertical infection (from mother-to-child), however, shows that the maxim of ART therapy being for life has frequently not been the case with regard to provisions of ART to pregnant women. The case study below, I suggest, is an example of how the prevention benefit of ART was initially prioritised above the healthcare of pregnant women with HIV.

The prevention of HIV transmission from mother to child (PMTCT) was the first instance of effective biomedical HIV prevention, achieved in 1994 by the ACTG 076 study (Connor et al. 1994). Famously, this breakthrough spawned a series of placebo-controlled trials in LMIC using less intensive, cheaper regimens (see Wade et al. 1998). This chapter will not delve into the ethical quagmire surrounding the use of placebos despite an effective preventative intervention having been established, as this has been exhaustively covered elsewhere (see Macklin 2001). Instead, this chapter will recount and analyse what occurred programmatically in PMTCT following the results of the HIVNET 012 Trial, which established that a single dose of the ART drug nevirapine to both mother and infant reduced transmission in the first 14–16 weeks of life by nearly 50% in a breastfeeding population (Guay et al. 1999). This regimen, while not as effective as the ACTG 076 regimen, was considered to be a major breakthrough for LMIC. Unlike ACTG 076, it did not require Caesarian section, it did not require treatment uptake in mid pregnancy, it did not require intravenous ART during delivery, and it appeared to work in breastfeeding populations. All of these factors made it significantly more feasible to implement at scale in LMIC. (Of note, when the Food and Drug Administration looked at the data from this trial, it found serious anomalies in the conduct of the trial. Accordingly questions remain regarding the validity of this study's results (Cohen 2004; Institute of Medicine Committee 2005).

One of the issues with the early WHO guidelines that recommended ART treatment only for people with signs of immune damage and/or HIV disease was the problem it created regarding pregnant women with HIV. Despite pregnant women in high income countries achieving excellent health and prevention outcomes with early ART, it meant that pregnant women in LMIC without clinical signs of HIV disease and with CD4 counts above levels recommended for treatment were deemed not to require ART for their own health, despite knowledge that ART would reduce transmission to infants. This created an artificial distinction between the treatment use of ART and prophylactic use in pregnant women – prophylactic use only was recommended. In other words, a pregnant woman with HIV but in otherwise good health would get access to ART to protect her infant, but this would be short-term.

Despite its appeal in terms of feasibility, the nevirapine single-dose[1] regimen had a very specific problem. Although a potent ART drug, nevirapine as noted earlier has a low genetic barrier to resistance, and a long half-life. Thus the drug persists in the blood stream for a long time after a dose, but at concentrations insufficient to fully suppress viraemia. This creates a good environment for the development of drug resistance, and a single dose is enough for this to occur. Exposing women and their infants to this regimen could thus potentiate the development of drug resistance, which might reduce the efficacy of the intervention for any subsequent pregnancies, and limit treatment options for the mother and potentially for the infant, should the infant be HIV infected despite the use of nevirapine prophylaxis.

The publication of the long-term results HIVNET 012 trial was accompanied by a controversial commentary by Karen Palmore Beckerman (2003) that argued that the implementation of single-dose nevirapine would leave 'between 20–100% of women who received prophylaxis resistant to [the class of drugs to which nevirapine belongs]'. While the claim that up to 100% would develop resistance was hyperbolic (Wilfert 2003), the issues she raised were prescient. Beckerman argued that pregnant women with HIV should be treated with effective ART regimens both for their own sake and to enable their survival – citing the devastating example that three women who participated in HIVNET 012 died of AIDS within 56 days of delivery. She suggested that adding a combination ART 'tail' to the nevirapine regimen could reduce the likelihood of resistance (a suggestion later taken up in WHO guidelines in 2010), and that the primary focus be on sustained and sustainable ART treatment.

Beckerman's (2003) article built on an earlier commentary of hers (Beckerman 2002) where – again in response to the publication of short-course trial to reduce mother-to-child transmission – she argued that the risks of programs using single or

[1] This regimen is referred to in the literature as 'single dose' though it in fact involves two doses – one to mother and one to infant. For simplicity's sake I'm adopting the common usage.

dual ART drugs were increasing as the prospect of good treatment access in LMIC grew, given that women who had used short-course ART would be more likely to experience treatment failure due to drug resistance. With limited treatment options available, failing first line ART options would increase the risk of the mother dying, which would in turn increase risk for surviving children, Beckerman argued.

There is a considerable literature on the clinical implications of nevirapine resistance, with much focus on whether or not it 'fades' over time such that subsequent introduction of an ART regimen containing nevirapine might still have clinical utility as either treatment or prophylaxis (Johnson et al. 2005; Lockman et al. 2007, McConnell et al. 2007; Stringer et al. 2010). Regardless of whether or not resistance 'fades' to a level that would result in nevirapine-based combination being effective in women exposed to single-dose PMTCT, it is clear that, as others have noted, the prevention of transmission to infants took precedence over the health security of women with HIV, at least for a time when these single-dose nevirapine programs were widespread (Eyakuze et al. 2008). As noted in a meta-analysis, these programs ultimately resulted in a high burden of drug resistance in women and children, with significant potential to contribute to increase failure of first line ART therapy (Arrivé et al. 2007; Samuel et al. 2016).

From 2003, WHO guidance recognised that pregnant women should not be prescribed ART regimens likely to result in drug resistance, and had specifically provided a warning about the single-dose nevirapine regimen. By 2012 the policy of women cycling on and off ART with successive pregnancies was superseded by 'Option B+'[2] – a recommendation that pregnant women with HIV should be prescribed fully suppressive ART regimens, and kept on them for life, regardless of CD4 cell count or HIV disease stage. While Option B+ has not been fully implemented in all LMIC, it is the only PMTCT option that fully applies the 'rules' of effective ART treatment – that regimens should be fully suppressive, and taken for life. Ironically, there have been reports of significant loss to follow up with these programs, perhaps because women with HIV had being educated to accept intermittent therapy unless they themselves were in poor health (Tenthani et al. 2014)

Reflecting on the history of PMTCT, there are tensions between the prevention imperative, emerging knowledge about optimal timing of ART, the status of women's health, equity, and the constraints of the early stages of implementation of the morally praiseworthy but hugely ambitious goal of universal access. In the late 90s and early 2000s, the nevirapine single-dose regimen had appeal in terms of its simplicity, its low drug burden, and the fact that it could be implemented during

[2] Option B+ was added to two previous options, option A and Option B. Briefly, Under Option A, women received ARV prophylaxis prenatally and during delivery, along with an antiretroviral postpartum "tail" regimen to reduce risk of drug resistance, and their infants received postpartum antiretroviral prophylaxis throughout the duration of breastfeeding. With Option B, all pregnant and lactating women with HIV were offered ARV – beginning in the antenatal period and continuing throughout the duration of breastfeeding. At the end of breastfeeding those women deemed to not yet require ARV for their own health would discontinue the prophylaxis and continue to monitor their CD4 count, eventually re-starting ARV when their CD4 cell count fell below 350 cells.

delivery. In short, it had been shown to be better than nothing at a time when 'nothing' was still seen in some quarters as an acceptable comparator. While the shift away from the single dose regimen happened relatively quickly (at least in terms of normative guidance, if not in practice), its impacts are likely to live on in the form of suboptimal response to first line ART regimens and transmitted drug resistance (Kébé et al. 2014).

It took 6 years from the initial reporting of the SMART study – which showed that starting and stopping ART was detrimental – for PMTCT guidance to recommend life-long treatment for women who initiated ART due to pregnancy. On the one hand, this seems shocking. On the other hand, due to PMTCT programs even with their limitations, women in LMIC tended to access ART earlier than men, and hence have had lower risk of death from HIV disease than men (Beckham et al. 2016; Taylor-Smith et al. 2010), so further strengthening care access for women may have seemed inequitable in some contexts. It could be argued that the history of PMTCT in LMIC demonstrates a programmatic emphasis on prevention without adequate regard for the potential development of drug resistance, and subsequent drug failure in mothers and pregnant women with HIV. It is probably more reasonable, however to say that the complexity of implementing best practice PMTCT in the midst of programmatic scale up of ART access in a context where knowledge about ART changed significantly made compromise and incremental steps forward hard to avoid, if not inevitable. Nevertheless, exposure to sub-optimal therapy through PMCTC programs has left a legacy of drug resistance in some settings (Rowley et al. 2016; Cambiano et al. 2013).

Now that lifelong ART from the point of diagnosis is the WHO recommendation for everyone, exponentially more people will be accessing ART prior to any clinical indications of HIV. That number will be expected to keep increasing, as ART access should enable people with HIV to live normal lifespans. In this context the risk of the development of drug resistance must necessarily increase, given the difficulties of maintaining good-enough adherence for large populations over long periods of time. While the low-level clinical monitoring approach to HIV disease had an important role in enabling the 'public health' roll out of ART in LMIC, this approach would not be sustainable in populations accessing treatment much earlier in HIV disease.

Addressing ART Resistance

Addressing the risk of drug resistance requires strategic action at many levels. Action is required at the community and local levels, to develop and sustain programs that support individual adherence and that work to address systemic problems that can affect adherence (by improving systems of clinic appointments and transport and drug access, for example). Scaling up monitoring and investing in viral load testing will become critical so that people who are on failing regimens – for whatever reason – are identified quickly and either supported to improve adherence or switched to second line therapy. Development of viral load and CD4 testing technologies that are better adapted to use in remote and/or resource constrained settings, and which do not require highly trained laboratory staff, should obviously be prioritised to reduce the dependence of remote and under-resourced clinics on distant laboratory services. Research and development into new effective ART that are well tolerated and are effective against current common resistance patterns in HIV – and new modes of delivery, such as periodic injectables – are of course highly desirable.

While some commentators have suggested withdrawing or withholding ART from non-adherent people rather than providing practical support and transitioning them as necessary to second line ART, this perspective positions poor adherence as an individual (and moral) issue (Chawana & Bogaert 2011). A perspective of adherence that is informed by public health and human rights, on the other hand, recognises that while adherence is an individual behaviour, it is highly determined by structural factors and social context, which can and should be modified to make adherence as simple and as socially acceptable and socially desirable as possible. There is evidence that people in certain demographics (such as young people) may have more trouble with adherence (Haire 2015). Withholding or withdrawing ART on the basis of poor adherence from young people, for example, would not only remove the benefits of early treatment from the demographic with the most to gain, it would also remove the prevention benefit from a population group highly likely to be sexually active. Accordingly, it would seriously undermine global targets for universal access. Recognising, working with, and seeking to ameliorate adherence problems in the social groups that experience them, while advocating for ART that provide different delivery options such as periodic injection, makes sense from a public health and human rights perspective. Universal access goals aim for 90% of people with HIV knowing their status, 90% of those being on ART and 90% of those having undetectable viral loads by 2020 (UNAIDS 2017). Using 2017 figures, this would require more than 14 million more people to be on ART within 2 years – considerable investment in supportive and responsive programming to achieve, support and sustain adherence must be factored into such ambitious plans.

Biomedical Prevention and Drug Resistance

Biomedical prevention is the use of antiretroviral drugs to prevent HIV transmission. It includes ART use after exposure to prevent transmission (post-exposure prophylaxis or PEP), ART use prior to exposure in HIV negative people at high risk of HIV acquisition to prevent transmission (pre-exposure prophylaxis or PrEP), and ART use in HIV positive people to fully supress HIV replication, preventing onward transmission to sexual/injecting partners ('treatment-as-prevention'). The latter two strategies are highly effective and well supported by both RCT and observational data (data on PEP is less robust as it has not been tested in an RCT). PMTCT programs contain elements of two biomedical approaches: maternal viral load is reduced to reduce infectiousness, like treatment as prevention, and infants receive

ART to prevent or abort HIV acquisition, similar to PrEP and PEP. The preventative aspect of early ART treatment is one aspect (in addition to the clinical benefit for the person with HIV) that makes implementation of ART programs in people immediately after diagnosis attractive to governments and donors – it has the potential to reduce onward infection. Similarly, while investment in PrEP programs has been slow, there is a steady increase in availability (AVAC n.d.).

In adherent participants, both PrEP and treatment -as -prevention have shown close to 100% protection in trials (Grant et al. 2014; Anderson et al. 2012; Bavinton et al. 2018; Rodgers et al. 2016, 2018; Cohen et al. 2011). There has however been at least one verified example of HIV transmission occurring in an adherent PrEP-taker, due to being exposed to HIV that was resistant to both the drugs used in the PrEP combination (Knox et al. 2016). With regard to treatment -as -prevention, having a lowered viral pool in a population would be expected to translate into fewer transmissions at population level. To have confidence in treatment -as -prevention at an individual level, however, the sexual partner with HIV needs to be confident that his/her viral load is sustained at an undetectable level, and that requires access to viral load tests at regular intervals. A combination of PrEP and treatment-as-prevention is being trialled in LMIC in serodiscordant couples, where the HIV positive partner is initiated on ART and the negative partner on PrEP, until such time as the positive partner has a sustained undetectable viral load. For this to succeed programmatically, viral load monitoring is required for the ongoing protection of the negative partner (should the positive partner be non-adherent, the negative partner would run the risk of acquiring HIV, and possibly drug resistant HIV), and to maintain the efficacy of the regimen for the positive partner. In this new era of biomedical prevention and all people with HIV being eligible for ART, the need to implement viral load monitoring at scale is increasingly being recognised (WHO 2016).

Monitoring Drug Resistance Beyond the Individual

In high income countries, when people are diagnosed with HIV, a blood sample is sent to a laboratory for genotypic testing – a form of analysis that provides information of whether the person has been infected with a strain of HIV that is resistant (or less susceptible) to particular ART drugs. The person is then prescribed an appropriate regimen that will be effective against the person's HIV.[3]

In LMIC surveillance of HIV drug resistance includes country specific surveys of HIV genotypes to determine incidence of transmitted drug resistance in

[3] Genotyping HIV also has some risks in high income countries, such as the potential to use these data to track 'infection trees' – map pathways of infection. This is ethically problematic in terms of maintaining an enabling environment, as it uses information gleaned from people who test positive for HIV intended to maximise their health outcomes for a purpose that could potentially lead to criminalisation.

populations, through a WHO network of designated laboratories (Bertagnolio et al. 2008). In LMIC this information is directed towards making country or region-wide decisions about first line treatment, and other programs such as the drugs used in post-exposure prophylaxis. In addition, early warning indicators provide information about critical aspects of whether/how people are accessing ART. These include on-time pill pickup; retention in care at 12 months following ART initiation; whether pharmacies experience stock-outs; prescribing practices (whether regimens prescribed meet national or international guidance regarding adequate viral suppression); and, in settings where viral load testing is implemented, viral load suppression at 12 months following ART initiation. These early warning indicators are well designed to signal structural problems, like interruptions in drug supply and poor prescriber compliance with guidelines, and access issues such as whether drug collection systems are 'good enough' (reliable and convenient) for people to be able to pick up pills on time. In 2017, WHO reported 'brisk' implementation of these systems, with 26 countries having completed or currently completing surveys, and 14 having reported data (WHO 2017). Of note, in countries or regions where drug stock outs are frequent, the benefit of putting people with high CD4 counts onto ART would need to be weighed against the individual and public health concern of the development of resistance, should ART be repeatedly started and stopped (for people with CD4 counts lowered by HIV, the clinical benefit of the ART is likely to outweigh the risk). Ideally, of course, the stock out issues should be addressed effectively.

Conclusion

Although hope and hype about vaccines and cures for HIV circulate, ART is currently the most effective tool for the elimination of HIV as a public health threat, both in terms of treatment and prevention (in combination with or as an adjunct to condoms). Preventing the emergence of drug resistance at levels that compromises treatment efficacy and ART based prevention is crucial.

With PMTCT programs, the emphasis on the simplest and cheapest regimens, maintained well after the implications for drug resistance were apparent, has already compromised optimal response to ART for too many women and children. This cannot be repeated in the expansion of ART access. Standardised first, second and third line ART has facilitated the rapid scale up of ART in LMIC, and saved many lives. To build on this, a highly strategic approach to monitoring drug resistance in populations and individuals needs to be taken, with viral load monitoring supporting more rapid change to second and third line therapies as required, rather than running the risk of keeping people on failing regimens. Supporting adherence at health service, community, family and individual levels also requires investment – investment in research, to find context-appropriate solutions that work, in communities to provide labour, and in systems to streamline the medical and dispensing processes and practices that can facilitate or hinder access and adherence. While refinements in drug development may make adherence simpler in years to come, the challenge is to ensure that programming now is responsive to problem of resistance, and that existing drugs and monitoring are carefully deployed to optimise longevity of tools currently available.

References

Anderson, P.L., D.V. Glidden, A. Liu, S. Buchbinder, J.R. Lama, J.V. Guanira, et al. 2012. Emtricitabine-tenofovir concentrations and pre-exposure prophylaxis efficacy in men who have sex with men. *Science Translational Medicine* 4 (151): 151ra125.

Arrivé, E., M.-L. Newell, D.K. Ekouevi, M.-L. Chaix, R. Thiebaut, B. Masquelier, et al. 2007. Prevalence of resistance to nevirapine in mothers and children after single-dose exposure to prevent vertical transmission of HIV-1: a meta-analysis†. *International Journal of Epidemiology* 36 (5): 1009–1021.

Arts, E.J., and D.J. Hazuda. 2012. HIV-1 antiretroviral drug therapy. *Cold Spring Harbor Perspectives in Medicine* 2 (4): a007161. https://doi.org/10.1101/cshperspect.a007161.

AVAC. PrEP Watch. Scaling up country updates. http://www.prepwatch.org/scaling-up/country-updates

Bavinton, B.R., A.N. Pinto, N. Phanuphak, et al. 2018. Viral suppression and HIV transmission in serodiscordant male couples: An international, prospective, observational, cohort study. *Lancet*. Published online July 16.

Beckerman, K.P. 2002. Mothers, orphans, and prevention of paediatric AIDS. *The Lancet* 359 (9313): 1168–1169.

———. 2003. Long-term findings of HIVNET 012: The next steps. *The Lancet* 362 (9387): 842–843.

Beckham, S.W., C. Beyrer, P. Luckow, M. Doherty, E.K. Negussie, and S.D. Baral. 2016. Marked sex differences in all-cause mortality on antiretroviral therapy in low- and middle-income countries: A systematic review and meta-analysis. *Journal of the International AIDS Society* 19 (1): 21106.

Bertagnolio, S., I. Derdelinckx, M. Parker, J. Fitzgibbon, H. Fleury, M. Peeters, et al. 2008. World Health Organization/HIVResNet drug resistance laboratory strategy. *Antiviral Therapy* 13 (Suppl 2): 49–57.

Cambiano, V., S. Bertagnolio, M.R. Jordan, J.D. Lundgren, and A. Phillips. 2013. Transmission of drug resistant HIV and its potential impact on mortality and treatment outcomes in resource-limited settings. *The Journal of Infectious Diseases* 207 (Suppl 2): S57–S62.

Chawana, R., and D.K. van Bogaert. 2011. Risk management in HIV/AIDS: Ethical and economic issues associated with restricting HAART access only to adherent patients. *African Journal of AIDS Research* 10 (sup1): 369–380.

Cohen, Jon. 2004. Allegations raise fears of backlash against AIDS prevention strategy. *Science* 306 (5705): 2168–2169. https://doi.org/10.1126/science.306.5705.2168.

Cohen, M.S., Y.Q. Chen, M. McCauley, T. Gamble, M.C. Hosseinipour, N. Kumarasamy, et al. 2011. Prevention of HIV-1 infection with early antiretroviral therapy. *The New England Journal of Medicine* 365 (6): 493–505.

Connor, E.M., R.S. Sperling, R. Gelber, P. Kiselev, G. Scott, M.J. O'Sullivan, et al. 1994. Reduction of maternal-infant transmission of human immunodeficiency virus type 1 with Zidovudine treatment. *The New England Journal of Medicine* 331 (18): 1173–1180.

DART Trial Team. 2010. Routine versus clinically driven laboratory monitoring of HIV antiretroviral therapy in Africa (DART): A randomised non-inferiority trial. *The Lancet* 375 (9709): 123–131. https://doi.org/10.1016/S0140-6736(09)62067-5.

Eyakuze, C., D.A. Jones, A.M. Starrs, and N. Sorkin. 2008. From PMTCT to a more comprehensive aids response for women: A much-needed shift. *Developing World Bioethics* 8 (1): 33–42.

Grant, R.M., P.L. Anderson, V. McMahan, A. Liu, K.R. Amico, M. Mehrotra, et al. 2014. Uptake of pre-exposure prophylaxis, sexual practices, and HIV incidence in men and transgender women who have sex with men: A cohort study. *The Lancet Infectious Diseases* 14 (9): 820–829.

Guay, L.A., P. Musoke, T. Fleming, D. Bagenda, M. Allen, C. Nakabiito, et al. 1999. Intrapartum and neonatal single-dose nevirapine compared with zidovudine for prevention of mother-to-child transmission of HIV-1 in Kampala, Uganda: HIVNET 012 randomised trial. *The Lancet* 354 (9181): 795–802.

Gulick, Roy M., Heather J. Ribaudo, Cecilia M. Shikuma, Stephanie Lustgarten, Kathleen E. Squires, William A. Meyer III, Edward P. Acosta, Bruce R. Schackman, Christopher D. Pilcher, Robert L. Murphy, William E. Maher, Mallory D. Witt, Richard C. Reichman, Sally Snyder, Karin L. Klingman, and Daniel R. Kuritzkes. 2004. Triple-Nucleoside regimens versus Efavirenz-containing regimens for the initial treatment of HIV-1 infection. *New England Journal of Medicine* 350 (18): 1850–1861. https://doi.org/10.1056/NEJMoa031772.

Haire, B. 2015. Preexposure prophylaxis-related stigma: Strategies to improve uptake and adherence – A narrative review. *HIV/AIDS – Research and Palliative Care* 7: 241–249. https://doi.org/10.2147/HIV.S72419.

Ho, David D. 1995. Time to hit HIV, early and hard. *New England Journal of Medicine* 333 (7): 450–451. https://doi.org/10.1056/nejm199508173330710.

Institute of Medicine (US) Committee on Reviewing the HIVNET 012 Perinatal HIV Prevention Study. 2005. *Review of the HIVNET 012 perinatal HIV prevention study*. National Academy of Sciences. Washington, DC: National Academies Press.

Johnson, J.A., Li J-f, L. Morris, N. Martinson, G. Gray, J. McIntyre, et al. 2005. Emergence of drug-resistant HIV-1 after Intrapartum administration of single-dose Nevirapine is substantially underestimated. *The Journal of Infectious Diseases* 192 (1): 16–23.

Kaufmann, G.R., H. Furrer, B. Ledergerber, L. Perrin, M. Opravil, P. Vernazza, M. Cavassini, E. Bernasconi, M. Rickenbach, B. Hirschel, and M. Battegay. 2005. Characteristics, determinants, and clinical relevance of CD4 T cell recovery <500 Cells/μL in HIV type 1 – Infected individuals receiving potent antiretroviral therapy. *Clinical Infectious Diseases* 41 (3): 361–372. https://doi.org/10.1086/431484.

Kébé, K., L. Bélec, H.D. Ndiaye, S.B. Gueye, A.A.M. Diouara, S. Ngom, et al. 2014. The case for addressing primary resistance mutations to non-nucleoside reverse transcriptase inhibitors to treat children born from mothers living with HIV in sub-Saharan Africa. *Journal of the International AIDS Society* 17 (1): 18526.

Knox, D.C., D.H. Tan, P.R. Harrigan, and P.L. Anderson. 2016. *HIV-1 infection with multiclass resistance despite Preexposure Prophylaxis (PrEP). 169aLB.* In Conference on retro viruses and opportunistic infections, 22–25 February 2016, Boston, Massachusetts.

Lockman, S., R.L. Shapiro, L.M. Smeaton, C. Wester, I. Thior, L. Stevens, F. Chand, J. Makhema, C. Moffat, A. Asmelash, P. Ndase, P. Arimi, E. van Widenfelt, L. Mazhani, V. Novitsky, S. Lagakos, and M. Essex. 2007. Response to antiretroviral therapy after a single, peripartum dose of nevirapine. *New England Journal of Medicine* 356 (2): 135–147. https://doi.org/10.1056/NEJMoa062876.

Luber, A.D. 2005. Genetic barriers to resistance and impact on clinical response. *Medscape General Medicine* 7 (3): 69.

Macklin, R. 2001. After Helsinki: Unresolved issues in international research. *Kennedy Institute of Ethics Journal* 11 (1): 17–36. Project MUSE. https://doi.org/10.1353/ken.2001.0005.

———. 2004. *Ethics and equity in access the HIV treatment 3 by 5 initiative: Background paper consultation on ethics and equitable access to treatment and care for HIV/AIDS*. http://www.who.int/ethics/background-macklin2.pdf

McConnell, M.S., J.S.A. Stringer, A.P. Kourtis, P.J. Weidle, and S.H. Eshleman. 2007. Use of single-dose nevirapine for the prevention of mother-to-child transmission of HIV-1: Does development of resistance matter? *American Journal of Obstetrics & Gynecology* 197 (3): S56–S63.

Mellors, J.W., C.R. Rinaldo, P. Gupta, R.M. White, J.A. Todd, and L.A. Kingsley. 1996. Prognosis in HIV-1 infection predicted by the quantity of virus in plasma. *Science* 272 (5265): 1167–1170.

Mellors, J.W., A. Munoz, J.V. Giorgi, et al. 1997. Plasma viral load and CD4+ lymphocytes as prognostic markers of HIV-1 infection. *Annals of Internal Medicine* 126 (12): 946–954.

Moore, R.D., and R.E. Chaisson. 1999. Natural history of HIV infection in the era of combination antiretroviral therapy. *AIDS* 13 (14): 1933–1942.. PMID 10513653. https://doi.org/10.1097/00002030-199910010-00017.

Pharmacychecker. 2017. https://www.pharmacychecker.com/generic/price-comparison/zidovudine/300+mg. Accessed 29 July 2017.

Rodger AJ et al. for the PARTNER Study Group. 2016. Sexual activity without condoms and risk of HIV transmission in serodifferent couples when the HIV-positive partner is using suppressive antiretroviral therapy. *JAMA* 316 (2): 1–11. https://doi.org/10.1001/jama.2016.5148. http://jama.jamanetwork.com/article.aspx?doi=10.1001/jama.2016.5148. Accessed 12 July 2016.

Rodger AJ, V. Cambiano, T. Bruun, et al. 2018. *Risk of HIV transmission through condomless sex in MSM couples with suppressive ART: The PARTNER2 Study extended results in gay men*. In 22nd International AIDS conference (AIDS 2018), Amsterdam, the Netherlands. Oral Abstract WEAX0104LB.

Rosen, S., and M.P. Fox. 2011. Retention in HIV care between testing and treatment in Sub-Saharan Africa: A systematic review. *PLOS Medicine* 8 (7): e1001056.

Rowley, C.F., I.J. MacLeod, D. Maruapula, B. Lekoko, S. Gaseitsiwe, M. Mine, et al. 2016. Sharp increase in rates of HIV transmitted drug resistance at antenatal clinics in Botswana demonstrates the need for routine surveillance. *Journal of Antimicrobial Chemotherapy* 71 (5): 1361–1366.

Samuel, R., M.N. Julian, R. Paredes, R. Parboosing, P. Moodley, L. Singh, et al. 2016. HIV-1 drug resistance by ultra-deep sequencing following short course zidovudine, single-dose nevirapine, and single-dose tenofovir with emtricitabine for prevention of mother-to-child transmission. *JAIDS Journal of Acquired Immune Deficiency Syndromes* 73 (4): 384–389.

Severe, Patrice, Marc Antoine Jean Juste, Alex Ambroise, Ludger Eliacin, Claudel Marchand, Sandra Apollon, Alison Edwards, Heejung Bang, Janet Nicotera, Catherine Godfrey, Roy M. Gulick, Warren D. Johnson Jr., Jean William Pape, and Daniel W. Fitzgerald. 2010. Early versus standard antiretroviral therapy for HIV-infected adults in Haiti. *New England Journal of Medicine* 363 (3): 257–265. https://doi.org/10.1056/NEJMoa0910370.

Smart, T. 2006. *PEPFAR and Global Fund both highly effective, but is the funding sustainable?* AIDSMAP. http://www.aidsmap.com/PEPFAR-and-Global-Fund-both-highly-effective-but-is-the-funding-sustainable/page/1424121. Accessed 23 June 2006.

Strategies for Management of Antiretroviral Therapy Study Group, Sean Emery, Jacqueline A. Neuhaus, Andrew N. Phillips, Abdel Babiker, Calvin J. Cohen, Jose M. Gatell, Pierre-Marie Girard, Birgit Grund, Matthew Law, Marcelo H. Losso, Adrian Palfreeman, and Robin Wood. 2008. Major clinical outcomes in antiretroviral therapy (ART)-naive participants and in those not receiving ART at baseline in the SMART study. *The Journal of Infectious Diseases* 197 (8): 1133–1144. https://doi.org/10.1086/586713.

Stringer, J.S.A., M.S. McConnell, J. Kiarie, O. Bolu, T. Anekthananon, T. Jariyasethpong, et al. 2010. Effectiveness of non-nucleoside reverse-transcriptase inhibitor-based antiretroviral therapy in women previously exposed to a single intrapartum dose of nevirapine: A multi-country, prospective cohort study. *PLOS Medicine* 7 (2): e1000233.

Taylor-Smith, K., H. Tweya, A. Harries, E. Schoutene, and A. Jahn. 2010. Gender differences in retention and survival on antiretroviral therapy of HIV-1 infected adults in Malawi. *Malawi Medical Journal: The Journal of Medical Association of Malawi* 22 (2): 49–56.

Tenthani, Lyson, Andreas D. Haas, Hannock Tweya, Andreas Jahn, Joep J. van Oosterhout, Frank Chimbwandira, Zengani Chirwa, Wingston Ng'Ambi, Alan Bakali, Sam Phiri, Landon Myer, Fabio Valeri, Marcel Zwahlen, Gilles Wandeler, and Olivia Keiser. 2014. Retention in care under universal antiretroviral therapy for HIV infected pregnant and breastfeeding women ("Option B+") in Malawi. *AIDS* 28 (4): 589–598. https://doi.org/10.1097/QAD.0000000000000143.

The INSIGHT START Study Group. 2015. Initiation of antiretroviral therapy in early asymptomatic HIV infection. *New England Journal of Medicine* 373 (9): 795–807. https://doi.org/10.1056/NEJMoa1506816.

UNAIDS. 2017. *90–90–90 – An ambitious treatment target to help end the aids epidemic*. http://www.unaids.org/en/resources/documents/2017/90-90-90

Wade, N.A., G.S. Birkhead, B.L. Warren, T.T. Charbonneau, P.T. French, L. Wang, et al. 1998. Abbreviated regimens of zidovudine prophylaxis and perinatal transmission of the human immunodeficiency virus. *New England Journal of Medicine* 339 (20): 1409–1414.

Wilfert, C.M. 2003. HIVNET 012 and Petra. *The Lancet* 363 (9404): 244–245.

World Health Organization. 2003a. *3 by 5 Strategy: Making it happen*. http://www.who.int/3by5/publications/documents/en/3by5StrategyMakingItHappen.pdf

———. 2003b. *Scaling up antiretroviral therapy in resource-limited settings: Treatment guidelines for a public health approach*. http://www.who.int/hiv/pub/prev_care/en/ARTrevision2003en.pdf?ua=1

———. 2006. *Antiretroviral therapy for HIV infection in adults and adolescents: Recommendations for a public health approach (2006 revision)*. http://www.who.int/hiv/pub/ART/adult/en

———. 2009. *Rapid advice: antiretroviral therapy for HIV infection in adults and adolescents*. http://www.who.int/hiv/pub/arv/rapid_advice_art.pdf

——— 2016. *Global Action Plan on HIV Drug Resistance 2017–2021*. https://www.who.int/hiv/drugresistance/hivdr_darft_gap.pdf

———. 2017. *HIV drug resistance report 2017*. Geneva: World Health Organization. http://apps.who.int/iris/bitstream/handle/10665/255896/9789241512831-eng.pdf;jsessionid=9AFD8EB2096DEF42908467A854A90A9E?sequence=1

———. 2018. *WHO HIV data and statistics*. http://www.who.int/hiv/data/en

3

Hospital Infection Prevention and Control (IPC) and Antimicrobial Stewardship (AMS): Dual Strategies to Reduce Antibiotic Resistance (ABR) in Hospitals

Gwendolyn L. Gilbert and Ian Kerridge

Abstract In this chapter we review the development of hospital infection prevention and control (IPC) since the nineteenth century and its increasingly important role in reducing the spread of antibiotic resistance (ABR). Excessive rates of hospital-acquired infection (HAI) fell dramatically, towards the end of the nineteenth century, because of improved hygiene and surgical antisepsis, but treatment remained rudimentary until effective antibiotics became widely available in the mid-twentieth century. While antibiotics had profound clinical benefits, their widespread appropriate and inappropriate use in humans and animals inevitably led to the emergence of antibiotic resistance (ABR). Within 50 years, this could no longer be offset by a reliable supply of new drugs, which slowed to a trickle in the 1980s. In hospitals, particularly, high rates of (often unnecessary) antibiotic use and ABR are exacerbated by person-to-person transmission of multi-drug resistant organisms (MDRO), which have, so far, largely resisted the introduction of antimicrobial stewardship (AMS) programs and repeated campaigns to improve infection prevention and control (IPC). Despite clear evidence of efficacy in research settings, both AMS and IPC programs are often ineffective, in practice, because of, *inter alia,* insufficient resourcing, poor implementation, lack of ongoing evaluation and failure to

G. L. Gilbert (✉)
Sydney Health Ethics, University of Sydney, Sydney, NSW, Australia

Marie Bashir Institute for Emerging Infections and Biosecurity, University of Sydney, Sydney, NSW, Australia
e-mail: lyn.gilbert@sydney.edu.au

I. Kerridge
Sydney Health Ethics, University of Sydney, Sydney, NSW, Australia

Department of Haematology, Royal North Shore Hospital, Sydney, NSW, Australia consult frontline staff. In this chapter we review reasons for the relatively low priority given to preventive programs despite the ethical obligation of healthcare organisations to protect current and future patients from preventable harm. The imminent threat of untreatable infections may provide an impetus for a shared organisational and professional commitment to promoting the cultural and behavioural changes needed to successfully reduce the burdens of ABR and drug-resistant HAIs.

Keywords Medicine and public health · Infectious diseases · History of medicine · Infection prevention and control · Antimicrobial resistance · Antimicrobial stewardship

Introduction

Antibiotic resistance (ABR[1]) has been described as a "slowly emerging disaster" (Viens and Littmann 2015). The risk of acquired ABR was recognised before the first antibiotics were widely used and its dire consequences have been understood by experts for many years, but the magnitude of the threat and the urgent need for radical solutions to limit its impact have been widely acknowledged only recently. In this chapter, we argue that it is not too late to mitigate the disaster and check its progress, at least in hospital settings, if certain contributory factors are acknowledged and addressed without delay. These factors, we suggest, include naïve optimism, ignorance, hubris and nihilism on the part of pharmaceutical companies, healthcare professionals (mainly prescribing doctors) and health administrators, among others.

By the first half of the twentieth century, improvements in living conditions in industrialised countries contributed to rapidly falling infectious disease mortality (Armstrong et al. 1999). At the same time, surgical antisepsis, clean wards, hand washing by clinicians and skilled nursing care (Larson 1989; Gill and Gill 2005), had diminished the risk of death in hospitals from puerperal or postoperative sepsis (Gawande 2012). But the remedies for serious infections, such as bleeding, purging or toxic infusions of arsenic, mercury or opiates, probably hastened, more than they postponed, death (Funk et al. 2009).

Antibiotics changed all that. From the beginning they were hailed as miracle drugs. Doctors embraced their use, not only to cure once life-threatening diseases, but also, because they seemed so free of adverse effects, to treat minor infections or even a perceived risk of infection. But, as early as 1945, Alexander Fleming, who shared a Nobel Prize for the discovery of penicillin, warned: "...the public will demand [penicillin]...then will begin an era...of abuses. The microbes are educated to resist penicillin and a host of penicillin-fast organisms is bred out which can be

[1] Most of what follows applies to antimicrobial resistance (AMR), generally, but antibiotics are by far the most commonly prescribed antimicrobials, in human medicine, which is the focus of this chapter; therefore, our discussion will mainly focus on ABR.

passed to other individuals ......In such a case the thoughtless person playing with penicillin treatment is morally responsible for the death of the man who finally succumbs to infection with the penicillin-resistant organism. " (A. Fleming, 1945,[2] quoted in (Bartlett et al. 2013)) And, indeed, within a few years most hospital isolates of previously susceptible *Staphylococcus aureus* were penicillin resistant (Barber and Rozwadowska-Dowzenko 1948).

Although they recognised that overuse would promote resistance, pharmaceutical companies aggressively promoted the benefits and safety of antibiotics to doctors and directly to the public. And, in the 1950s they recognised an even larger market when Thomas Jukes, at Lederle laboratories, demonstrated the growth-promoting effect of antibiotics in food-producing animals: "Animals receiving 10 ppm of chlortetracycline in the diet developed resistance in their intestinal bacteria in less than two days...[but] their growth rate increased. ....we concluded that if [resistant pathogens] appeared ... usefulness of the antibiotic supplement would vanish and farmers would stop feeding it. ...The [company] decision was strongly opposed by the veterinarians at Lederle, but their wishes were abruptly denied by Dr. Malcolm [Lederle President], who made an individual decision to go ahead. Competition was right on our heels..." (Jukes 1985). And it soon caught up: "The power of the calliope in the antibiotic bandwagon increased spectacularly during the [1950s] while poultry, pigs, and patients danced to its tune." (T. D. Luckey, 1959,[3] quoted in (Podolsky 2017)).

By the mid-twentieth century, it was predicted that antibiotics (and vaccines) would put an end to infectious diseases. "[T]he belief that infectious diseases had been successfully overcome was pervasive in biomedical circles - including ... a Nobel Laureate, medical Dean, and other thought leaders - from as early as 1948........" (Spellberg and Taylor-Blake 2013). It was widely assumed that if bacteria developed resistance to one drug, as they often did, there would soon be better ones to replace it; and, for many years, there were. Indeed there was such confidence that infections could be easily cured, that preventing them became a lower priority. But by the 1970s there was mounting disquiet about the emergence of ABR. Methicillin resistant *S. aureus* (MRSA) (Jevons et al. 1963) and transmissible resistance in Gram-negative bacteria (Datta and Pridie 1960) had emerged in the 1960s and their prevalence was increasing, especially in hospitals (Chambers 2001; Aminov 2010; Ventola 2015). The first International Conference on Nosocomial Infections, in 1970, was followed by the Study on the Efficacy of Nosocomial Infection Control (SENIC), in the USA (Forder 2007); in Australia, the handbook of "Antibiotic Guidelines" was published for the first time, in 1978 (Harvey et al. 2003). Anxiety that antibiotics would progressively lose efficacy, became more acute in the 1980s, when the seemingly unlimited flow of new antibiotics slowed to

[2] Alexander Fleming. Penicillin''s finder assays its future. New York Times 26 June 1945: 21

[3] Luckey TD. Antibiotics in nutrition. In: Goldberg HS, ed. Antibiotics: Their Chemistry and Non-Medical Uses. Princeton: D. Van Nostrand; 1959:174–321.

a trickle, and pharmaceutical companies turned their attention to more profitable projects.

Antibiotic use is no longer regarded as an unquestioned good. Antimicrobial resistance (AMR) is now seen as a threat to global health security and the "end of the antibiotic era" predicted; it is broadly accepted that urgent measures are needed to salvage what we can of the "antibiotic miracle": more prudent use of existing antimicrobial agents; novel strategies to promote development of new ones; and greater attention to preventing the spread of drug resistance organisms (WHO 2012; CDC 2013).

Hospital Infection in the "Pre-Antibiotic Era"

In nineteenth century Europe, medical science advanced rapidly; there was increasing demand for new hospitals, where university-trained doctors could develop and experiment with new remedies and advance their knowledge. Anaesthetics increased the scope of surgery (Gawande 2012) and pregnant women were more likely to be admitted to 'lying-in' hospitals, where advances in obstetrics offered relief from excessively long, difficult labour (Loudon 1986). But hospitals were overcrowded, dirty and poorly ventilated; infectious disease outbreaks were common and maternal mortality from childbed fever much higher in hospitals than in the community.

Alexander Gordon, an Aberdeen physician, had recognised puerperal fever as a "specific contagion or infection" that could be carried between parturient women on the hands of her attendants, in 1795 (Gordon 1795), but his work was ignored until the 1840s, when James Young Simpson, in Edinburgh (Selwyn 1965), Oliver Wendell Holmes, in Boston (Holmes 2001), and Ignaz Semmelweis (Nuland 1979; Carter 1981), in Vienna, independently came to similar conclusions. Simpson also recognised that puerperal and surgical fevers were "intercommunicable" and coined the term "hospitalism" to describe outbreaks of surgical infection, which he believed were so serious that "…every patient placed upon an operating table … is in … greater danger than a soldier entering one of the bloodiest and most fatal battlefields" (J. Y. Simpson, 1859 quoted in (Selwyn 1965)).

In Vienna, Semmelweis was troubled by the much higher maternal mortality, in a clinic staffed by doctors and medical students, than in an otherwise similar clinic staffed by midwives. After months of investigation, he realised that the only significant difference between the clinics was that, unlike the midwives, the students and doctors frequented the mortuary, dissecting the bodies of women who had died from childbed fever. When they returned to the clinic, they carried on their hands "cadaver particles which are not entirely removed by the ordinary method of washing the hands with soap....[Therefore] the hands of the examiner must be cleansed with chlorine, not only after handling cadavers, but likewise after examining patients" (Semmelweis 1983). After he enforced this strict hand washing regime, the maternal mortality in the doctors' clinic rapidly fell to a level similar to that in the midwives' clinic (Nuland 1979). Despite the evidence, Semmelweis' findings lacked a conceptual basis, 20 years in advance of Pasteur's germ theory of disease, and were largely rejected by his peers. His accusation that anyone who did not follow his recommendations would be 'murderers', undoubtedly contributed to their antagonism (Pittet 2004; Saint et al. 2010a).

During the Crimean war, in 1854, the British public was scandalised by a newspaper report of deplorable conditions in the British Army hospital at Scutari. When Florence Nightingale was sent to investigate, she found vermin- and lice-infested wards, excreta on walls and floors, injured soldiers in dirty, bloodstained clothes and frequent infectious disease outbreaks. Nightingale believed that disease was caused by filth and foul air (miasmas); she overcame bitter opposition from the military surgeons and formidable logistic barriers to implement a strict regime - immediate wound care; clean dressings, clothes and bedding; nutritious food; and regular cleaning and ventilation of wards. Her meticulous records showed that soldiers were far more likely to die from preventable infection than war wounds. In the January–March quarter of 1855, the mortality at Scutari was 33%, by the July–September quarter it was 2%. While critics have belittled her achievements, her methods remain the basis of good nursing care and hospital infection control (Larson 1989; Gill and Gill 2005).

In the 1860s, Joseph Lister's knowledge of Pasteur's germ theory informed his belief that the almost inevitable (and often fatal) suppuration that complicated compound fractures and amputations was due to "minute organisms suspended in [the atmosphere], which owed their energy to their vitality" (Lister 1867). By liberal use of carbolic acid to soak wound dressings and disinfect his hands, instruments and the operative site, he was able to manage most compound fractures without amputation and the post-amputation mortality fell from 46% (16/35) in 1864–6 to 15% (6/40) in 1867–9 (Newsom 2003). Many of his compatriots ridiculed his methods, but they were gradually accepted, particularly in Europe. His acknowledged place as the "father of antiseptic surgery" owes much to its basis in the germ theory, which gave it an authority that Semmelweis' earlier work lacked.

As antisepsis and later asepsis, environmental hygiene and skilled nursing care were gradually incorporated into hospital practice, hospital infection rates fell and hospitals became places of healing rather than dying.

The Antibiotic Era

Acquired antibiotic resistance (ABR), of bacterial pathogens that affect humans, is mainly due to nearly 75 years' of both appropriate and inappropriate antibiotic use in human medicine and dissemination of resistant organisms. Antibiotic use in agriculture and veterinary practice and environmental contamination are also implicated, but their contributions are contested and vary from region to region (Landers et al. 2012; Marshall and Levy 2011; Chang et al. 2015). The dynamics are complex and incompletely understood (Turnidge and Christiansen 2005) but, in general, exposure of bacteria to antibiotics exerts powerful selection pressure; the greater the total amount and the broader the antibacterial spectra of antibiotics used in any setting, such as a hospital (Willemsen et al. 2009; Xu et al. 2013) or community (Goossens et al. 2005; Bell et al. 2014), the higher the prevalence of ABR. More antibiotics (by weight) are prescribed for non-human animals than people and environmental contamination is a major contributor to ABR. Nevertheless, although inappropriate prescribing is probably the main contributor to drug resistant infections humans, it is now accepted that control of AMR/ABR requires a One Health approach (Robinson et al. 2016). However, the focus of this chapter is on ABR in hospitals, where multidrug resistant organisms (MDROs)[4] are most obvious and prevalent[5] and preventive measures most likely to be effective.

Most life-threatening infections are treated in hospitals, where the greatest variety of antibiotics is used, in repeated courses or for prolonged periods. In hospitals, busy healthcare professionals often carry MDROs on their hands, exposing patients to the risk of healthcare-associated infection (HAI) or colonisation with an MDRO. Hospital laboratory reports increase prescribers' awareness of ABR and, perhaps, promote a (mistaken) perception that it is ubiquitous; this may encourage defensive prescribing – e.g. of multiple or broad-spectrum agents - to avert treatment failure. Paradoxically, increased awareness of ABR is not necessarily reflected in increased adherence to measures designed to prevent it. Now that it is recognised that profligate antibiotic use promotes ABR and inadequate infection prevention and control (IPC) facilitates transmission, the challenge is to break these intersecting vicious cycles, particularly in hospitals, where they are most apparent.

Antibiotic Use and Stewardship in Hospitals

Antibiotics are prescribed very frequently in hospitals; studies in USA and Australia have shown that more than 50% of hospital patients receive at least one antibiotic and up to 50% of prescriptions are unnecessary or inappropriate, according to prescribing guidelines (Turnidge et al. 2016; Baggs et al. 2016; Reddy et al. 2015). Making the right antibiotic prescribing decision is difficult, even for an experienced practitioner, particularly when the diagnosis is uncertain. For patients with sepsis - especially those most at risk of life-threatening infections, e.g. who are neutropenic or immune-compromised - delay can lead to serious complications or death from septic shock (Kumar et al. 2006). But antibiotics prescribed empirically are often continued, even after an alternative diagnosis is made, or not reviewed, despite laboratory results that indicate the empirical choice was ineffective or unnecessarily

[4] MDROs are resistant to more than one - usually several – classes of antibiotic; they include methicillin resistant *Staphylococcus aureus* (MRSA), vancomycin-resistant enterococci (VRE) and extended spectrum β lactamase- and carbapenemase-producing (ESBL and CPE, respectively) Enterobacteriaceae.

[5] In countries where antibiotics can be used in humans or animals without restriction, high rates of ABR occur in the community and in hospitals.

broad-spectrum (Braykov et al. 2014). Antibiotics are also often given in combination, in the wrong dose, by the wrong route or for too short or too long a period (Dryden et al. 2011; Gilbert 2015). Any of these errors can contribute to ABR, without concomitant benefit to the patient herself and, potentially, with significant harm including an increased risk of *Clostridium difficile* infection, MDRO acquisition or prolonged disruption of the gut microbiome, with potentially serious adverse effects (Dingle et al. 2017; Becattini et al. 2016).

Diagnostic uncertainty is not the only, or even the most common, reason for inappropriate prescribing. The prescriber's rational concern can transform into excessive risk aversion, without regard for antibiotic conservation or potential adverse effects on the patient. A junior hospital doctor may consider ABR "morally and professionally important..." but "of limited concern at the bedside" (Broom et al. 2014). Fear of missing something or being criticised, by peers or superiors, outweighs consideration of long-term risks to future patients or the environment. She may prescribe an antibiotic, even if she thinks it unnecessary or futile, because of inexperience, her consultant's routine practice or a duty of benevolence towards her patient that makes her want to do something. Junior doctors are required to make complicated prescribing decisions, often in the face of conflicting, inconsistent (or no) advice or feedback (Mattick et al. 2014). Broom et al. (Broom et al. 2014) concluded that "..social risks, including the peer-based and hierarchical reputational consequences associated with 'not doing enough'" are far more potent than the risk of ABR (Broom et al. 2014).

Over the past 10 years, programs have been introduced into hospital practice in many countries with the aim of minimising inappropriate antibiotic therapy. Antimicrobial stewardship (AMS) programs aim to ensure that patients are given antibiotics when they need them – "the right drug, at the right time, in the right dose and for the right duration" (Dryden et al. 2011; Doernberg and Chambers 2017) – with the least possible selection pressure. They consist of 'bundles' of interventions, including: restrictions on the use of certain key antibiotics, except with specific authorisation; prescriber education and academic detailing; audit of prescribing patterns, with feedback to prescribers; optimisation of laboratory testing, including rapid diagnostics; and technological support such as electronic access to microbiology results and computerised decision support systems (Davey et al. 2017).

AMS programs depend on multidisciplinary teams - including infectious disease physicians, clinical microbiologists, specialist antimicrobial pharmacists and/or IPC professionals - whose complementary expertise and spheres of influence provide mutual support and greater authority than each has, individually. The specialist pharmacist's expertise in drug dosing, interactions and administration and her role in implementing regulations, such as automatic stop orders or restricted drug authorisation, and auditing prescribing records, are critical to an AMS program. Nevertheless, even the most experienced pharmacist or AMS team can encounter resistance from a senior specialist who may regard their advice as a threat to her autonomy and clinical experience (Broom et al. 2016).

How effective an AMS program will be depends on what it includes and how it is implemented. A recent systematic review (Davey et al. 2017) showed that providing advice and feedback to clinicians improved prescribing and reduced overall antibiotic use more than simply imposing rules and restrictions, suggesting that AMS programs that support prescribers help to mitigate the fear of censure or litigation that often drives inappropriate prescribing. Overall, studies of AMS show that it can reduce inappropriate prescribing, pharmacy costs and avoidable drug reactions; improve therapeutic drug monitoring; shorten hospital length of stay by an average of 2 days; and may reduce rates of *C. difficile,* fungal and MDRO infections (Davey et al. 2013; Baur et al. 2017). Although some studies have confirmed the cost-effectiveness of AMS, more high-quality research is needed (Coulter et al. 2015).

Clearly, eliminating inappropriate antibiotic use is necessary, but not sufficient, to reduce the impact of ABR, which is exacerbated by hospital spread of MDROs.

Hospital Infection Prevention and Control (IPC) and ABR

Healthcare-Associated Infectionsand Their Consequences

According to WHO ".....HAI is the most frequent adverse event in health care [but] its true global burden remains unknown because of the difficulty in gathering reliable data" (WHO 2011). A systematic review of HAIs in high and middle/low-income countries showed that 3.5%–12% of hospitalised patients develop at least one HAI (WHO 2011), of which 50%, or more, are potentially preventable (Harbarth et al. 2003; Umscheid et al. 2011). The estimated number of people, globally, who die from drug-resistant infections each year – currently at least 700,000 - is predicted to increase to ten million by 2050 (O'Neill 2016). HAIs caused by MDROs are more difficult to treat, more likely to be fatal and more costly than comparable HAIs due to antibiotic-susceptible pathogens (Cosgrove 2006; de Kraker et al. 2011). HAI risks are associated with patient factors: severity of illness and co-morbidities such as chronic organ failure, malnutrition, immune-suppression, serious trauma or contaminated surgery; and organisational factors: bed occupancy rate; staff workload; hospital environment and infrastructure; prevalence of endemic or introduced MRDO pathogens; adherence of healthcare workers to basic hygiene principles (Clements et al. 2008; Daud-Gallotti et al. 2012; Scheithauer et al. 2017). Hospital IPC policies are designed to minimise these risks and the burden of HAIs and ABR. Unlike other adverse hospital events, MDRO colonisation and HAIs are not confined to individuals; they are communal threats that affect other patients, hospital staff and the wider community and add to the burden of AMR.

Even without clinically significant infection, MDRO colonisation has significant impacts. Patients colonised with certain high-impact MDROs[6] are identified by active admission screening and isolated in single rooms, with contact precautions.[7] These are expensive measures and they can adversely affect patient care and wellbeing. Patients in contact isolation are, on average, visited by healthcare workers less often and for shorter periods; less likely to be examined by a doctor; more likely to suffer non-infectious adverse effects, such as falls, pressure sores and fluid and electrolyte imbalance; and more likely to express dissatisfaction with their hospital care, than other patients (Saint et al. 2003; Stelfox et al. 2003; Morgan et al. 2014). They may feel stigmatised and anxious about risks to family members; they and their visitors are often inadequately informed or given conflicting information about the implications of MDRO colonisation and how to protect themselves and others (Wyer et al. 2015; Seibert et al. 2017). Contact isolation is also burdensome to healthcare workers. Compliance with hand hygiene and use of personal protective equipment (and, thus, the effectiveness of contact isolation) is often relatively poor and likely to deteriorate as the number of isolated patients increases (Clock et al. 2010; Dhar et al. 2014).

Moreover, there is conflicting evidence (Cohen et al. 2015; Morgan et al. 2017), as to whether active screening and contact isolation prevent MDRO transmission more effectively than less expensive and burdensome measures such as strict adherence to standard precautions[8] (Huskins et al. 2011) and/or targeted contact isolation of patients with other risk factors (e.g. diarrhoea, open wounds) (Djibre et al. 2017). This raises the question as to whether these practices are ethically justified, based on the precautionary principle - i.e. that they might prevent harm to others - or cost-effective. Patients are rarely asked for their consent to be screened or informed of the consequences of a positive result, although contact isolation will restrict their liberty for others', but not their own, benefit. It is arguable that these measures *are* ethically justifiable if: the specific MRDO for which they are implemented is particularly dangerous; patients are fully informed, before they are screened, of the reasons, implications and benefits of MDRO colonisation; and there is adequate staffing to ensure they are implemented with optimal effectiveness and minimal risk. An alternative approach would be to promote strict adherence to standard precautions, by all staff, behind a "veil of ignorance" by assuming that any patient might be MDRO-colonised and engaging patients - when their condition permits - and their visitors as active participants in IPC (Ahmad et al. 2016). If given an opportunity and adequate information, patients can make positive contributions to IPC, including how to minimise MDRO transmission and the adverse effects of contact isolation (Wyer et al. 2015).

---

[6] MDROs for which special control measures are used are chosen according to criteria such as: extent of resistance, transmissibility, virulence and local prevalence: e.g. they often include MRSA, VRE and CPE.

[7] Contact precautions include routine use of gown and gloves when caring for patients in isolation, in addition to standard precautions, which include hand hygiene as the main component, and use of personal protective equipment when exposure to patient's blood or body fluid is anticipated

[8] Mainly strict compliance with hand hygiene.

Hospital IPC Programs

Given the adverse individual and communal effects and excess costs of HAIs and MDRO colonisation, healthcare organisations and professionals have an unequivocal duty-of-care and ethical responsibility to take appropriate measures to prevent them. Hospital IPC programs include, *inter alia*: hand hygiene; appropriate use of personal protective equipment; aseptic technique for invasive procedures; environmental hygiene; air flow; bundles of measures to prevent certain HAI syndromes, such as device-related blood stream infections; surveillance of selected HAIs and feed-back of data to clinicians; and isolation of infected and MDRO-colonised patients, with the caveats outlined above (Sydnor and Perl 2011).

It is usually impossible to trace an HAI or MRDO transmission event to a specific action, omission or individual healthcare worker, because there are inevitable time gaps and multiple factors and people involved (McLaws 2015). HAIs "do not carry fingerprints ... to identify the offending healers who failed the patient." (Palmore and Henderson 2012).

The effectiveness of an IPC program depends on organisational commitment, adequate resources and participation of everyone in the hospital community. Despite the compelling ethical imperative to "do no harm", the economic burden of HAIs (Stone 2009) and proven cost-effectiveness (Dick et al. 2015) of IPC programs, they often struggle to attract the necessary support and resources. Their beneficiaries, like those of any preventive program, are unknown "statistical lives" whose demands are far less compelling than those of known "identified lives" who need immediate, often expensive, interventions (Cookson et al. 2008; Beauchamp and Childress 2009). The typically low priority of IPC is reflected in a vicious cycle of inadequate resources, poor compliance - and, hence, limited effectiveness - which can then seem to justify further cost cutting.

The basic principles of hospital IPC were recognised in the nineteenth century and incorporated into routine hospital policy in the latter part of the twentieth, when it became clear that antibiotics, alone, could not prevent morbidity and mortality from HAIs. Nevertheless, implementation and maintenance of IPC programs remain a major challenge. Variation in HAI rates, between otherwise comparable hospitals, presumably reflects differences in organizational cultures, policies, working conditions (Daud-Gallotti et al. 2012; Krein et al. 2010) and professional attitudes, behaviours and leadership (Saint et al. 2010a), suggesting that improvement is possible.

The Central Role of Hand Hygiene in IPC

"In the absence of the possibility to directly link individual infectious outcomes to individual hand hygiene failures... hand hygiene performance remains the only measure to judge the degree of system safety...." (Stewardson et al. 2011). Despite the proven effectiveness of hand hygiene in preventing MDRO transmission (Pittet et al. 2000; Johnson et al. 2005), compliance is often poor. The discovery, about

20 years ago, that it could be improved by use of alcohol-based hand rub (ABHR), was a major breakthrough. ABHR has significant advantages over traditional hand washing with soap and water: it takes less time, is less irritant to hands, accessible at the point-of-care and in settings without access to clean water and has more rapid and potent antibacterial action (Pittet et al. 2000; Widmer 2000). In 2007, "My Five Moments of Hand Hygiene" was introduced to improve healthcare worker training and standardise monitoring and reporting of hand hygiene compliance (Sax et al. 2007); in 2009, the "Five Moments" were incorporated into WHO hand hygiene guidelines. Since then, there have been numerous studies and reviews of factors affecting compliance and interventions to improve it (Erasmus et al. 2009; Huis et al. 2012; Neo et al. 2016; Kingston et al. 2016).

One review reported an overall average compliance of 40%; it was lower in ICUs (30–40%) than other settings (50–60%); among doctors (32%) than nurses (48%) and for moment one (before patient contact; 21%) than moment four (after patient contact; 47%). Performing dirty tasks, availability of ABHR, and performance feedback were associated with better compliance (Erasmus et al. 2009). A review of interventions reported an average pre-intervention compliance of 34% with variable, but modest improvements (8–31%) and mean post-intervention compliance of 57%. Multimodal interventions included various combinations of staff education, facility design and planning, HAI surveillance and/or compliance monitoring with feedback, financial incentives and active support by clinical champions and hospital administrations (Kingston et al. 2016).

These studies illustrate the enormous effort entailed in achieving even modest, often short-term, improvements. They contrast with the, apparently, much better compliance achieved by the Australian National Hand Hygiene Initiative, which was established in 2009 as a "standardised hand hygiene culture-change program throughout all Australian hospitals to improve ... compliance among Australian health care workers; establish a validated system of ...auditing to allow local, national and international benchmarking..." (Grayson et al. 2011). Between 2009 and June 2017, overall compliance increased, steadily, from 63% to 85%, which clearly represents major improvement, to above the national benchmark (70%) (http://www.hha.org.au/). But it obscures significant variation (e.g. between hospitals, professional groups and moments) and sampling biases, suggesting aggregated national data can be misleading. Moreover, the estimated auditing cost is AU$2.2 million per annum for an annual improvement (adjusted for sampling) of 1% compliance (Azim and McLaws 2014).

How should these data be interpreted? Routine audits, by direct observation, necessarily involve short periods of observation (20–30 minutes) at times of convenience and so are not representative of 24 hour/whole-of-hospital activity; it was estimated that <2% of total daily hand hygiene opportunities are sampled during a 60-minute audit (Fries et al. 2012). Auditing by direct observation is subject to the Hawthorne effect[9] (Srigley et al. 2014) and observer bias; it does not assess whether hand hygiene is performed correctly and, when compared with continuous

[9] Hawthorne effect: individuals modify their behaviour in response to awareness of being observed.

automated monitoring, overestimates compliance (Kwok et al. 2016). Furthermore, there is no consensus as to what target compliance rate is necessary or realistic (Mahida 2016). Video or electronic monitoring systems would reduce workload, measure compliance more consistently and could improve it, by providing rapid feedback and prompts (Srigley et al. 2015), but experience with their use is limited and there are many logistic, industrial, and ethical challenges (Palmore and Henderson 2012; Conway 2016). There is clearly a need to establish realistic compliance targets, more accurate, less labour intensive auditing methods and a more holistic approach to IPC monitoring.

Doctors and IPC

There is extensive evidence than doctors' hand hygiene compliance is consistently less than that of nurses, overall, albeit highly variable (Pittet et al. 2004; Cantrell et al. 2009). In one hospital it was more than 80% among physicians and paediatricians but only 30% among surgeons and anaesthetists (Pittet et al. 2004). Compliance has been associated with an emotional, outcome-oriented, rather than a 'rational', thinking style – typically associated with nurses and doctors, respectively (Sladek et al. 2008) - and inversely correlated with professional education level i.e. senior doctors were less compliant than junior doctors or nurses (Duggan et al. 2008). These differences matter: senior doctors have status and power within hospital communities and their attitudes and behaviours disproportionately influence those of other staff (Lankford et al. 2003). Poorly compliant, peripatetic junior doctors can act as "super-spreaders", with many opportunities to transmit pathogens between the numerous individual patients they encounter each day (Temime et al. 2009; Hornbeck et al. 2012). Doctors are more likely to perform hand hygiene *after* patient contact, to avoid a perceived personal risk, than *before* contact, to protect patients (Scheithauer et al. 2011). Many believe these are equivalent, but overlook the many opportunities for contamination of their hands, from bed curtains, patient notes, door handles, computer keyboards etc., between patients. In a focus-group study of hospital staff, most non-physician participants said they noticed the hand hygiene practices of other staff and rated doctors least compliant. Doctors were confident of their hand hygiene knowledge but discounted its importance before patient contact. They rarely noticed the practices of others, apart from their senior colleagues; medical students said that senior doctors' hand hygiene practices influenced their own (Jang et al. 2010a, 2010b).

The reasons for some doctors' apparent lack of commitment to IPC may lie in the medical practice model, which focuses on individual patient's clinical problems, which require investigation, decision-making, intervention, often with tangible results. IPC policies fit poorly with this model; they lack obvious utility, since they do not, meaningfully, influence clinical practice. The common perception that HAIs and MDRO acquisition are rare, but unavoidable, can promote a sense of nihilism – that they are inevitable features of contemporary healthcare. Often this is attributable to ignorance of the impacts of HAIs and benefits of IPC, which is partly because of inadequate surveillance and feedback to clinicians.

Some doctors' apparent indifference or even hostility towards IPC may also reflect aspects of professional and organisational cultures. Traditionally, IPC has been a nursing responsibility; the role of infection control practitioners' (usually nurses) is to implement IPC policies on behalf of hospital management, who have to report, against mandatory IPC performance indicators, to a central authority (e.g. Ministry of Health). Responsibility for monitoring these indicators, such as hand hygiene compliance, is often devolved to nurse managers, who are held to account if targets are not met. But they have little influence over doctors, who choose to ignore rules they see as unnecessary or excessive or who object, on principle, to any regulation, imposed by nurses or managers. "Senior doctors consider themselves exempt from following policy and practice within a culture of perceived autonomous decision-making that relies more on personal knowledge and experience than formal policy" (Charani et al. 2013). This professional antipathy to IPC, may also reflect the historical - but gradually changing - gender distribution between nursing, which has been a largely female profession, and medicine, traditionally dominated by men, particularly in senior positions. Doctors' attitudes to IPC are consistent with a more general failure - there are many exceptions - to engage in quality improvement activities or comply with organisational policies, which have been linked to an entrenched medical culture (Jorm and Kam 2004) and/or to the perceived loss of professional autonomy and dominance associated with managerialism (Davies and Harrison 2003).

How widespread these attitudes are and how the hospital management handles them will determine the success or failure of hospital-wide quality improvement programs such as IPC or AMS. If they are tolerated or seen as "too hard" to address, the morale of other staff and the success of the program will be compromised and recalcitrant doctors' skepticism about its relevance, reinforced. On the other hand, some IPC rules *are* unnecessarily rigid and officiously enforced. They may seem straightforward to their authors, but poor compliance is sometimes due to clinicians' finding them confusing, incompatible with the realities of frontline practice or inappropriate in some settings (Hor et al. 2017). There are faults on both sides when, ideally, all "sides" should be working collaboratively to promote patient safety. The issues need to be addressed if healthcare management and staff are to fulfil their moral responsibility to support and participate in programs that promote patient safety. Individuals "are not somehow 'outside' and separate from 'systems': they create, modify and are subject to the social forces that are an inescapable feature of any organizational system; each element acts on the other" (Aveling et al. 2016). The success of any program is likely to hang on the extent to which the values and goals of all of its members – particularly the most influential - align with, and contribute to, those of the organisation.

The Organization's Role in IPC/AMS Programs

Government and private healthcare funding bodies generally mandate that each hospital has established IPC and AMS programs and reports regularly, sometimes publicly, against mandatory performance targets. This does not necessarily guarantee the programs' success; there are wide variations in practices and outcomes between apparently similar hospitals. Most studies of successful IPC/AMS interventions have focused on "what" works, rather than "why" it works. The components of organisational culture likely to determine the success or failure of program implementation are leadership, shared vision and values, inter-professional relationships, resources and service priorities (Krein et al. 2010). Successful implementation of IPC/AMS, requires commitment by hospital management, strong clinical leadership (Saint et al. 2010b), highly motivated champions (Damschroder et al. 2009) and interdisciplinary departmental teams. The goals, benefits and measures of success of the programs need to be clearly defined, but flexible enough to allow local modification, based on the knowledge and experience of frontline staff. Imposing cultural change from without is less likely to be sustainable than allowing frontline staff to discover how to change it from within (Iedema et al. 2015; Zimmerman et al. 2013). Measures of success should be defined, monitored and rewarded, at least by timely feedback, if not more tangible recognition.

Conclusions

AMR is an acknowledged threat to global health security and will not be adequately addressed by development of new antibiotics. The most urgent priority is to curtail the inappropriate use of antibiotics and spread of MDROs, which are most prevalent in hospitals where they are also most amenable to control. Despite evidence that properly implemented hospital AMS/IPC programs can reduce the burden of ABR, the increasing prevalence of preventable HAIs, show that many healthcare organisations have either not recognised, or failed to meet, the challenge. In this chapter, we have identified some of the barriers to successful implementation of AMS/IPC programs; although they are usually mandatory, in hospitals, their quality and outcomes vary. The organisational characteristics most likely to assure successful implementation include: commitment to a shared vision and values; strong leadership, governance and systems; respectful, collaborative inter-professional relationships and fair, cost-effective resource allocation.

Healthcare organisations and hospital managers have ethical and legal responsibilities to protect existing patients, employees and the public – and future patients whose treatment will be compromised by a lack of effective antimicrobial therapy - from preventable harm originating in hospital facilities or activities. Unfortunately, preventive programs are often a low priority because their beneficiaries are unknown future persons whose claims are eclipsed by known, present persons and powerful professional or commercial interests. Preventive programs also generally lack the solid, cost-effectiveness data that administrators demand before committing resources, especially if it is at the expense of therapies. A case for adequate resources to sustain AMS/IPC programs would, ideally, include *local,* as well as published, statistics on current rates, costs and adverse consequences of HAIs and ABR and personal histories of known patients who have suffered adverse effects from an HAI, contact isolation or inappropriate antibiotic administration.

Successful AMS/IPC policies will be adaptable to unit/department-specific requirements rather than rigidly imposed rules and restrictions, which fail to account for variable, unpredictable clinical exigencies and so are liable to be ignored or circumvented. Effective policy implementation needs frontline ownership of "practice-based guidelines", based on local knowledge, including potential patient participation.

Policies and implementation plans often fail to clearly define their goals or how success will be measured. Evidence of success that can be rapidly fed back to staff is a strong motivator of adherence, but many hospital managers fail to invest in HAI surveillance and feedback to clinicians that is relevant, accessible and timely enough to motivate improvement. Despite the importance of hand hygiene compliance, its prominence as a single (often inaccurate) measure of IPC practice risks neglecting other important cultural and behavioural factors – teamwork, interdisciplinary co-operation and motivation – that determine the effectiveness of a hospital's AMS/IPC programs.

Securing the commitment, of an often small, but powerful, minority of senior medical staff, who regard AMS/IPC programs as a threat to professional autonomy and status, remains a challenge for many hospitals. It requires, as a minimum, respectful consultation during program planning, recruitment of clinical leaders and champions and, once a decision is made to adopt it, clarity that all staff are expected to support and participate in programs to which the organisation is committed.

References

Ahmad, R., et al. 2016. Defining the user role in infection control. *The Journal of Hospital Infection* 92 (4): 321–327.

Aminov, R.I. 2010. A brief history of the antibiotic era: Lessons learned and challenges for the future. *Frontiers in Microbiology* 1: 134.

Armstrong, G.L., L.A. Conn, and R.W. Pinner. 1999. Trends in infectious disease mortality in the United States during the 20th century. *JAMA* 281 (1): 61–66.

Aveling, E.L., M. Parker, and M. Dixon-Woods. 2016. What is the role of individual accountability in patient safety? A multi-site ethnographic study. *Sociology of Health & Illness* 38 (2): 216–232.

Azim, S., and M.L. McLaws. 2014. Doctor, do you have a moment? National Hand Hygiene Initiative compliance in Australian hospitals. *The Medical Journal of Australia* 200 (9): 534–537.

Baggs, J., et al. 2016. Estimating National Trends in inpatient antibiotic use among US hospitals from 2006 to 2012. *JAMA Internal Medicine* 176 (11): 1639–1648.

Barber, M., and M. Rozwadowska-Dowzenko. 1948. Infection by penicillin-resistant staphylococci. *Lancet* 2 (6530): 641–644.

Bartlett, J.G., D.N. Gilbert, and B. Spellberg. 2013. Seven ways to preserve the miracle of antibiotics. *Clinical Infectious Diseases* 56 (10): 1445–1450.

Baur, D., et al. 2017. Effect of antibiotic stewardship on the incidence of infection and colonisation with antibiotic-resistant bacteria and Clostridium difficile infection: A systematic review and meta-analysis. *The Lancet Infectious Diseases* 17 (9): 990–1001.

Beauchamp, T.L., and James F. Childress. 2009. *Principles of biomedical ethics*. 7th ed. New York: Oxford University Press.

Becattini, S., Y. Taur, and E.G. Pamer. 2016. Antibiotic-induced changes in the intestinal microbiota and disease. *Trends in Molecular Medicine* 22 (6): 458–478.

Bell, B.G., et al. 2014. A systematic review and meta-analysis of the effects of antibiotic consumption on antibiotic resistance. *BMC Infectious Diseases* 14: 13.

Braykov, N.P., et al. 2014. Assessment of empirical antibiotic therapy optimisation in six hospitals: An observational cohort study. *The Lancet Infectious Diseases* 14 (12): 1220–1227.

Broom, A., J. Broom, and E. Kirby. 2014. Cultures of resistance? A Bourdieusian analysis of doctors' antibiotic prescribing. *Social Science & Medicine* 110: 81–88.

Broom, A., et al. 2016. A qualitative study of hospital pharmacists and antibiotic governance: Negotiating interprofessional responsibilities, expertise and resource constraints. *BMC Health Services Research* 16: 43.

Cantrell, D., et al. 2009. Hand hygiene compliance by physicians: Marked heterogeneity due to local culture? *American Journal of Infection Control* 37 (4): 301–305.

Carter, K.C. 1981. SemmelWeis and his predecessors. *Medical History* 25 (1): 57–72.

CDC. 2013. *Antibiotic threats in the USA*..

Chambers, H.F. 2001. The changing epidemiology of Staphylococcus aureus? *Emerging Infectious Diseases* 7 (2): 178–182.

Chang, Q., et al. 2015. Antibiotics in agriculture and the risk to human health: How worried should we be? *Evolutionary Applications* 8 (3): 240–247.

Charani, E., et al. 2013. Understanding the determinants of antimicrobial prescribing within hospitals: The role of "prescribing etiquette". *Clinical Infectious Diseases* 57 (2): 188–196.

Clements, A., et al. 2008. Overcrowding and understaffing in modern health-care systems: Key determinants in meticillin-resistant Staphylococcus aureus transmission. *The Lancet Infectious Diseases* 8 (7): 427–434.

Clock, S.A., et al. 2010. Contact precautions for multidrug-resistant organisms: Current recommendations and actual practice. *American Journal of Infection Control* 38 (2): 105–111.

Cohen, C.C., B. Cohen, and J. Shang. 2015. Effectiveness of contact precautions against multidrug-resistant organism transmission in acute care: A systematic review of the literature. *The Journal of Hospital Infection* 90 (4): 275–284.

Conway, L.J. 2016. Challenges in implementing electronic hand hygiene monitoring systems. *American Journal of Infection Control* 44 (5 Suppl): e7–e12.

Cookson, R., C. McCabe, and A. Tsuchiya. 2008. Public healthcare resource allocation and the rule of rescue. *Journal of Medical Ethics* 34 (7): 540–544.

Cosgrove, S.E. 2006. The relationship between antimicrobial resistance and patient outcomes: Mortality, length of hospital stay, and health care costs. *Clinical Infectious Diseases* 42 (Suppl 2): S82–S89.

Coulter, S., et al. 2015. The need for cost-effectiveness analyses of antimicrobial stewardship programmes: A structured review. *International Journal of Antimicrobial Agents* 46 (2): 140–149.

Damschroder, L.J., et al. 2009. The role of the champion in infection prevention: Results from a multisite qualitative study. *Quality & Safety in Health Care* 18 (6): 434–440.

Datta, N., and R.B. Pridie. 1960. An outbreak of infection with Salmonella typhimurium in a general hospital. *The Journal of Hygiene (London)* 58: 229–240.

Daud-Gallotti, R.M., et al. 2012. Nursing workload as a risk factor for healthcare associated infections in ICU: A prospective study. *PLoS One* 7 (12): e52342.

Davey, P., et al. 2013. Interventions to improve antibiotic prescribing practices for hospital inpatients. *Cochrane Database of Systematic Reviews* 4: CD003543.

———. 2017. Interventions to improve antibiotic prescribing practices for hospital inpatients. *Cochrane Database of Systematic Reviews* 2: CD003543.

Davies, H.T., and S. Harrison. 2003. Trends in doctor-manager relationships. *BMJ* 326 (7390): 646–649.

de Kraker, M.E., et al. 2011. Mortality and hospital stay associated with resistant Staphylococcus aureus and Escherichia coli bacteremia: Estimating the burden of antibiotic resistance in Europe. *PLoS Medicine* 8 (10): e1001104.

Dhar, S., et al. 2014. Contact precautions: More is not necessarily better. *Infection Control and Hospital Epidemiology* 35 (3): 213–221.

Dick, A.W., et al. 2015. A decade of investment in infection prevention: A cost-effectiveness analysis. *American Journal of Infection Control* 43 (1): 4–9.

Dingle, K.E., et al. 2017. Effects of control interventions on Clostridium difficile infection in England: An observational study. *The Lancet Infectious Diseases* 17 (4): 411–421.

Djibre, M., et al. 2017. Universal versus targeted additional contact precautions for multidrug-resistant organism carriage for patients admitted to an intensive care unit. *American Journal of Infection Control* 45 (7): 728–734.

Doernberg, S.B., and H.F. Chambers. 2017. Antimicrobial stewardship approaches in the intensive care unit. *Infectious Disease Clinics of North America* 31 (3): 513–534.

Dryden, M., et al. 2011. Using antibiotics responsibly: Right drug, right time, right dose, right duration. *The Journal of Antimicrobial Chemotherapy* 66 (11): 2441–2443.

Duggan, J.M., et al. 2008. Inverse correlation between level of professional education and rate of handwashing compliance in a teaching hospital. *Infection Control and Hospital Epidemiology* 29 (6): 534–538.

Erasmus, V., et al. 2009. A qualitative exploration of reasons for poor hand hygiene among hospital workers: Lack of positive role models and of convincing evidence that hand hygiene prevents cross-infection. *Infection Control and Hospital Epidemiology* 30 (5): 415–419.

Forder, A.A. 2007. A brief history of infection control - past and present. *South African Medical Journal* 97 (11 Pt 3): 1161–1164.

Fries, J., et al. 2012. Monitoring hand hygiene via human observers: How should we be sampling? *Infection Control and Hospital Epidemiology* 33 (7): 689–695.

Funk, D.J., J.E. Parrillo, and A. Kumar. 2009. Sepsis and septic shock: A history. *Critical Care Clinics* 25 (1): 83–101. viii.

Gawande, A. 2012. Two hundred years of surgery. *The New England Journal of Medicine* 366 (18): 1716–1723.

Gilbert, G.L. 2015. Knowing when to stop antibiotic therapy. *The Medical Journal of Australia* 202 (11): 571.

Gill, C.J., and G.C. Gill. 2005. Nightingale in Scutari: Her legacy reexamined. *Clinical Infectious Diseases* 40 (12): 1799–1805.

Goossens, H., et al. 2005. Outpatient antibiotic use in Europe and association with resistance: A cross-national database study. *Lancet* 365 (9459): 579–587.

Gordon, A.. 1795. *Treatise on the Epidemic Puerperal Fever of Aberdeen*. Internet archive open knowledge commons and Harvard Medical School ed. 1795, London: G.G. & J. Robinson.

Grayson, M.L., et al. 2011. Outcomes from the first 2 years of the Australian National Hand Hygiene Initiative. *The Medical Journal of Australia* 195 (10): 615–619.

Harbarth, S., H. Sax, and P. Gastmeier. 2003. The preventable proportion of nosocomial infections: An overview of published reports. *The Journal of Hospital Infection* 54 (4): 258–266. quiz 321.

Harvey, K., J. Dartnell, and M. Hemming. 2003. Improving antibiotic use: 25 years of antibiotic guidelines and related initiatives. *Communicable Diseases Intelligence Quarterly Report* 27 (Suppl): S9–S12.

Holmes, O.W. 2001. *The contagiousness of puerperal fever*. New York: P.F. Collier & Son, 1909–14; Bartleby.com, 2001. http://www.bartleby.com/38/5/. [Date of Printout]. The Harvard Classics ed. The Harvard Classics. Vol. XXXVIII, part 5. New York: P.F. Collier & Son.

Hor, S.Y., et al. 2017. Beyond hand hygiene: A qualitative study of the everyday work of preventing cross-contamination on hospital wards. *BMJ Quality and Safety* 26 (7): 552–558.

Hornbeck, T., et al. 2012. Using sensor networks to study the effect of peripatetic healthcare workers on the spread of hospital-associated infections. *The Journal of Infectious Diseases* 206 (10): 1549–1557.

Huis, A., et al. 2012. A systematic review of hand hygiene improvement strategies: A behavioural approach. *Implementation Science* 7: 92.

Huskins, W.C., et al. 2011. Intervention to reduce transmission of resistant bacteria in intensive care. *The New England Journal of Medicine* 364 (15): 1407–1418.

Iedema, R., S.-Y. Hor, M. Wyer, G.L. Gilbert, C. Jorm, C. Hooker, and M.V.N. O'Sullivan. 2015. An innovative approach to strengthening health professionals' infection control and limiting hospital-acquired infection: video-reflexive ethnography. *BMJ Innovations* 1: 157–162.

Jang, J.H., et al. 2010a. Focus group study of hand hygiene practice among healthcare workers in a teaching hospital in Toronto, Canada. *Infection Control & Hospital Epidemiology* 31 (2): 144–150.

———. 2010b. Physicians and hand hygiene practice: A focus group study. *The Journal of Hospital Infection* 76 (1): 87–89.

Jevons, M.P., A.W. Coe, and M.T. Parker. 1963. Methicillin resistance in staphylococci. *Lancet* 1 (7287): 904–907.

Johnson, P.D., et al. 2005. Efficacy of an alcohol/chlorhexidine hand hygiene program in a hospital with high rates of nosocomial methicillin-resistant Staphylococcus aureus (MRSA) infection. *The Medical Journal of Australia* 183 (10): 509–514.

Jorm, C., and P. Kam. 2004. Does medical culture limit doctors' adoption of quality improvement? Lessons from Camelot. *Journal of Health Services Research & Policy* 9 (4): 248–251.

Jukes, T.H. 1985. Some historical notes on chlortetracycline. *Reviews of Infectious Diseases* 7 (5): 702–707.

Kingston, L., N.H. O'Connell, and C.P. Dunne. 2016. Hand hygiene-related clinical trials reported since 2010: A systematic review. *The Journal of Hospital Infection* 92 (4): 309–320.

Krein, S.L., et al. 2010. The influence of organizational context on quality improvement and patient safety efforts in infection prevention: A multi-center qualitative study. *Social Science & Medicine* 71 (9): 1692–1701.

Kumar, A., et al. 2006. Duration of hypotension before initiation of effective antimicrobial therapy is the critical determinant of survival in human septic shock. *Critical Care Medicine* 34 (6): 1589–1596.

Kwok, Y.L., C.P. Juergens, and M.L. McLaws. 2016. Automated hand hygiene auditing with and without an intervention. *American Journal of Infection Control* 44 (12): 1475–1480.

Landers, T.F., et al. 2012. A review of antibiotic use in food animals: Perspective, policy, and potential. *Public Health Reports* 127 (1): 4–22.

Lankford, M.G., et al. 2003. Influence of role models and hospital design on hand hygiene of healthcare workers. *Emerging Infectious Diseases* 9 (2): 217–223.

Larson, E. 1989. Innovations in health care: Antisepsis as a case study. *American Journal of Public Health* 79 (1): 92–99.

Lister, J. 1867. Antiseptic principles in the practice of surgery. *British Medical Journal* (Sept, 21): 246–248.

Loudon, I. 1986. Deaths in childbed from the eighteenth century to 1935. *Medical History* 30 (1): 1–41.

Mahida, N. 2016. Hand hygiene compliance: Are we kidding ourselves? *The Journal of Hospital Infection* 92 (4): 307–308.

Marshall, B.M., and S.B. Levy. 2011. Food animals and antimicrobials: Impacts on human health. *Clinical Microbiology Reviews* 24 (4): 718–733.

Mattick, K., N. Kelly, and C. Rees. 2014. A window into the lives of junior doctors: Narrative interviews exploring antimicrobial prescribing experiences. *The Journal of Antimicrobial Chemotherapy* 69 (8): 2274–2283.

McLaws, M.L. 2015. The relationship between hand hygiene and health care-associated infection: it's complicated. *Infection and Drug Resistance* 8: 7–18.

Morgan, D.J., K.S. Kaye, and D.J. Diekema. 2014. Reconsidering isolation precautions for endemic methicillin-resistant Staphylococcus aureus and vancomycin-resistant enterococcus. *JAMA* 312 (14): 1395–1396.

Morgan, D.J., R.P. Wenzel, and G. Bearman. 2017. Contact precautions for endemic MRSA and VRE: Time to retire legal mandates. *JAMA* 318 (4): 329–330.

Neo, J.R., et al. 2016. Evidence-based practices to increase hand hygiene compliance in health care facilities: An integrated review. *American Journal of Infection Control* 44 (6): 691–704.

Newsom, S.W. 2003. Pioneers in infection control-Joseph Lister. *The Journal of Hospital Infection* 55 (4): 246–253.

Nuland, S.B. 1979. The enigma of Semmelweis--an interpretation. *Journal of the History of Medicine and Allied Sciences* 34 (3): 255–272.

O'Neill, J. 2016. Tackling drug-resistant infections globally: final report and recommendations. In *The review on antimicrobial resistance*, ed. J. O'Neill. London, UK.

Palmore, T.N., and D.K. Henderson. 2012. Big brother is washing...Video surveillance for hand hygiene adherence, through the lenses of efficacy and privacy. *Clinical Infectious Diseases* 54 (1): 8–9.

Pittet, D. 2004. The Lowbury lecture: Behaviour in infection control. *The Journal of Hospital Infection* 58 (1): 1–13.

Pittet, D., et al. 2000. Effectiveness of a hospital-wide programme to improve compliance with hand hygiene. Infection Control Programme. *Lancet* 356 (9238): 1307–1312.

———. 2004. Hand hygiene among physicians: Performance, beliefs, and perceptions. *Annals of Internal Medicine* 141 (1): 1–8.

Podolsky, S.H. 2017. Historical perspective on the rise and fall and rise of antibiotics and human weight gain. *Annals of Internal Medicine* 166 (2): 133–138.

Reddy, S.C., et al. 2015. Antibiotic use in US hospitals: Quantification, quality measures and stewardship. *Expert Review of Anti-Infective Therapy* 13 (7): 843–854.

Robinson, T.P., et al. 2016. Antibiotic resistance is the quintessential one health issue. *Transactions of the Royal Society of Tropical Medicine and Hygiene* 110 (7): 377–380.

Saint, S., et al. 2003. Do physicians examine patients in contact isolation less frequently? A brief report. *American Journal of Infection Control* 31 (6): 354–356.

Saint, S., J.D. Howell, and S.L. Krein. 2010a. Implementation science: How to jump-start infection prevention. *Infection Control and Hospital Epidemiology* 31 (Suppl 1): S14–S17.

Saint, S., et al. 2010b. The importance of leadership in preventing healthcare-associated infection: Results of a multisite qualitative study. *Infection Control and Hospital Epidemiology* 31 (9): 901–907.

Sax, H., et al. 2007. 'My five moments for hand hygiene': A user-centred design approach to understand, train, monitor and report hand hygiene. *The Journal of Hospital Infection* 67 (1): 9–21.

Scheithauer, S., et al. 2011. Suspicion of viral gastroenteritis does improve compliance with hand hygiene. *Infection* 39 (4): 359–362.

———. 2017. Workload even affects hand hygiene in a highly trained and well-staffed setting: A prospective 365/7/24 observational study. *The Journal of Hospital Infection* 97 (1): 11–16.

Seibert, G., et al. 2017. What do visitors know and how do they feel about contact precautions? *American Journal of Infection Control.*

Selwyn, S. 1965. Sir James Simpson and Hospital cross infection. *Medical History* 9: 241–248.

Semmelweis, I. 1983. *The etiology, concept and prophylaxis of childbed fever*, Wisconsin Publications in the History of Science and Medicine. London: University of Wisconsin Press.

Sladek, R.M., M.J. Bond, and P.A. Phillips. 2008. Why don't doctors wash their hands? A correlational study of thinking styles and hand hygiene. *American Journal of Infection Control* 36 (6): 399–406.

Spellberg, B., and B. Taylor-Blake. 2013. On the exoneration of Dr. William H. Stewart: debunking an urban legend. *Infectious Diseases of Poverty* 2 (1): 3.

Srigley, J.A., et al. 2014. Quantification of the Hawthorne effect in hand hygiene compliance monitoring using an electronic monitoring system: A retrospective cohort study. *BMJ Quality and Safety* 23 (12): 974–980.

———. 2015. Hand hygiene monitoring technology: A systematic review of efficacy. *The Journal of Hospital Infection* 89 (1): 51–60.

Stelfox, H.T., D.W. Bates, and D.A. Redelmeier. 2003. Safety of patients isolated for infection control. *JAMA* 290 (14): 1899–1905.

Stewardson, A., et al. 2011. Back to the future: Rising to the Semmelweis challenge in hand hygiene. *Future Microbiology* 6 (8): 855–876.

Stone, P.W. 2009. Economic burden of healthcare-associated infections: An American perspective. *Expert Review of Pharmacoeconomics & Outcomes Research* 9 (5): 417–422.

Sydnor, E.R., and T.M. Perl. 2011. Hospital epidemiology and infection control in acute-care settings. *Clinical Microbiology Reviews* 24 (1): 141–173.

Temime, L., et al. 2009. Peripatetic health-care workers as potential superspreaders. *Proceedings of the National Academy of Sciences of the United States of America* 106 (43): 18420–18425.

Turnidge, J., and K. Christiansen. 2005. Antibiotic use and resistance--proving the obvious. *Lancet* 365 (9459): 548–549.

Turnidge, J.D., et al. 2016. Antimicrobial use in Australian hospitals: How much and how appropriate? *The Medical Journal of Australia* 205 (10): S16–S20.

Umscheid, C.A., et al. 2011. Estimating the proportion of healthcare-associated infections that are reasonably preventable and the related mortality and costs. *Infection Control and Hospital Epidemiology* 32 (2): 101–114.

Ventola, C.L. 2015. The antibiotic resistance crisis: Part 1: Causes and threats. *P T* 40 (4): 277–283.

Viens, A.M., and J. Littmann. 2015. Is antimicrobial resistance a slowly emerging disaster? *Public Health Ethics* 8 (3): 255–265.

WHO. 2011. *Report on the burden of endemic health care-Associated infection worldwide*. Geneva: WHO.

———, The evolving threat of antimicrobial resistance. Options for action. 2012 WHO: Geneva.

Widmer, A.F. 2000. Replace hand washing with use of a waterless alcohol hand rub? *Clinical Infectious Diseases* 31 (1): 136–143.

Willemsen, I., et al. 2009. Correlation between antibiotic use and resistance in a hospital: Temporary and ward-specific observations. *Infection* 37 (5): 432–437.

Wyer, M., et al. 2015. Involving patients in understanding hospital infection control using visual methods. *Journal of Clinical Nursing* 24 (11–12): 1718–1729.

Xu, J., et al. 2013. Surveillance and correlation of antimicrobial usage and resistance of Pseudomonas aeruginosa: A hospital population-based study. *PLoS One* 8 (11): e78604.

Zimmerman, B., et al. 2013. Front-line ownership: Generating a cure mindset for patient safety. *Healthcare Papers* 13 (1): 6–22.

4

Preventive Therapy for Multidrug Resistant Latent Tuberculosis Infection: An Ethical Imperative with Ethical Barriers to Implementation?

Binh Nguyen, Greg J. Fox, Paul H. Mason, and Justin T. Denholm

Abstract Multidrug resistant tuberculosis (MDR-TB) has a substantial impact on individuals and communities globally, including lengthy, expensive and burdensome therapy with high rates of treatment failure and death. Strategies to prevent disease are well established for those who acquire latent tuberculosis infection (LTBI) after exposure to drug susceptible TB (DS-TB). However, there has been limited research or programmatic experience regarding the prevention of MDR-TB. Accordingly, while global recommendations strongly emphasize the need to deliver LTBI therapy after TB exposure, most programs do not do so where MDR LTBI is identified.

The paucity of prospective randomized trial evidence for the effectiveness of MDR LTBI therapy, and concerns regarding its adverse effects, have been used to justify a reluctance to scale up programmatic interventions to prevent MDR-TB, or to participate in research evaluating such strategies. However, such a response fails to adequately balance potential risks of therapy with the substantial harms associ-

B. Nguyen
Woolcock Institute of Medical Research, University of Sydney, Sydney, NSW, Australia

G. J. Fox
Woolcock Institute of Medical Research, University of Sydney, Sydney, NSW, Australia

Faculty of Medicine, University of Sydney, Sydney, NSW, Australia

P. H. Mason
Woolcock Institute of Medical Research, University of Sydney, Sydney, NSW, Australia

School of Social Sciences, Monash University, Melbourne, VIC, Australia

J. T. Denholm (✉)
Department of Microbiology and Immunology, University of Melbourne, Melbourne, VIC, Australia

Victorian Tuberculosis Program at the Doherty Institute, Melbourne, VIC, Australia
e-mail: justin.denholm@mh.org.au

ated with inaction. Furthermore, the cost of inaction falls disproportionately on the most vulnerable members of society, including children. Delays in implementing proven preventive strategies may also mask hidden programmatic concerns, particularly regarding the financial cost and other burdens of treating drug resistant infection. Reticence to engage with preventative therapy for MDR-TB, even in the absence of high-level evidence, may run counter to the best interests of individuals who have been exposed to MDR-TB.

This chapter will explore ethical tensions raised by expanding access to preventative therapies for MDR-TB, and consider how ethically optimal responses to this adverse condition may be evaluated. An ethical perspective on evidentiary burden will be addressed, emphasizing how MDR LTBI research may both offer, and be shaped by, paradigmatic insights into human research ethics more generally. Emerging research and illustrations from the authors programmatic engagement in Vietnam are offered as case examples, because social and community expectations and norms may challenge, or support, implementation of therapy for drug-resistant infection. Such circumstances prompt consideration of the broader questions of social impact, such as the potential for widespread preventive therapy to accelerate the development of antimicrobial resistance.

Keywords Bioethics · Infectious diseases · Public health · Social justice · Equality and human rights · Asian culture

Background

Multidrug resistant tuberculosis (MDR-TB) is a global pandemic disease, characterised as 'Ebola with wings' by public health experts due to its airborne transmission and significant patient mortality (Voelker 1998). With more than 450,000 cases reported in 2015, MDR-TB has become an established global health emergency (World Health Organization 2013a, 2015a, 2016; Hoang et al. 2015a). While treatment for drug-susceptible (DS)-TB typically involves multiple antibiotic tablets for a period of 6 months, standard MDR-TB treatment involves up to 2 years of both oral and injected antibiotics. These toxic regimens frequently cause nausea, liver damage and irreversible hearing loss, and may also require surgery or other invasive procedures (Fox et al. 2016; Torun et al. 2005). Despite the availability of these intensive regimens, MDR-TB therapy is successful in only around half of cases globally, with a high risk of treatment failure and death (Orenstein et al. 2009). In addition, the burden of MDR-TB extends far beyond its medical impact. The prolonged illness, and its associated treatment, has major financial implications for patients and their families - incurring significant financial and housing instability (Tanimura et al. 2014). In short, MDR-TB is costly, prolonged, and complex for both individuals and health care services (Keal et al. 2013).

As TB is a contagious infectious disease, those who live in close contact with affected individuals are themselves at a high risk of developing disease - around 10% of contacts with latent (asymptomatic) TB infection (LTBI) due to *M. tuberculosis* will subsequently develop disease (Marks et al. 2000). Current strategies to prevent the spread of MDR-TB mainly focus upon interrupting the transmission of infection, by identifying and treating patients with active disease (World Health Organization 2011, 2013b; Fox et al. 2013a). Such strategies are important for individuals with MDR-TB, but have limited impact on preventing disease in those around them who are likely to have already been infected prior to the diagnosis of the treated patient. Transmission studies indicate that close contacts of MDR-TB patients have an elevated risk of infection. Not only are contacts exposed directly to the recognised patient, but they also share socio-economic determinants of disease (World Health Organization 2014; Grandjean et al. 2011; Fox et al. 2017a). This confers an increased risk of exposure to other affected individuals, and susceptibility to developing this dangerous and burdensome disease (Fox et al. 2013b).

Given the high risk of developing active disease after infection with either DS- or MDR-TB, interventions to reduce risk among close contacts are of considerable clinical and public health importance (Trauer et al. 2016). In cases of DS-TB exposure, international guidelines recommend screening of exposed contacts, and a period of antibiotic therapy to prevent progression for those at highest risk of disease progression – such as children under 5 years of age, or those with HIV infection (World Health Organization 2015b). The effectiveness of preventative chemoprophylaxis for DS-TB is well established, including through randomized controlled trials in a variety of global settings (Lobue and Menzies 2010; Sterling et al. 2011). The importance of strategies for preventing MDR-TB has recently been summarised in national and international guidelines for the programmatic management of drug-resistant TB based on the risks of transmission, high morbidity and mortality, and the further development of drug resistance (World Health Organization 2014, 2015c; Ministry of Health 2015; European Centre for Disease Prevention and Control 2012). However, most guidelines have not recommended the routine use of targeted chemopreventive therapy for contacts of MDR-TB (Fox et al. 2017b), citing insufficient evidence of effectiveness in preventing disease, instead recommending programmatic surveillance of contacts. While such surveillance may lead to earlier identification of those developing disease, it fails to reduce the risk of disease among infected contacts, and hence does not prevent the consequent social and economic hardship caused by drug-resistant disease. Thus, current approaches to MDR-TB contacts recognise the high risk of disease among contacts, but do not offer routine use of preventive therapy in most settings, including Vietnam.

Discussion

Ongoing and Proposed Clinical Trials to Evaluate Antibiotic Therapy to Prevent Drug-Resistant Infection

In this section, we will introduce ongoing and planned clinical trials that aim to establish the effectiveness of preventive therapy for MDR-TB in order to highlight ethical issues arising from this research and reflect upon possible solutions. The first of these is the V-QUIN MDR Trial - a randomised placebo-controlled trial among infected contacts of patients with MDR-TB. Contacts are recruited from district tuberculosis clinics (DTUs) where MDR-TB treatment is delivered, throughout the Southeast Asian nation of Vietnam. The trial is underway within the Programmatic Management of Drug Resistant TB (PMDT) program at 132 clinics across 10 Provinces of the country. The primary aim of the VQUIN MDR Trial is to evaluate the effectiveness of levofloxacin (a fluoroquinolone antibiotic) in the prevention of active TB among household contacts of patients with MDR-TB with latent tuberculosis infection. Adult contacts will receive either levofloxacin or placebo daily for 6 months. In accordance with international recommendations, contacts will then be monitored for disease progression over a further 2 years to detect incident TB disease.

Vietnam has the twelfth highest TB burden in the world, and is listed among the top 27 countries with the highest burden of MDR-TB (WHO 2015). The country applies regimens recommended by WHO for the treatment of MDR-TB in Vietnam, including at least 19 months of treatment. This comprises, a minimum of 6 months of intensive phase treatment (including a second line injectable antibiotic, kanamycin or capreomycin) and 13 months of continuation phase therapy. Antibiotic treatment is provided free of charge for patients meeting the eligibility criteria for the program.

Despite having a nation-wide TB Program network and a structured, well-organized health service, and reporting impressive rates of treatment completion (WHO 2015), Vietnam still faces many challenges in implementing effective MDR-TB screening and treatment. Ongoing difficulties include a lack of communication and consistency in implementing policy changes, a lack of integration between general district hospitals and the National TB Program network, and limited resources. These health-system factors contribute to a significant gap between the estimated number of cases and the number of patients commencing treatment (Hoang et al. 2015b).

In the hope of gaining more data for evidence of effective regimens in MDR-TB contacts, two other clinical trials are planned, TB-CHAMP and PHOENIx (ACTG A5300) (Clayden et al. 2015; ACTG and IMPAACT Networks 2015). Similar to V-QUIN MDR Trial using levofloxacin and placebo for intervention and control groups, TB-CHAMP study is aimed to test levofloxacin as chemoprevention in children recruited from four clinical sites in South Africa. In this trial, children under five who are household contacts of MDR-TB patients are randomized into two groups taking levofloxacin or placebo every day for 6 months and followed-up for up to 2 years (Tuberculosis child multidrug-resistant preventive therapy: TB CHAMP trial 2016). PHOENIx (ACTG A5300) run by AIDS Clinical Trials Group (ACTG) and International Maternal Pediatric Adolescent AIDS Clinical Trials Network (IMPAACT) presents another different approach in which it aims to assess the efficacy of delamanid which is a new TB drug treatment for MDR-TB and XDR TB (Xavier and Lakshmanan 2014) in treating LTBI for high risk groups of household contacts of MDR-TB patients by comparing its daily use in 6 months with isoniazid preventive therapy then follow up study subjects in 2 years. The trial is planned to be conducted in Africa, South America and Asia (ACTG and IMPAACT Networks 2015).

Observational studies of LTBI treatment are limited. The three randomized controlled clinical trials on LTBI treatment in MDR-TB contacts that we outline here could well be the only research projects currently designed to address this research gap (Mitnick et al. 2016). In the following section, we will present issues and challenges in more detail, informed by our work in Vietnam and discussion with other research teams and experts in the field. Programmatic and research ethics are contextual, and specific settings may provide useful insights into the range of issues which consideration of MDR LTBI generates. In this chapter, we aim to draw on Vietnamese experience to illustrate and reflect on key ethical issues, which may be more broadly applicable in other contexts.

Challenges in the Use of Antibiotics as a Research Intervention in LTBI Treatment

How to Balance Between Uncertainties and Risk of Harm: A Common Issue in Public Health Practice

Medical decision-making for LTBI is replete with medical uncertainty. Diagnostic tools with the capacity to identify resistance patterns in LTBI are unavailable. Similarly, diagnostic tools capable of identifying which cases of LTBI will progress to TB disease are lacking. Developing appropriate responses with this diagnostic repertoire requires reflective engagement with medical uncertainty and the ethical challenges of emerging practices (Mason 2014a; Mason 2014b). An effective treatment for LTBI may well be the best method to stop progression to active disease (World Health Organization 2011; Hill et al. 2008), but puzzling questions persist about who should receive treatment for LTBI. The problem is complex enough for LTBI cases where the index patient has drug sensitive TB, but even more complicated for MDR LTBI, where high risk of progression is recognized but uncertainty regarding potential side effects of the drugs and the impact of preventative therapy persists. For LTBI cases who have been exposed to MDR-TB, there is little consensus to guide clinicians and programs towards the risk/benefit of MDR LTBI treatment. In contexts where existing programmatic guidelines recommend against MDR LTBI treatment on the basis of such uncertainty, additional difficulties are faced for researchers seeking to establish a study protocol, which may not align to traditional clinical views and practices in a study country site even if evidentiary equipoise is present.

In the balance between benefits and harms to receivers of MDR-TB preventive treatment, a default approach of 'surveillance' is frequently assumed in which "strict clinical observation and close monitoring for the development of active TB disease for at least two years is preferred over the provision of preventive treatment for contacts with MDR-TB cases" (World Health Organization 2015c). However, such a conclusion perhaps does not follow reasonably from the available evidence and resource availability in resource-limited settings. First, strict observation and close monitoring in order to early detect active TB disease requires many resources for TB screening, diagnosis and case follow-up at a community level over a long period of time. In resource-limited settings where there is a lack of healthcare staff, diagnostic tools and competency, this approach is likely neither feasible nor sustainable. Even if such an approach to surveillance were in place, some may argue in support of providing additional chemoprophylactic agents such as isoniazid (INH) for contacts exposed to MDR-TB patients, thus raising a question of ethical acceptability for study protocols which use a placebo as a control arm.

Based on the fact that INH or RIF has been proven to reduce the risk of developing active TB by at least 60%, and widely adopted in international and national guidelines for LTBI as a standard treatment for those exposed to TB (World Health Organization 2015c; Ministry of Health 2015), the argument in favour of giving INH for MDR-TB contacts involves three rationales. The first reason is that a proportion of contacts with LTBI will have been infected previously, or infected by another index patient, and so will benefit from the therapy. The second is that giving INH is recommended as the standard of care in many countries, and that it would be inappropriate to deprive people of that option because even if it is less effective, it still will be somewhat effective. The third reason is INH is a relatively safe drug, particularly for those under 35 years. For small children, on the balance of risks and benefits, using INH is preferred where the risk of untreated infection leading to disseminated disease is high. However, considering that equipoise may be present given the lack of evidence to guide LTBI treatment for MDR-TB contacts, randomized controlled trials using placebo with periodic follow-ups could be considered ethical for the following reasons: (a) INH is unlikely to be effective, given the most proximate exposure is with MDR-TB; (b) in settings where there is a high rate of INH resistant TB—for example, in Vietnam, at least 17% of all newly diagnosed TB is INH resistant (Nhung et al. 2015)—the effectiveness will be less even if the person has been infected by non-MDR-TB; (c) the current standard of care for adults is either passive case-finding or screening for prevalent TB, (d) INH has a degree of toxicity associated with its use (Denholm et al. 2014). If a drug is toxic, ineffective, and unlikely to benefit patients, then it cannot be ethically administered. Given the diagnostic and therapeutic tools available, serial follow-up by chest Xray is a preferable form of active intervention that exceeds the current standard of care, and will detect cases early enough to reduce serious consequences and allow referral for free treatment.

Recognising that MDR-TB preventive treatment is important, more efforts should be made in finding out effective therapies when there is no standard treatment, or when no proven effective and safe treatment is known to exist. This brings us to our second theme about assessing the effectiveness of LTBI treatment in MDR-TB contacts. Systematic reviews highlight the lack of data and limits of studies conducted in assessing the effectiveness of LTBI regimens available in relevant settings (Fraser et al. 2006; van der Werf et al. 2012). Small observational studies on LTBI regimens have reported promising results. In these studies, a combination of first and second-line TB medications, including a fluoroquinolone antibiotic, is prescribed to both adult and child contacts as preventive therapy from 2 to 12 months with post treatment follow-up mean periods less than 2 years comparing with placebo or no intervention. High rates of treatment completion, low rates of incident TB disease with low rates of adverse events and good tolerability are reported from the studies (Lobue and Menzies 2010; Seddon et al. 2013; Bamrah et al. 2010). Put together, this evidence suggests that LTBI treatment may be beneficial and further research on LTBI alternative therapies is necessary in producing more comprehensive data on both effectiveness and safety on LTBI therapies.

As the risk of developing MDR-TB is acknowledged to be high in recent contacts, the risk of serious adverse effects from any preventative treatment would need to outweigh the potential benefits in order to justify withholding treatment. While sensible responses to identified MDR-TB exposure should prioritise those at highest risk, the institution of a surveillance strategy instead of provision of treatment with potential adverse effects would preferentially advantage those at lowest risk of developing disease. On this basis, despite imperfect objective estimation of the risks and benefits of different therapeutic options, we would argue that programs may default towards provision of potentially effective therapy for those with MDR LTBI, provided reasonable measures to minimize harms (such as pharmacovigilance programs to identify adverse effects) are in place. In parallel, however, it is also contingent on clinicians and programs continuing to strengthen knowledge of both risks and benefits associated with MDR LTBI therapy, so that future care may be optimally targeted and individuals appropriately informed.

Development of Acquired Drug Resistance during Preventive Therapy

Research collaborators and infectious disease clinicians participating in the VQUIN MDR-TB Trial raised valid concerns about administering drugs with unknown effectiveness and the potential harm of selecting new strains of drug resistant TB. The use of antibiotics whose effectiveness has not been demonstrated raises potential problems for individuals and the community. An ineffective regimen may fail to protect the individual, or even result in acquired drug resistance if taken infrequently. Consequently, acquired drug resistance, particularly fluoroquinolone resistance, may then lead to transmission of more advanced strains of drug resistant TB. In the case of the VQUIN MDR-TB Trial, concern hinged on two issues. First, fluoroquinolones (such as levofloxacin) are a part of the backbone of the standard regimen used to treat MDR-TB. Treatment of active TB requires effective multidrug therapy, in order to prevent resistance. If active disease is not excluded prior to commencing preventive therapy, single drug therapy could lead to acquired drug resistance. This concern underpins the reluctance of some physicians to use single-antibiotic preventive therapy in these patients. Second, in settings where LTBI is not routinely managed, clinicians and patients report reluctance to prescribe treatment in the absence of symptoms. In high-burden, low-income settings such as Vietnam, LTBI is not perceived as a disease or condition requiring treatment. Such concerns are compounded by lack of programmatic experience with the use of LTBI therapies more generally in resource-limited settings, as clinicians have few opportunities to confidently exclude active disease and develop experience with preventative therapies.

Responding to perceptions of risk in relation to amplification of drug resistance is challenging, particularly when public health messaging regarding good antimicrobial stewardship emphasizes the need to avoid unnecessary antibiotic use to preserve drug effectiveness (Doron and Davidson 2011). Some evidence suggests that isoniazid monotherapy to treat drug-susceptible LTBI is unlikely to contribute to drug resistance (Balcells et al. 2006). In fact, modeling data suggest that preventive therapy may actually reduce the overall prevalence of resistance in a population by its secondary effect of reduced propagation among cases that would otherwise have been generated (Fox et al. 2015). One priority is clear: assisting clinicians and community members to appropriately distinguish active from latent TB is an important issue if preventive therapy is to be scaled up. This requires concerted efforts to provide education, clear guidelines and updated knowledge of TB management and research.

Challenge in Conducting Research Using Fluoroquinolone in Children

A significant challenge in conducting research using levofloxacin to treat LTBI in contacts of MDR-TB patients is that fluoroquinolones are generally contraindicated in children and growing adolescents by drug manufacturers and cautiously prescribed by doctors, due to theoretical concerns about the toxicity of the drug class (Goldman and Kearns 2011). In Vietnam, the study proposal to use levofloxacin to treat MDR LTBI in children under 15 years old has caused some controversy among local scientists and members of national ethics committee in considering appropriate assessment of risks and benefits to conducting the research on children. Scientifically, the debate mainly revolves around possible adverse effects of levofloxacin to tendon and musculoskeletal system of children. This concern originated from an association between fluoroquinolone use and irreversible joint cartilage defects in juvenile animals (Ingham et al. 1977) and reversible musculoskeletal events in children (Schaaf et al. 2006). Considering that children have an increased risk of both developing active disease and more severe disseminated forms of disease, and only indirect evidence for a link between fluoroquinolones and musculoskeletal harm exists, there is a strong argument for the inclusion of children in studies such as VQUIN. However, while strategies to deal with potential risks have been considered, including enhanced adverse effect monitoring of younger participants, at present the study has only been approved for adult contacts of MDR-TB.

Poor Understanding about LTBI and the Use of Diagnostic Tests

LTBI is generally poorly understood (Colson et al. 2010). Interviews with community members in a variety of contexts consistently identify confusion regarding the difference between latent and active TB, the extent of risk associated with infection, and the availability of treatment to prevent progression to disease (Wieland et al. 2012). A lack of knowledge about LTBI and its attendant risks of progression to disease presents difficulties for the introduction of preventative therapies, particularly where they involve prolonged treatment with some potential adverse effects.

Such uncertainty exists among healthcare workers as well as in the general community. In the research of LTBI therapy given to contacts of MDR-TB patients in Provincial Hospitals and District TB Units in Vietnam, we have identified particular issues including low level of knowledge of LTBI and a general lack of knowledge of treatment options for both active MDR-TB and suspected MDR LTBI. While TB is commonly known as a transmissible airborne infection, the pathways to active disease following exposure are still poorly understood by most healthcare staff. Uncertainties have been repeatedly expressed over the use of diagnostic tests for LTBI, the type and duration of LTBI treatment, presumably reflecting a lack of familiarity with preventative therapies in this context.

Challenges in Obtaining Informed Consent and Following-up Study Participants

The requirement to obtain informed consent is central to the ethical conduct of research involving human subjects. As clinical research has become more global, bringing with it a requirement to obtain consent in different places where many disparate values are held, the obtaining of valid consent increasingly raises a range of challenges. Consent practices in resource-limited settings may be impacted by time constraints for researchers to provide detailed research information, the lack of familiarity with medical research, traditionally paternalistic doctor-patient power dynamics and communication styles, involvement of family members and community members in the decision making process, conflict of duty of healthcare provider acting as researcher (Cheah and Parker 2014; Nguyen 2016), not to mention the significant cultural dimensions involved in adapting (and asserting) this research practice in settings where it is a foreign concept (Mason et al. 2017). Suffice to say that obtaining consent in research on LTBI treatment presents complex issues posed by its research context and clinical practice in addition to the complexities of explaining LTBI to a naïve audience.

Based on our experience in conducting research on LTBI therapy given to contacts of MDR-TB patients in Vietnam, we outline challenges generated by different understandings about research and preventive treatment. When the term "research" is translated directly into Vietnamese, it arouses commonly-held negative perceptions within the lay Vietnamese population. Healthcare workers also often express concerns that patients will decline to participate in research studies due to these negative associations, and prefer to avoid the term. An inability to refer to a study as being "research" may obstruct appropriate consent practices, since participants may not be aware of the experimental nature of the involved procedures. This difficulty is further complicated by differing understandings about LTBI and the appropriateness of preventive treatment.

The practical experience of obtaining consent in Vietnam for this study has been explored in series of research staff interviews, highlighting misperceptions about preventive therapy and the low priority people give to it. A staff member who worked on the community studies of the V-QUIN TB screening commented:

> "Our Vietnamese common perception is that "no disease, no treatment". Preventive treatment is not a priority to our people, especially people in farming regions. Their educational level is low so they don't think about preventive treatment. They only buy drugs when they get sick" (Study staff – N01).

With limited information about LTBI treatment in national guidelines, and specific recommendations against MDR LTBI treatment, challenges to effective consent and study participation are likely. In the traditionally hierarchical Vietnamese healthcare system, the existence of guidelines recommending against MDR LTBI treatment is a strong disincentive to both clinicians and community members' participation in research. Research into MDR LTBI treatment may be perceived as being in opposition to existing recommendations, despite the limited evidence on which they are based.

Stigmatization

The stigmatization of TB may impact upon the management of and research into LTBI. In research practice, we experienced that some MDR-TB patients are self stigmatised, or are isolated by their family members due to their disease status. Such patients may want to hide the disease from household contacts and neighbors (therefore prefer going to a private clinic to keep their privacy) and have poor medical adherence. Those most concerned about stigma may also avoid providing accurate information about their household contacts. Study staff in collaboration with local healthcare providers have to explore the information on household contacts by gradually building the relationship between patients and their care-giver, if there is any. This can be achieved through talking with them and providing them more information about TB, LTBI and preventive treatment in clinical assessments performed at hospitals or district tuberculosis clinics. The same stigma may drive healthy household contacts with LTBI to avoid sharing their infection status with neighbors and friends. As a result, these infected individuals do not want any home visit made by NTP staff/study staff, and do not want to be contacted and asked about the patient. This can create difficulties and challenges in approaching potential study subjects who may participate in the research. It also impedes monitoring of drug adherence and post-treatment following up. As expressed by a study staff about stigmatization in TB:

> "TB is a social disease. It makes participant feel ashamed of getting infection, and thus not wanting to talk about their disease status or being followed up for a long period of time in the study to have their health checked. They also avoid their neighbors knowing about the disease" (Study staff – S01).

Solutions for Identified Ethical Problems and Challenges

So far, we have attempted to map out a range of issues arising in the prevention of MDR-TB, current approaches to MDR LTBI therapy and in the context of doing a randomized controlled trial in LTBI with our experiences in Vietnam as an exemplary case of high burden TB and limited resource countries. What we will propose as solutions in this chapter accordingly will be general solutions to be considered in providing LTBI treatment and in doing MDR LTBI research. They are put forward in light of the nature of the problems, challenges occurring in the research practice and practical conditions in the setting.

Developing a Comprehensive LTBI Research Agenda

Clinical studies are crucial in advancing medical care. They are needed to produce systematic information on pathogenesis, clinical course, potential interventions and response to treatment. Especially in LTBI, it is important to address a key ethical challenge which is balancing between uncertainties and risk of harm involved in screening and treatment provision, and from that to derive lessons and possible ways to scale up interventions at the community level. Any new scientific information or breakthroughs can bring about alterations to current accounts of scientific and ethical considerations about existing interventions. Concerns about how best to apply systematic screening of LTBI and its related accounts of risk and benefit with beneficiaries (Degeling et al. 2017) is an example which can be expected to be resolved via promising outcome of studies on new LTBI diagnostic methods and indicators of reactivation risk (Dodd and Schlesinger 2017). From our experience drawn in the setting as outlined above, we argue that systematic research, especially randomized clinical trials in evaluating the effectiveness of preventive therapy for LTBI in the contacts of patients with MDR-TB are imperative to better inform clinical decisions, to benefit future infected people and the public in general.

Collaboration

Efforts toward the elimination of tuberculosis call for wide collaboration of various stakeholders including, but not limited to, clinicians in both public and private sectors, public health practitioners (Hauck and Panchal 2009; Taylor et al. 2005), researchers of all groups of expertise, funders, research communities and the public (Sablan 2009). This would serve as a ground for developing a comprehensive and balanced research agenda to inform clinical and public health practice, and to create sustainable research and public health platforms with long term facilities and community support. This type of collaboration can be conducted through the format of national and international collaborative research networks, for example, The Tuberculosis Network European Trials group (TBNET) (Giehl et al. 2012), The Australasian Clinical Tuberculosis Network (ACTnet), The Union World Conference on Lung Health, and the involvement of research community, public and mass media. The primary aim of such collaborations is to engage relevant stakeholders from the beginning of a research initiative to translating research findings into practice in community level on the basis of mutual understanding of a shared account of vision and mission and benefit generating for afflicted population.

While collaborations are recognized as crucial to successful research schemes, effective collaborations, in our view, need to be characterized by 'openness' in which collaborative partners see each other having supplementary role rather competitors, and a shared common interest that is to contribute to the knowledge of the disease for the public good through sharing data and samples. Contributing to the framework of global health, such an open form of collaboration is aimed to protect the common interest towards the global health and stress on the duty to protect affected members of the public and the public good.

Provide Education and Raise Community Awareness of LTBI

Provide necessary scientific training to healthcare workers and study staff.

In order to help ensure success in LTBI treatment program and research initiatives, given the issues related to the lack of knowledge of current LTBI diagnostic methods and therapies which we have outlined above, training on scientific knowledge of LTBI and the role of research in producing systematic information to inform practice is necessary. It is importantly required for frontline health workers who directly provide healthcare to patients and communities where are most needed. These can include pharmacists, nurses, clinicians, and public health officers who serve in hospitals and community clinics. As the first and sometimes the only link to essential healthcare services in limited resource settings, this group of experts hold great potential to make a direct impact on individual and community health through supporting research activities, delivering good healthcare services and community consultation. Studies and our experience have shown that interaction and communication between health workers/study doctors and patients/study participants brings significant effect to the level of recruitment, medication adherence and treatment outcomes (Horne 1999; Dwamena et al. 2012; Sumartojo 1993). In this case of LBTI and TB control, it is knowledge of current approaches for TB control and prevention available locally and internationally, important health implications of LTBI, the need to provide LTBI treatment, and associated adverse events and their management that needs to be provided and updated to health workers and study staff to equip them in delivering healthcare services at the best level and standard.

Public education.

When research participants are subject to possible sources of vulnerability, the consent process with consideration of some additional protections should aim to protect the safety and the rights of research participants and benefits of afflicted population. This duty should be taken on by ethics committees, physician-researchers, local and international research institutions and other entities involved in the research in designing, reviewing and implementing research projects. At the same time, the consent process should be developed in a way that will enhance "voluntary actions that are intended to help or benefit another individual or group of individuals" (Eisenberg and Mussen 1989a) of research participants, family members and community.

In addressing the key issues in consent and the awareness of LTBI and the role of MDR LTBI treatment in the prevention of TB, we propose that educating the public about the nature of research and its necessity for the improvement and advancement of science in medicine as an overarching plan to make people understand more about the meaning of research and therefore to encourage their participation. For the purpose of raising community awareness of LTBI and the importance of doing more research on this subject, along with the general public education as mentioned above, it also requires providing education programs about clinical research and LTBI to the population and disseminating information about LTBI treatment in the forms of national guidelines with references to international guidelines, health promotional materials and community consultation. This form of education should be carried out on a long term and regular basis. Specific aims of these plans would be (1) to change negative attitude towards research, e.g. 'being a Guinea Pig'; (2) to let people have a better understanding of research, scientific methods in treatment and healthcare, and the role of research in support of medicine; and (3) to maintain trust and nurture pro-social behavior that will enhance "voluntary actions that are intended to help or benefit another individual or group of individuals" in society (Eisenberg and Mussen 1989b) for research and public health agenda.

Strengthen Communication Between Research Ethics Committees (RECs) and Researchers

Facilitating cooperation between RECs and scientists/researchers is necessary for mutual understanding and a rapid response in LTBI research context. One way to achieve this is to establish and maintain communication between researchers and RECs throughout research scheme. On the part of RECs, effective communication strategies with researchers will help the RECs to improve transparency in their decisions, understand practical challenges in doing research in the local context, develop expertise in a particular topic area, understand researchers' perspectives and make researchers mutually understand the challenges and duties of RECs. This mutual understanding would eventually place both RECs and researchers in an engaged process whereby research participants are better protected and research can be conducted effectively without being subject to unnecessary delays, misunderstanding and uncertainties.

Conclusion

In this chapter, we have outlined key issues in preventative therapies for MDR-TB and challenges in conducting research to assess potentially effective MDR LTBI therapies. We have raised possible solutions, derived from our own work in the Vietnamese setting in juxtaposition with broader ethical considerations. We have argued that preventive therapy for MDR-TB should be a high priority. There is a need for appropriately conducted systematic research to address the spread of MDR-TB in limited-resource settings globally. Engagement with local cultural norms and priorities is critical for ensuring that such research is conducted in both ethical and effective fashion.

References

ACTG and IMPAACT Networks. 2015. *A5300B/IMPAACT2003B: Protecting Households On Exposure to Newly Diagnosed Index Multidrug Resistant Tuberculosis Patients (PHOENIx)*. Available from: http://impaactnetwork.org/studies/IMPAACT2003B.asp.

Balcells, M.E., et al. 2006. Isoniazid preventive therapy and risk for resistant tuberculosis. *Emerging Infectious Diseases* 12 (5): 744–751.

Bamrah, S., et al.. 2010. *An ounce of prevention: Treating MDR-TB contacts in a resource-limited setting*, in *International Union of Tuberculosis and Lung Disease Conference* 2010: Berlin, Germany, 11–15 November, 2010. p. FA-1- 656-14:S180.

Cheah, P.Y., and M. Parker. 2014. Consent and assent in paediatric research in low-income settings. *BMC Medical Ethics* 15 (1): 22.

Clayden, P., et al. 2015. *Pipeline report: HIV, hepatitis C virus (HCV), and tuberculosis (TB). Drugs, diagnostics, vaccines, preventive technologies, research towards a cure, and immune-based and gene therapies in development*. New York: Treatment Action Group.

Colson, P.W., et al. 2010. Tuberculosis knowledge, attitudes, and beliefs in foreign-born and US-born patients with latent tuberculosis infection. *Journal of Immigrant and Minority Health* 12 (6): 859–866.

Degeling, C., et al. 2017. Eliminating latent tuberculosis in low-burden settings: Are the principal beneficiaries to be disadvantaged groups or the broader population? *Journal of Medical Ethics* 43: 632–636.

Denholm, J.T., et al. 2014. Adverse effects of isoniazid preventative therapy for latent tuberculosis infection: A prospective cohort study. *Drug, Healthcare and Patient Safety* 6: 145–149.

Dodd, C.E., and L.S. Schlesinger. 2017. New concepts in understanding latent tuberculosis. *Current Opinion in Infectious Diseases* 30 (3): 316–321.

Doron, S., and L.E. Davidson. 2011. Antimicrobial stewardship. *Mayo Clinic Proceedings* 86 (11): 1113–1123.

Dwamena, F., et al. 2012. Interventions for providers to promote a patient-centred approach in clinical consultations. *Cochrane Database of Systematic Reviews* 12: CD003267.

Eisenberg, N., and P.H. Mussen. 1989a. *The roots of prosocial behavior in children*. Cambridge: Cambridge University Press.

———. 1989b. *The roots of prosocial behavior in children (Cambridge studies in social and emotional development)*, 208. Cambridge: Cambridge University Press.

European Centre for Disease Prevention and Control. 2012. *Management of contacts of MDR TB and XDR TB patients*. Stockholm: ECDC.

Fox, G.J., et al. 2013a. Contact investigation for tuberculosis: A systematic review and meta-analysis. *European Respiratory Journal* 41: 134–150.

———. 2013b. Contact investigation for tuberculosis: A systematic review and meta-analysis. *The European Respiratory Journal* 41 (1): 140–156.

Fox, G.J., O. Oxlade, and D. Menzies. 2015. *Fluoroquinolone Therapy for the Prevention of Multidrug-Resistant Tuberculosis in Contacts. A Cost-Effectiveness Analysis.* (1535–4970 (Electronic)).

Fox, G.J., et al. 2016. Surgery as an adjunctive treatment for multidrug-resistant tuberculosis: An individual patient data Metaanalysis. *Clinical Infectious Diseases* 62 (7): 887–895.

———. 2017a. Latent tuberculous infection in household contacts of multidrug-resistant and newly diagnosed tuberculosis. *The International Journal of Tuberculosis and Lung Disease* 21 (3): 297–302.

———. 2017b. Preventing the spread of multidrug-resistant tuberculosis and protecting contacts of infectious cases. *Clinical Microbiology and Infection* 23 (3): 147–153.

Fraser, A., et al. 2006. Drugs for preventing tuberculosis in people at risk of multiple-drug-resistant pulmonary tuberculosis. *Cochrane Database of Systematic Reviews* 2: CD005435.

Giehl, C., et al. 2012. TBNET – Collaborative research on tuberculosis in Europe. *European Journal of Microbiology & Immunology* 2 (4): 264–274.

Goldman, J.A., and G.L. Kearns. 2011. *Flouroquinolone Use in Paediatrics: Focus on Safety and Place in Therapy - A commissioned work for the Guidelines Group for the Revision of the "Guidance for National Tuberculosis Programmes on the Management of Tuberculosis in Children", World Health Organization, 30-31* March 2010, Geneva, Switzerland. 2011.

Grandjean, L., et al. 2011. Tuberculosis in household contacts of multidrug-resistant tuberculosis patients. *International Journal of Tuberculosis & Lung Disease* 15 (9): 1164–1169.

Hauck, F.R., and A.S. Panchal. 2009. Latent tuberculosis infection: The physician's role in tuberculosis control. *American Family Physician* 79 (10): 845–846.

Hill, L., et al. 2008. *Multi-level barriers to LTBI treatment: a research note.* (1557–1920 (Electronic)).

Hoang, T.T.T., et al. 2015a. Challenges in detection and treatment of multidrug resistant tuberculosis patients in Vietnam. *BMC Public Health* 15 (1): 980.

———. 2015b. Challenges in detection and treatment of multidrug resistant tuberculosis patients in Vietnam. *BMC Public Health* 15: 980.

Horne, R. 1999. Patients' beliefs about treatment: The hidden determinant of treatment outcome? *Journal of Psychosomatic Research* 47 (6): 491–495.

Ingham, B., et al. 1977. Arthropathy induced by antibacterial fused n-alkyl-4-pyrodoine-3-carboxylic acids. *Toxicology Letters* 1: 21–26.

Keal, J., et al. 2013. P97 multi-drug resistant tuberculosis: The first UK guideline for treatment monitoring. *Thorax* 68 (Suppl 3): A119.

Lobue, P., and D. Menzies. 2010. Treatment of latent tuberculosis infection: An update. *Respirology* 15 (4): 603–622.

Marks, G.B., et al. 2000. Incidence of tuberculosis among a cohort of tuberculin-positive refugees in Australia: Reappraising the estimates of risk. *American Journal of Respiratory & Critical Care Medicine* 162 (5): 1851–1854.

Mason, P.H. 2014a. The liminal body: Comment on "Privacy in the Context of 'Re-emergent' Infectious Diseases" by Justin T. Denholm and Ian H. Kerridge. *Journal of Bioethical Inquiry* 11 (4): 565–566.

———. 2014b. *The liminal body: Comment on "Privacy in the context of 're-emergent' infectious diseases" by Justin T. Denholm and Ian H. Kerridge.* (1176–7529 (Print)).

Mason, P.H., I. Kerridge, and W. Lipworth. 2017. The global in Global Health is not a given. *The American Journal of Tropical Medicine and Hygiene* 96 (4): 767–769.

Ministry of Health. 2015. *Guidelines for tuberculosis diagnosis, treatment and prevention.*

Mitnick, C.D., et al. 2016. Programmatic management of drug-resistant tuberculosis: An updated research agenda. *PLoS One* 11 (5).

Nguyen, T.C.B. 2016. The ethics of research in rapidly evolving epidemics: an international perspective. In *Kellogg*. Oxford: University of Oxford.

Nhung, N.V., et al. 2015. The fourth national anti-tuberculosis drug resistance survey in Viet Nam. *The International Journal of Tuberculosis and Lung Disease* 19 (6): 670–675.

Orenstein, E.W., et al. 2009. Treatment outcomes among patients with multidrug-resistant tuberculosis: Systematic review and meta-analysis. *The Lancet Infectious Diseases* 9 (3): 153–161.

Sablan, B. 2009. An update on primary care management for tuberculosis in children. *Current Opinion in Pediatrics* 21 (6): 801–804.

Schaaf, H., et al. 2006. Childhood drug-resistant tuberculosis in the Western Cape Province of South Africa. *Acta Paediatrica* 95 (5): 523–528.

Seddon, J.A., et al. 2013. Preventive therapy for child contacts of multidrug-resistant tuberculosis: A prospective cohort study. *Clinical Infectious Diseases* 57 (12): 1676–1684.

Sterling, T.R., et al. 2011. Three months of rifapentine and isoniazid for latent tuberculosis infection. *The New England Journal of Medicine* 365 (23): 2155–2166.

Sumartojo, E. 1993. When tuberculosis treatment fails. A social behavioral account of patient adherence. *The American Review of Respiratory Disease* 147 (5): 1311–1320.

Tanimura, T., et al. 2014. Financial burden for tuberculosis patients in low- and middle-income countries: A systematic review. *The European Respiratory Journal* 43 (6): 1763–1775.

Taylor, Z., C.M. Nolan, and H.M. Blumberg. 2005. Controlling tuberculosis in the United States. Recommendations from the American Thoracic Society, CDC, and the Infectious Diseases Society of America. *MMWR Recommendations and Reports* 54 (RR-12): 1–81.

Torun, T., et al. 2005. Side effects associated with the treatment of multidrug-resistant tuberculosis. *The International Journal of Tuberculosis and Lung Disease* 9 (12): 1373–1377.

Trauer, J.M., et al. 2016. Risk of active tuberculosis in the five years following infection … 15%? *Chest* 149 (2): 516–525.

Tuberculosis child multidrug-resistant preventive therapy: TB CHAMP trial. 2016. Available from: http://www.isrctn.com/ISRCTN92634082.

van der Werf, M.J., et al. 2012. Lack of evidence to support policy development for management of contacts of multidrug-resistant tuberculosis patients: Two systematic reviews. *The International Journal of Tuberculosis and Lung Disease* 16 (3): 288–296.

Voelker, R. 1998. Ebola with wings. *JAMA* 280 (14): 1216–1216.

WHO. 2015. *World Health Organization global tuberculosis report, 2015*. Geneva: WHO.

Wieland, M.L., et al. 2012. Perceptions of tuberculosis among immigrants and refugees at an adult education center: A community-based participatory research approach. *Journal of Immigrant and Minority Health* 14 (1): 14–22.

World Health Organization. 2011. *Guidelines for the programmatic management of drug-resistant tuberculosis – 2011 update*. Geneva: WHO.

———. 2013a. *Global tuberculosis report 2013*. Geneva: World Health Organization.

———. 2013b. *Systematic screening for active tuberculosis: principles and recommendations*. Geneva: WHO.

———. 2014. *Companion handbook to the WHO guidelines for the programmatic management of drug-resistant tuberculosis*. Geneva: WHO.

———. 2015a. *Global tuberculosis report 2015*. Geneva: World Health Organization.

———. 2015b. *Guidelines on the management of latent tuberculosis infection*. Geneva: WHO.

———. 2015c. *Guidelines on the management of latent tuberculosis infection*. Geneva: WHO. WHO/HTM/TB/2015.01. 38.

———. 2016. *Global tuberculosis report 2016*. Geneva: WHO.

Xavier, A.S., and M. Lakshmanan. 2014. Delamanid: A new armor in combating drug-resistant tuberculosis. *Journal of Pharmacology and Pharmacotherapeutics* 5 (3): 222–224.

5

Ethics and Antimalarial Drug Resistance

Phaik Yeong Cheah, Michael Parker, and Nicholas P. J. Day

Abstract There has been impressive progress in malaria control and treatment over the past two decades. One of the most important factors in the decline of malaria-related mortality has been the development and deployment of highly effective treatment in the form of artemisinin-based combination therapies (ACTs). However, recent reports suggest that these gains stand the risk of being reversed due to the emergence of ACT resistance in the Greater Mekong Subregion and the threat of this resistance spreading to Africa, where the majority of the world's malaria cases occur, with catastrophic consequences. This chapter provides an overview of strategies proposed by malaria experts to tackle artemisinin-resistant malaria, and some of the most important practical ethical issues presented by each of these interventions. The proposed strategies include mass antimalarial drug administrations in selected populations, and mandatory screening of possibly infected individuals prior to entering an area free of artemisinin-resistant malaria. We discuss ethical issues such as tensions between the wishes of individuals versus the broader goal of

P. Y. Cheah (✉)
Mahidol Oxford Tropical Medicine Research Unit (MORU), Faculty of Tropical Medicine, Mahidol University, Bangkok, Thailand

Centre for Tropical Medicine and Global Health, Nuffield Department of Clinical Medicine, University of Oxford, Oxford, UK

The Ethox Centre, Nuffield Department of Population Health, University of Oxford, Oxford, UK
e-mail: Phaikyeong@tropmedres.ac

M. Parker
The Ethox Centre, Nuffield Department of Population Health, University of Oxford, Oxford, UK

Wellcome Centre for Ethics and Humanities, Nuffield Department of Population Health, University of Oxford, Oxford, UK
e-mail: michael.parker@ethox.ox.ac.uk

N. P. J. Day
Mahidol Oxford Tropical Medicine Research Unit (MORU), Faculty of Tropical Medicine, Mahidol University, Bangkok, Thailand

Centre for Tropical Medicine and Global Health, Nuffield Department of Clinical Medicine, University of Oxford, Oxford, UK malaria elimination, and the risks of harm to interventional populations, and conclude by proposing a set of recommendations.

The Problem, Context and Background

Malaria is the most important parasitic disease of man. It remains a major cause of death in tropical countries, and an important cause of illness, particularly in childhood. There were an estimated 435,000 deaths from malaria in 2017, of which over 90% were in Africa (Global Malaria Programme, World Health Organization 2018). Although there has been impressive progress in malaria control and treatment over the past two decades in recent years progress has stalled and there has been a resurgence of malaria in Southeast Asia, where antimalarial drug resistance is increasingly prevalent (Global Malaria Programme, World Health Organization 2018). One of the most important factors in the decline of malaria related mortality since the 1990s has been the development and deployment of highly effective treatment in the form of artemisinin-based combination therapies (ACTs) (Bhatt et al. 2015). ACTs are currently the mainstay of antimalarial treatment throughout the world, recommended by the World Health Organization as the first line treatment globally for falciparum malaria (World Health Organization 2016a). Their widespread deployment, along with the expanded use of insecticide treated bed nets, accounts for a large part of the reduction in malaria deaths in Africa over the past decade (White et al. 2014).

The effectiveness of current and future interventions are, however, at risk from the emergence of new forms of drug resistance. In the early 2000s malaria parasites that were partially resistant to the artemisinins emerged in Western Cambodia. The problem was identified and characterised in 2008 (Dondorp et al. 2009; Noedl et al. 2008). The hallmark of infection by these resistant parasites was slow parasite clearance rather than outright treatment failure (Dondorp et al. 2009). These slow clearing infections were associated with mutations in the *PfKelch13* gene, with multiple *PfKelch13* mutations described (though each parasite only carried one) (Ariey et al. 2014). By 2014 slow clearing malaria infections caused by *PfKelch13* mutation-carrying artemisinin resistant parasites could be found in Myanmar, Laos, Thailand, Vietnam and Yunnan province in China, and by 2016 *Pfkelch13* mutants were identified in Arunachal Pradesh state in northeastern India (Ashley et al. 2014; Tun et al. 2016; Mishra et al. 2016).

The initial response to the emergence of artemisinin resistance had two aspects. The major concerns were that: i. artemisinin resistance might lead to or combine with partner drug resistance resulting in resistance to ACTs. That is, to the loss of the drug combinations that are the mainstay of malaria treatment; and ii. that were this to be the case, artemisinin resistance and then ACT resistance then has the potential to spread from Southeast Asia to Africa, where the majority of the world's malaria cases occur, with catastrophic consequences. There are precedents for this latter concern; in the last 60 years first chloroquine resistance and then sulfadoxine-pyrimethamine resistance arose in Western Cambodia and subsequently spread to Africa, leading to millions of deaths (Verdrager 1986; Roper et al. 2004; Trape et al. 1998).

Recognizing the risks and consequences of spread to Africa, the World Health Organization initially developed a plan to contain rather than eliminate the problem (World Health Organization 2011). However, this approach was criticized by some at the time who called for initiatives aimed at eliminating all malaria in the Greater Mekong Subregion, on the grounds that the resistant parasites were in fact already at that stage contained (Dondorp et al. 2017). They argued that the view that elimination would be an appropriate strategy was supported by mathematical modelling that showed that as malaria was controlled and transmission fell, the proportion of infections that were resistant would increase – the 'last man standing' would be resistant (Maude et al. 2012). This modelling suggested that resistance could not be eliminated without eliminating all malaria in the affected regions.

Bolstered by advocacy for global malaria eradication by the Bill and Melinda Gates Foundation, the WHO did eventually change its policy from containment to one of elimination (Global Malaria Programme WHO 2015), but the discovery through molecular studies that *PfKelch13* mutations had arisen spontaneously and independently multiple times within the Greater Mekong Subregion (GMS) led to what some saw as a reduction in the urgency to eliminate malaria to prevent the 'spread' of resistant parasites (Takala-Harrison et al. 2015). Surveillance for resistance and an aim to eliminate malaria *everywhere* was now the policy of WHO (World Health Organization 2017; Global Malaria Programme WHO 2016). This necessarily spread resources more widely and reduced the focus on drug resistance. Despite this there has been considerable investment in malaria control and elimination efforts in the GMS, with at least initially substantial reductions in malaria transmission (Dondorp et al. 2017). These successes have, however, to some extent masked the continued threat of increasingly drug resistant malaria parasites emerging and spreading in the region – as the mathematical modelling had predicted (Maude et al. 2009) – with outbreaks of artemisinin-resistant malaria occurring in areas previously considered malaria free (Imwong et al. 2015).

In the 10 years since the first description of artemisinin resistance the concern that ACT resistance and failure would develop has come to pass, with rising mefloquine resistance on the Thai-Myanmar border and piperaquine resistance in Cambodia, Thailand, Southern Laos and Viet Nam (Phyo et al. 2016a; Amaratunga et al. 2016; Imwong et al. 2017). Recent evidence that most of the resistance to dihydroartemisinin-piperaquine is due to the geographical *spread* of a particularly fit artemisinin-resistant parasite clone which has picked up piperaquine resistance has rekindled the debate about whether urgent focus should be placed on an accelerated effort to eliminate artemisinin-resistant malaria in Southeast Asia, with the aim of preventing the spread of ACT resistance to Africa (World Health Organization 2016b).

Although the global pipeline for new malaria drugs in development is healthier than it has been for decades, all the most promising candidates (schizonticidals, that kill the asexual blood stage of the parasite which causes the clinical manifestations of malaria) are at least five years away from being available in the market (Phyo et al. 2016b). The RTS,S/AS01 malaria vaccine which recently received a favourable scientific opinion from the European Medicines Agency (EMA) is only partially protective (Vandoolaeghe and Schuerman 2018). This means that protecting the efficacy of the currently available antimalarial drugs is of global importance. The spread of ACT resistance to Africa would threaten the loss of millions of lives, especially those of young African children. This will be a global health issue – untreatable malaria worldwide arising from resistance in Southeast Asia. A problem arising in a specific location that has the potential to threaten global health is not unique to malaria. Many 'global health problems' arise in low-income settings, for example outbreaks of Ebola in West Africa and Zika in South America, and are recognized as having worldwide implications. In the case of Ebola and Zika the World Health Organization formally declared a 'Public Health Emergency of International Concern' (PHEIC), but for the emergence of artemisinin resistant malaria in Southeast Asia WHO has as of 2018 declined to do this despite some experts calling for it to do so (World Health Organization 2016b; Talisuna et al. 2012).

How Should the Problem of Artemisinin Resistant Malaria be Tackled?

There is now broad agreement amongst experts that to prevent the spread of artemisinin-resistant *P. falciparum* it is necessary to completely interrupt *P. falciparum* transmission (Maude et al. 2009), and that a programme of accelerated malaria elimination is warranted in the GMS and surrounding areas. The scientific consensus is that a combination of strategies is required to achieve this (Dondorp et al. 2017; World Health Organization 2017). These include:

1. *Ongoing surveillance* with a network of village malaria workers (VMWs) in endemic areas trained and equipped to provide early detection and treatment of malaria cases.

2. *Targeting of the asymptomatic malaria reservoir* in so called malaria 'hotspots', identified through surveys of healthy individuals employing highly sensitive methods of parasite detection such as large volume quantitative PCR and highly sensitive rapid diagnostic tests (RDTs). This may take two forms:

   a. *Mass drug administration* (MDA) -WHO agrees that targeted mass antimalarial drug administration may play an important role in malaria elimination (World Health Organization, Global Malaria Programme 2015a).
   b. *Mass screening and treatment* (MSAT) using novel highly sensitive diagnostics.

3. *Vector control* with insecticide treated bed nets, despite these being less effective in the GMS than in Africa because of the biting habits of many of the vector species (biting in the forest rather than in houses, and in the early evening or morning).
4. *Targeting 'source' populations* such as forest workers and migrants, rather than 'sink' populations secondarily affected. This requires an understanding of transmission dynamics and population movements – important in the GMS where cross border movement/migration is common.
5. *Mandatory screening* may be necessary of possibly infected individuals entering an area free of artemisinin-resistant malaria (Houston and Houston 2015; Tatarsky et al. 2011).
6. Use of *effective antimalarial treatments*. Most currently approved ACTs consist of only two drugs (a fast acting short half-life artemisinin and a longer half-life partner drug) and are vulnerable to the development of resistance. The testing and deployment of new triple artemisinin-based combination therapies (TACTs) has been recommended, and several of these are currently being tested in the GMS and beyond (Dondorp et al. 2017).

In the face of the global threat posed by increasing ACT resistance, there is therefore now an emerging expert consensus that the combination of strategies outlined above is the most effective way of halting or slowing its international spread provide strong ethical arguments for their rapid adoption. Each of the interventions listed above present a wide range of interconnected challenges – including, scientific, technological, governmental, economic and ethical – all of which will need to be overcome if the elimination of malaria in the region is to be achieved. In addition to these practical scientific, and political challenges, the success of each of the interventions also depends upon the addressing of a number of important practical ethical questions, which need to be taken into account in their design and implementation. In the next section, we outline some of the most important practical ethical issues presented by each of the interventions proposed above.

Practical Ethical Issues Arising in These Interventions

Ongoing Surveillance

In many countries in the Greater Mekong Subregion, networks of VMWs are the cornerstone of malaria surveillance and the delivery of malaria-related interventions. These networks are usually run either directly by the national malaria control programmes (NMCPs) or by NGOs working with the NMCPs, but may also be put in place by private providers such as companies running palm oil plantations. The coverage of such networks has increased impressively in many areas in SEA, particularly in border areas, conflict zones and areas underserved by government health programmes. VMWs are consulted by villagers suffering from fever, and are equipped with RDTs and antimalarial treatments. Where a substantial proportion of febrile illnesses are indeed caused by malaria VMWs are a valuable resource for the local population. However, the success of malaria control and elimination efforts increasingly means that a diminishing proportion of the febrile illnesses they encounter are caused by malaria. Unfortunately, VMWs are not usually equipped to deal with these alternative causes of illness. This means that as malaria rates decline there is a risk that villagers will cease consulting VMWs as more of them are told that because their fever is not clinical malaria infection, no diagnosis or treatment of the cause of their illness is available or offered. Unless these village workers are retrained for a wider role as 'village *health* workers' able to manage other febrile illnesses or simple primary health problems, they will become increasingly irrelevant and demotivated. The consequences of this would be diminishing effectiveness of the malaria surveillance network itself, at the point in the elimination process when it is most needed and, in the absence of a wider role, for the goal of malaria elimination becoming a disincentive for the VMWs (and NMCPs), for many of whom being a VMW is a source of their livelihood. This suggests that, even if the elimination of malaria is the primary goal, there are strong arguments in favour of the provision of resources for access to health care beyond malaria in the region.

Mass Drug Administration (MDA)

MDA in the context of malaria elimination consists of mass treatment with a schizonticide to kill the asexual blood stage of the parasite which causes the clinical manifestations of malaria combined with a transmission blocking drug to kill gametocytes. Giving such treatment to all members of a community should eliminate the asymptomatic parasite reservoir and speed up the interruption of malaria transmission. Where and when it is warranted has been the subject of much debate, but the consensus is that MDA should be targeted at communities with high transmission and a large asymptomatic reservoir (World Health Organization 2011; von Seidlein and Dondorp 2015). This requires a functioning surveillance system to identify such communities, with surveys of healthy individuals with highly sensitive tests to estimate accurately the scale of the asymptomatic reservoir.

There are a number of important ethical considerations when determining when and where to use MDA. The first of these arises out of the fact that MDA by its nature involves administering drugs to individuals who will not benefit *directly* from the treatment, i.e. to healthy people in the interests of the wider community and the broader goal of elimination. In the case of transmission blocking drugs this is the entire community, and for the schizonticidal drugs this is the substantial proportion of the community who are not infected with malaria parasites. However, if the MDA is effective and malaria is eliminated from the area, all individuals will benefit *indirectly* by living in a malaria free community. In the GMS the schizonticide currently used in MDA is dihydroartemisinin-piperaquine (DP), which in the treatment of malaria is considered a safe drug. Studies of the safety of DP in this context have shown that DP is safe (Tripura et al. 2018), but widespread deployment of DP exposes much larger numbers of individuals such that its rare but serious side effects may occur (Cheah and White 2016). The transmission blocking drug currently used in MDA is primaquine, which targets the transmissible sexual gametocytes not killed by the schizonticide but has little or no impact on the asexual parasites which cause disease. Primaquine is an oxidative drug which causes haemolysis (the rupture of red blood cells) in G6PD-deficient individuals (median 8% of the population in malaria endemic areas) when given in the large doses needed to radically cure vivax malaria (killing the hypnozoites in the liver) (Howes et al. 2012). However to kill gametocytes (rather than cure malaria) a single much lower dose is required, one considered safe to be administered to all individuals without prior G6PD testing (World Health Organization, Global Malaria Programme 2015b; Bancone et al. 2016).

A second ethically significant consideration is a worry that there is a risk that with the widespread deployment of antimalarial drugs in MDA the resulting increased drug pressure may itself lead to drug resistance, particularly in the case where elimination is not achieved. It has been argued on theoretical grounds that this is unlikely, but the risk however low highlights the importance of achieving elimination in areas where MDA is deployed (White 2017). This suggests that the initiation of MDA is only ethically justified where there is a genuine commitment to complete the elimination task. Once the process of MDA has begun, important ethical issues are presented relating to the question of when such an initiative should be ended.

Thirdly, the effectiveness of MDA is predicated upon high population coverage (World Health Organization 2017; Newby et al. 2015). Achieving this is a challenge for several reasons: explaining the rationale for taking antimalarials when asymptomatic can be difficult in the absence of an understanding of the underlying scientific concepts, target communities are often remote with poor access and populations can be highly mobile. For these reasons, effective community engagement efforts are essential, so that individuals are informed of the risks and benefits of malaria elimination efforts in general and MDA in particular (Adhikari et al. 2016; Peto et al. 2018). For effective community engagement those implementing MDA need to understand and adapt the information they provide and the form of the engagement they adopt, to the cultural and practical requirements of each community. Engagement with community leaders is essential, and coverage can be promoted by offering healthcare alongside MDA (Sahan et al. 2017; Pell et al. 2017). Effective community engagement may also minimize risks of coercion or counterproductive misunderstanding of the aims of the public health authorities (Parker and Allen 2013). The ethical issues around these concerns are similar in some respects to those encountered in the context of vaccination campaigns.

Mass Screening and Treatment (MSAT)

Mass screening and treatment of village populations has been suggested as an alternative strategy to MDA for speeding up malaria elimination. Its advantage over MDA is that only those individuals with proven asymptomatic malaria infection will be exposed to antimalarial drugs and their attendant risks, negating many of the ethical concerns described in the MDA section above. However, the likely success of this is limited by the sensitivity of the tests available for detecting low levels of parasites in the blood. Because the current tests are laboratory based there is inevitably considerable delay between sampling and result, which appears to limit the effectiveness of MSAT (von Seidlein 2014). Highly sensitive rapid diagnostic tests have now been developed, but these are only now being tested in the field (Slater et al. 2015). Such tests have the potential to be much quicker but they are not as sensitive as the laboratory based tests, and it possible that up to half of asymptomatic carriers will be 'missed'. However, the contribution to malaria transmission of individuals with very low parasitaemias at the time of testing is uncertain, and the results of studies of the field effectiveness of MSAT with highly sensitive RDTs are awaited with interest. If MSAT with highly sensitive RDTs does turn out to be effective, effective community engagement will be as important as it is with MDA.

Vector Control

The distribution of insecticide treated nets (ITNs) in Africa has had a major impact on malaria there, and as a result it has become almost an article of faith in the global malaria community that ITNs should be considered the most important single intervention in the battle against malaria (Bhatt et al. 2015). In a WHO-sponsored meeting on tackling artemisinin resistant malaria in the GMS the chairman suggested that *all* the additional resources being made available to counter resistance in the region should be spent on ITNs (*NPJD personal communication*). Unfortunately, Southeast Asian malaria vectors and populations do not behave like African vectors and populations, with most transmission occurring in the forest rather than in dwellings (Gryseels et al. 2015; Smithuis et al. 2013a). Several studies have now confirmed the limited efficacy of bed nets in malaria elimination effort in this region (Smithuis et al. 2013b; Satitvipawee et al. 2012). An important ethical issue here is around resource allocation, and overcoming established (but not evidence-based) pro-ITN sentiment amongst international and national policy makers. ITNs do have an important role to play and are relatively cheap to deploy, but given the evidence of differences in vector behaviours in Africa and the GMS, the relative allocation of limited resources should be driven by evidence-based health economics studies (Drake et al. 2015).

Targeting 'Source' Populations

In the GMS, malaria transmission is concentrated in poor, hard-to-reach, highly mobile populations. Transmission is mainly occupationally related, highest among men who travel into forested areas to work. Many of the most at-risk populations are disenfranchised minority groups, often living in border regions, with little or no health infrastructure. Understanding the drivers of transmission in these populations entails acquiring better knowledge of population movement/migration, much of which is 'illegal'. Working with these populations requires sensitivity not only to the cultural contexts but also to the uncertain legal status of many of the individuals. Several of the more endemic areas are mired in armed conflicts, and many populations are vulnerable as refugees or economic migrants without papers. The area currently with the highest endemicity in the GMS, for example, is Rakhine State in Myanmar, currently undergoing considerable civil strife and large-scale movement of populations. NGOs, government workers and researchers have to work within their own externally determined constraints, limiting their ability to engage 'source' populations. Even if the not inconsiderable task of eliminating malaria from many of these areas were to be achieved, political difficulties, the mobile nature of these populations, and changes in the ability to access them would leave them vulnerable to the reintroduction of malaria. Furthermore, as immunity will have waned because of the intervention the public health consequences of this reintroduction could potentially be worse than if malaria had not been eliminated in the first place.

Mandatory Screening

There are a number of situations in which mandatory screening for asymptomatic malaria may be indicated to prevent individuals unwittingly spreading drug resistant malaria parasites. Following the disastrous importation of cholera into Haiti by African UN peacekeepers (leading to 8300 deaths), for example, a call has been made for Southeast Asian Peacekeepers to be screened for malaria before they travel to missions in Africa (Houston and Houston 2015). This would prevent peacekeepers from importing drug resistant malaria to a drug sensitive region, and could be implemented by the UN. Another situation where mandatory screening could potentially be introduced in the context of eliminating artemisinin-resistant malaria within the GMS, would be screening local people moving between areas where malaria has and has not been eliminated. Although practically difficult to implement, this has the potential to be of real importance in geographical locations with highly mobile populations – such as along the Thai-Myanmar Border. There are a number of practical barriers to implementing such a policy, which make it unlikely to be introduced at present. However, its possibility raises important ethical questions about the legitimacy of overriding personal autonomy in the global public interest and its limits.

Triple Artemisinin Combination Therapies (TACTs)

The rationale for TACTs is similar to that of triple or quadruple therapy in HIV, tuberculosis, leprosy and other infectious diseases – to prevent the development of resistance. Two TACTs are currently being studied in 16 sites in Asia and 1 site in Africa (web identifier: NCT02453308): dihydroartemisinin-piperaquine + mefloquine; and artemether-lumefantrine + amodiaquine. The combination of a short acting artemisinin with two long acting partner drugs ensures that parasites are less likely to encounter only one long acting partner drug at any one time, minimizing the chance of resistance developing. In addition, it is hypothesized that these triple therapies could exploit potential inverse relationships between the parasite molecular resistance mechanisms to the paired long-acting partner drugs. It is thought that the wide implementation of triple therapy in malaria will slow the spread of multidrug-resistant malaria in areas where artemisinin and partner drug resistance is well established, and slow down or prevent the emergence of drug resistance in areas where resistance has not yet emerged. It is in the latter case where TACTs should be most effective.

There are several ethical issues to be considered here. TACTs differ from other examples of combination therapy in that the objective is to prevent antimalarial drug resistance at the population rather than at the individual level. Unlike in chronic infections such as TB and HIV development of ACT resistance within an individual patient during treatment is rare. Hence individuals are potentially exposed to the additional side effects of three rather than two drugs for little or no benefit to themselves; it is against the interest of the individual patient (usually a child) to take three rather than two drugs. If the strategy works the benefit will be to the population, which will only indirectly benefit the individual. In addition, TACTs are expected to be most effective at countering resistance in areas where resistance has not yet developed to any of the components, so that the long acting partner drugs will protect each other from the development of resistance and both will protect the short acting artemisinin component. Hence the areas where they will be most effective will be the ones where currently ACTs remain highly effective at the individual level.

Preliminary evidence of triple therapy is promising but safety and efficacy data are not widely available yet. Even if evidence is available, populations where ACTs still work such as in Africa where the majority of malaria cases are in children under five, may not readily change their prescribing behaviours. Other practical problems might be access to the triple therapy, availability of co-formulated drugs and the problem of substandard and falsified drugs especially in the private and informal sectors (Liverani et al., Chap. 5, this volume).

Summary of Ethical Considerations

Above we have attempted to illustrate the ethical complexity of the implementation of the strategies widely agreed by experts to be necessary for the control of resistance to antimalarial drugs. It is clear that there are strong ethical arguments in favour of the implementation of such strategies in the global public interest. However, the considerations outlined above suggest that such interventions raise important ethical questions both about the nature and scope of implementation itself and about the obligations of countries both outside and within the region to those who are to bear its costs. The success of an elimination strategy based on these elements will depend upon these problems being addressed. In the remainder of this chapter, we summarise what we consider to be some of the most important ethical tensions and outline some preliminary thoughts about ways these might be addressed.

Autonomy and Consent Versus the Global Benefit

There are a number of different ways in which the implementation of the intervention strategies above raises important questions about respect for autonomy. In some cases, these interventions may lead to tensions between the interests and wishes of individuals and the global benefit. During implementation of each strategy, individuals in selected communities are subjected to interventions – 'treatment' or surveillance – not for their own good but for the common good of current and future populations both locally and internationally (see discussion on common goods in Chaps. 8 and 9) (Jamrozik and Selgelid, Chap. 1, this volume-a; Smith and Coast, Chap. 17, this volume). Under current circumstances, such interventions are voluntary: making MDA compulsory or imposing travel restrictions on people who have come from areas with artemisinin resistant malaria is not considered achievable or justified at present. However, it is possible that as in other global health contexts this judgement might change and that individuals may lose their right to opt out of, for example, MDA. Draconian measures have been taken to contain dangerous contagions such as H5N1 influenza, SARS, MERS-CoV, Ebola virus, Lassa fever, and multidrug-resistant tuberculosis, which involved restriction of liberty in order to protect the public. Were compulsory approaches to be considered in the context of malaria, this would present important questions about the legitimacy of restrictions of liberty per se but also questions about how this was in fact undertaken, and about the nature of the obligations of the wider global community – particularly wealthy countries – to those who are subjected to such interventions in the global health interest.

Questions about autonomy also arise in the context of voluntary approaches. Where individuals and their communities are being asked to decide about participation in the strategies outlined above, it is vital that best efforts are made to ensure that any consent they give is grounded in a good understanding of the implications. However, the evidence is that valid consent is likely to be difficult to achieve in such contexts. This places particular importance on the roles of wider communication, community participation, political involvement and other forms of public engagement preceding and during the intervention. It has to be acknowledged that even in the context of well-resourced, evidence-based approaches to consent and community engagement, understanding is likely to be partial given the complexities of malaria transmission and how these inventions work. This need not mean that the choice to participate is invalid but it does mean that the moral basis for the intervention cannot rest on consent alone, even when the choice to participate is voluntary. This suggests that those who are responsible for the conduct of such strategies have obligations to ensure that they are conducted to high ethical standards, and that appropriate protections, and possibly compensation, are in place.

Risk Benefit

The potential benefits of malaria elimination are substantial, including the direct burden averted and economic growth through improved educational attainment and productivity; these gains were estimated recently to far outstrip the costs required to achieve them (Purdy et al. 2013). That said it is clear from the discussion above that those who bear the consequences of malaria elimination efforts are not those who will benefit directly. The majority of the populations with the highest prevalence of resistant malaria and of submicroscopic malaria in Southeast Asia are poor and mobile forest workers (Phommasone et al. 2016; Tripura et al. 2017). This is unsurprising as vulnerability to malaria – as is also true of many other infectious diseases – is largely a consequence of social determinants of health such as poverty, malnutrition and insufficient access to healthcare. Malaria burden is both a consequence and an illustration of global inequities. These populations are already burdened by their circumstances and environments. Yet they are the very individuals who will likely to be shouldering the burdens of any global intervention to curb resistant malaria. In the case of MDA, entire communities are treated whether or not they are unwell with malaria. That means that many individuals who are neither ill nor carriers of the parasite will be asked (or required) to take drugs and therefore be at some risk of potential adverse drug reactions. This uneven distribution of individual risks and inconveniences – that is individuals in SEA shouldering the burden for the benefit of good health outcomes primarily in the interests of populations elsewhere – is a key moral challenge. Whilst at the macroeconomic level the costs of malaria elimination are outweighed by the benefits, this may well not be true at the level of the individuals involved. Important ethical questions concern the question of when, if at all, the imposition of risks of harm on (often vulnerable) individuals is legitimate in the interests of others and the limits of this. The ethical questions here concern not only those related to whether the imposition of such burdens is justified but also, where this is the case, both the approach adopted to such implementation and the nature and scope of our obligations to those upon whom it is imposed. Is there, for example, an obligation to compensate such populations?

Data and Sample Sharing

Ethical issues also arise with regard to the international collaboration required to ensure high scientific and public health standards in the interventions. This is important because it is the achievement of such high standards (and hence the potential for success) that justify the imposition of risks and restrictions of liberty on vulnerable populations. In order to make the most informed decisions about planning interventions to eliminate malaria, there is a need to ensure that there is access to as much good quality data as possible. That is, it depends crucially upon data sharing. However, there is generally a lack of transparency and confidence in the quality of available malaria data. This can be due to poor quality data and underreporting of cases, which can in turn be due to variable availability of diagnostic tools such as rapid diagnostic tests and blood slides, unsurprising given that data are frequently collected under resource-starved conditions. This contributes to the lack of trust in the data on antimalarial resistance, and in the data used in mathematical modeling and the resulting predictions. An additional key problem is that many national malaria control programmes do not readily share their malaria data for political, economic and national security reasons. Data related to population movement and migration that could aid interventions such as MDA and engagement with "source populations" are, for example, particularly difficult to access. Although there is advantage in data sharing, it is also acknowledged that it can pose a number of ethical challenges around issues of privacy, potential stigma and economic harms (Mishra et al. 2016; Bull et al. 2015; Cheah et al. 2015). This suggests that questions about the ethical tensions between the interests of individuals and the global health interest also arise at the level of institutions, health ministries, and countries.

Scientific Disagreement About the Best Way Forward

We outlined a number of proposed interventions above, and given the current state of the evidence there are valid debates in the scientific community about what action or actions are appropriate where. Interventions such as TACTs and MDA are still under study. An important, as yet unresolved, scientific debate is about the way resistance spreads or emerges. There are data supporting both sides of the argument – geographical spread of sporadic vs. spontaneous distributed emergence (Lu et al. 2017). However, there is also a limited window of opportunity to act. There are strong moral reasons for acting to prevent the spread of resistance both within and beyond Southeast Asia. Inaction will almost inevitably lead to a repeat of history – the loss of safe, inexpensive and highly effective treatments and an increase in cases of severe malaria and related deaths. It may also mean that a once in a generation opportunity, capitalizing on the combination of the availability of political will and effective tools to take a big step towards the eradication of malaria, will have been missed. There remains, however, a degree of scientific uncertainty. This raises ethical questions about the level of scientific consensus required for action. Understanding is likely to remain imperfect. Is it legitimate to initiate strategies such as those outlined above on the basis of good but imperfect understanding? The answer to this question cannot be 'never' because there is widespread agreement about the urgency of the situation and a residual degree of scientific uncertainty will always remain.

Conclusions

In this chapter, we have described practical ethical issues arising in currently proposed interventions (and the lack of them) to reduce the risk of the movement of resistance to the current best antimalarial drugs from Southeast Asia to Africa, as well as to prevent resistance emerging in Africa. Whilst strong ethical reasons for such interventions are provided by the seriousness and scale of the threat and the existence of a degree of scientific consensus on this strategy, its implementation is ethically complex. We have outlined some of the most important practical ethical problems presented by each of possible components of the proposed strategy, and have also argued that even if the various interventions were to be ethically justified this would not be the end of the ethical debate. We have argued that important ethical questions about the mode of implementation of the interventions and about the obligations of the wider community to those they affect would remain.

Some of the most important of such considerations are those relating to fairness in the selection of interventional populations. All populations which meet a set of criteria for an intervention, be it MDA, TACT or travel restrictions, should where practical have the same intervention. The intervention should be evidence-based and justified, and all relevant stakeholders should be involved in the decision-making process and have meaningful input into the deliberations. The manner and context in which decisions are made should be reasonable, fair and transparent.

In addition to ethical considerations relating to the selection of such populations, we have argued that important obligations exist for those countries and governments that can afford it to assist and perhaps to compensate those individuals who are subject to such interventions and may experience harms as a result of their participation (Upshur 2002). Meeting these obligations may call for the provision of compensation, for example where businesses suffer due to lack of mobility or where people suffer from side effects of MDA. Or perhaps, in the form of community level benefits such as improved healthcare facilities. An important aspect of the obligations of the wider world to those who live in the region is that any intervention is well-planned and adequately resourced. It is clear that curbing antimalarial resistance, similar to resistance of other antimicrobials, is both a global priority and a global responsibility (Jamrozik and Selgelid, Chap. 1, this volume-b). Both scientifically and in terms of effective public health interventions, solutions to this problem are inevitably going to be collaborative. In addition to the provision of adequate resources, communities, countries, researchers and funders must be encouraged to work together. It is our view that four key requirements for a successful and appropriate collaborative approach to addressing emerging ACT resistance, and hence ethically important requirements of those who propose such interventions, are as follows:

i. *Encouraging and funding more research.* Research should be conducted to address the gaps needed for each of the interventions proposed by the scientific community such as determining the safety of DP for MDA, the efficacy and safety of triple therapy, and determining the way resistance spreads. More evidence would help channel resources to the correct people and places, and facilitate a scientific consensus.

ii. *Retraining and supporting village malaria workers* so that they are able to manage other febrile diseases and hence remain relevant and retain community support. This could be provision of education and strengthening support from provincial health departments.

iii. *Encourage collection of quality malaria data, and sharing and pooling of these data.* A data sharing initiative, the WorldWide Antimalarial Resistance Network (www.WWARN.org) was established by malaria researchers in 2009 to facilitate collaborative study groups working to answer specific research questions using pooled analyses. WWARN has had considerable success in pooling individual-participant data from multiple clinical trials from academic groups and pharmaceutical companies, but has been less successful with NMCPs. Individual research groups have also established data sharing mechanisms via a managed access route (Cheah and Day 2017).

iv. *Engaging with affected communities in creative and sensitive ways.* Some work has already been conducted to engage forest workers, minority groups and mobile populations, and much more is needed (Lim et al. 2017). This will improve understanding of the science behind malaria and malaria elimination and will facilitate interventions such as MDAs and MSATs.

References

Adhikari, B., N. James, G. Newby, L. von Seidlein, N.J. White, N.P. Day, et al. 2016. Community engagement and population coverage in mass anti-malarial administrations: A systematic literature review. *Malaria Journal* 15 (1): 523.

Amaratunga, C., P. Lim, S. Suon, S. Sreng, S. Mao, C. Sopha, et al. 2016. Dihydroartemisinin-piperaquine resistance in Plasmodium falciparum malaria in Cambodia: A multisite prospective cohort study. *The Lancet Infectious Diseases* 16 (3): 357–365.

Ariey, F., B. Witkowski, C. Amaratunga, J. Beghain, A.C. Langlois, N. Khim, et al. 2014. A molecular marker of artemisinin-resistant Plasmodium falciparum malaria. *Nature* 505 (7481): 50–55.

Ashley, E.A., M. Dhorda, R.M. Fairhurst, C. Amaratunga, P. Lim, S. Suon, et al. 2014. Spread of artemisinin resistance in Plasmodium falciparum malaria. *The New England Journal of Medicine* 371 (5): 411–423.

Bancone, G., N. Chowwiwat, R. Somsakchaicharoen, L. Poodpanya, P.K. Moo, G. Gornsawun, et al. 2016. Single low dose primaquine (0.25 mg/kg) does not cause clinically significant haemolysis in G6PD deficient subjects. *PLoS One* 11 (3): e0151898.

Bhatt, S., D.J. Weiss, E. Cameron, D. Bisanzio, B. Mappin, U. Dalrymple, et al. 2015. The effect of malaria control on Plasmodium falciparum in Africa between 2000 and 2015. *Nature* 526 (7572): 207–211.

Bull, S., P.Y. Cheah, S. Denny, I. Jao, V. Marsh, L. Merson, et al. 2015. Best practices for ethical sharing of individual-level health research data from low- and middle-income settings. *Journal of Empirical Research on Human Research Ethics* 10 (3): 302–313.

Cheah, P.Y., and N.P.J. Day. 2017. Data sharing: Experience from a tropical medicine research unit. *Lancet* 390 (10103): 1642.

Cheah, P.Y., and N.J. White. 2016. Antimalarial mass drug administration: Ethical considerations. *International Health* 8 (4): 235–238.

Cheah, P.Y., D. Tangseefa, A. Somsaman, T. Chunsuttiwat, F. Nosten, N.P. Day, et al. 2015. Perceived benefits, harms, and views about how to share data responsibly: A qualitative study of experiences with and attitudes toward data sharing among research staff and community representatives in Thailand. *Journal of Empirical Research on Human Research Ethics* 10 (3): 278–289.

Dondorp, A.M., F. Nosten, P. Yi, D. Das, A.P. Phyo, J. Tarning, et al. 2009. Artemisinin resistance in Plasmodium falciparum malaria. *The New England Journal of Medicine* 361 (5): 455–467.

Dondorp, A.M., F.M. Smithuis, C. Woodrow, and L.V. Seidlein. 2017. How to contain artemisinin- and multidrug-resistant falciparum malaria. *Trends in Parasitology* 33 (5): 353–363.

Drake, T.L., S.S. Kyaw, M.P. Kyaw, F.M. Smithuis, N.P. Day, L.J. White, et al. 2015. Cost effectiveness and resource allocation of Plasmodium falciparum malaria control in Myanmar: A modelling analysis of bed nets and community health workers. *Malaria Journal* 14: 376.

Global Malaria Programme WHO. 2015. *World Malaria Report 2015*. Available from: http://apps.who.int/iris/bitstream/10665/200018/1/9789241565158_eng.pdf.

———. 2016. *World Malaria Report 2016*. Available from: http://apps.who.int/iris/bitstream/10665/254912/1/WHO-HTM-GMP-2017.4-eng.pdf.

Global Malaria Programme, World Health Organization. 2018. *World Malaria Report 2018*. Available from: https://www.who.int/malaria/publications/world-malaria-report-2018/report/en/.

Gryseels, C., L. Durnez, R. Gerrets, S. Uk, S. Suon, S. Set, et al. 2015. Re-imagining malaria: Heterogeneity of human and mosquito behaviour in relation to residual malaria transmission in Cambodia. *Malaria Journal* 14: 165.

Houston, S., and A. Houston. 2015. Screening and treating UN Peacekeepers to prevent the introduction of artemisinin-resistant malaria into Africa. *PLoS Medicine* 12 (5): e1001822.

Howes, R.E., F.B. Piel, A.P. Patil, O.A. Nyangiri, P.W. Gething, M. Dewi, et al. 2012. G6PD deficiency prevalence and estimates of affected populations in malaria endemic countries: A geostatistical model-based map. *PLoS Medicine* 9 (11): e1001339.

Imwong, M., T. Jindakhad, C. Kunasol, K. Sutawong, P. Vejakama, and A.M. Dondorp. 2015. An outbreak of artemisinin resistant falciparum malaria in Eastern Thailand. *Scientific Reports* 5: 17412.

Imwong, M., K. Suwannasin, C. Kunasol, K. Sutawong, M. Mayxay, H. Rekol, et al. 2017. The spread of artemisinin-resistant Plasmodium falciparum in the Greater Mekong subregion: A molecular epidemiology observational study. *The Lancet Infectious Diseases* 17 (5): 491–497.

Jamrozik, E., and M. Selgelid. 2020a. The ethics and politics of antimicrobial resistance: Moral responsibility and the justifications of policies to preserve antimicrobial effectiveness. In *Ethics and drug resistance: Collective responsibility for Global Public Health*. Cham: Springer.

———. 2020b. Drug-resistant infection: Causes, consequences, and responses. In *Ethics and drug resistance: Collective responsibility for Global Public Health*. Cham: Springer.

Lim, R., R. Tripura, T.J. Peto, M. Sareth, N. Sanann, C. Davoeung, et al. 2017. Drama as a community engagement strategy for malaria in rural Cambodia. *Wellcome Open Research* 2: 95.

Liverani, M.H.L., M. Khan, and R. Coker. this volume. Antimicrobial resistance and the private sector in Southeast Asia. In *Ethics and drug resistance: Collective responsibility for Global Public Health*. Cham: Springer.

Lu, F., R. Culleton, M. Zhang, A. Ramaprasad, L. von Seidlein, H. Zhou, et al. 2017. Emergence of indigenous artemisinin-resistant plasmodium falciparum in Africa. *The New England Journal of Medicine* 376 (10): 991–993.

Maude, R.J., W. Pontavornpinyo, S. Saralamba, R. Aguas, S. Yeung, A.M. Dondorp, et al. 2009. The last man standing is the most resistant: Eliminating artemisinin-resistant malaria in Cambodia. *Malaria Journal* 8: 31.

Maude, R.J., D. Socheat, C. Nguon, P. Saroth, P. Dara, G. Li, et al. 2012. Optimising strategies for Plasmodium falciparum malaria elimination in Cambodia: Primaquine, mass drug administration and artemisinin resistance. *PLoS One* 7 (5): e37166.

Mishra, N., R.S. Bharti, P. Mallick, O.P. Singh, B. Srivastava, R. Rana, et al. 2016. Emerging polymorphisms in falciparum Kelch 13 gene in Northeastern region of India. *Malaria Journal* 15 (1): 583.

Newby, G., J. Hwang, K. Koita, I. Chen, B. Greenwood, L. von Seidlein, et al. 2015. Review of mass drug administration for malaria and its operational challenges. *The American Journal of Tropical Medicine and Hygiene* 93 (1): 125–134.

Noedl, H., Y. Se, K. Schaecher, B.L. Smith, D. Socheat, M.M. Fukuda, et al. 2008. Evidence of artemisinin-resistant malaria in western Cambodia. *The New England Journal of Medicine* 359 (24): 2619–2620.

Parker, M., and T. Allen. 2013. Questioning ethics in global health. In *Ethics in the field: Contemporary challenges*, Studies of the Biosocial Society, ed. J. MacClancy and A. Fuentes, vol. 7, 24–41. New York: Berghahn Books.

Pell, C., R. Tripura, C. Nguon, P. Cheah, C. Davoeung, C. Heng, et al. 2017. Mass anti-malarial administration in western Cambodia: A qualitative study of factors affecting coverage. *Malaria Journal* 16 (1): 206.

Peto, T.J., R. Tripura, C. Davoeung, C. Nguon, S. Nou, C. Heng, et al. 2018. Reflections on a community engagement strategy for mass antimalarial drug administration in Cambodia. *The American Journal of Tropical Medicine and Hygiene* 98 (1): 100–104.

Phommasone, K., B. Adhikari, G. Henriques, T. Pongvongsa, P. Phongmany, L. von Seidlein, et al. 2016. Asymptomatic Plasmodium infections in 18 villages of southern Savannakhet Province, Lao PDR (Laos). *Malaria Journal* 15 (1): 296.

Phyo, A.P., E.A. Ashley, T.J.C. Anderson, Z. Bozdech, V.I. Carrara, K. Sriprawat, et al. 2016a. Declining efficacy of artemisinin combination therapy against P. Falciparum malaria on the Thai-Myanmar Border (2003-2013): The role of parasite genetic factors. *Clinical Infectious Diseases* 63 (6): 784–791.

Phyo, A.P., P. Jittamala, F.H. Nosten, S. Pukrittayakamee, M. Imwong, N.J. White, et al. 2016b. Antimalarial activity of artefenomel (OZ439), a novel synthetic antimalarial endoperoxide, in patients with Plasmodium falciparum and Plasmodium vivax malaria: An open-label phase 2 trial. *The Lancet Infectious Diseases* 16 (1): 61–69.

Purdy, M., M. Robinson, K. Wei, and D. Rublin. 2013. The economic case for combating malaria. *The American Journal of Tropical Medicine and Hygiene* 89 (5): 819–823.

Roper, C., R. Pearce, S. Nair, B. Sharp, F. Nosten, and T. Anderson. 2004. Intercontinental spread of pyrimethamine-resistant malaria. *Science* 305 (5687): 1124.

Sahan, K., C. Pell, F. Smithuis, A.K. Phyo, S.M. Maung, C. Indrasuta, et al. 2017. Community engagement and the social context of targeted malaria treatment: A qualitative study in Kayin (Karen) State, Myanmar. *Malaria Journal* 16 (1): 75.

Satitvipawee, P., W. Wongkhang, S. Pattanasin, P. Hoithong, and A. Bhumiratana. 2012. Predictors of malaria-association with rubber plantations in Thailand. *BMC Public Health* 12: 1115.

Slater, H.C., A. Ross, A.L. Ouedraogo, L.J. White, C. Nguon, P.G. Walker, et al. 2015. Assessing the impact of next-generation rapid diagnostic tests on Plasmodium falciparum malaria elimination strategies. *Nature* 528 (7580): S94–S101.

Smith, R.D., and J. Coast. this volume. The economics of resistance through an ethica lens. In *Ethics and drug resistance: Collective responsibility for Global Public Health*. Cham: Springer.

Smithuis, F.M., M.K. Kyaw, U.O. Phe, I. van der Broek, N. Katterman, C. Rogers, et al. 2013a. Entomological determinants of insecticide-treated bed net effectiveness in Western Myanmar. *Malaria Journal* 12: 364.

———. 2013b. The effect of insecticide-treated bed nets on the incidence and prevalence of malaria in children in an area of unstable seasonal transmission in western Myanmar. *Malaria Journal* 12: 363.

Takala-Harrison, S., C.G. Jacob, C. Arze, M.P. Cummings, J.C. Silva, A.M. Dondorp, et al. 2015. Independent emergence of artemisinin resistance mutations among Plasmodium falciparum in Southeast Asia. *The Journal of Infectious Diseases* 211 (5): 670–679.

Talisuna, A.O., C. Karema, B. Ogutu, E. Juma, J. Logedi, A. Nyandigisi, et al. 2012. Mitigating the threat of artemisinin resistance in Africa: Improvement of drug-resistance surveillance and response systems. *The Lancet Infectious Diseases* 12 (11): 888–896.

Tatarsky, A., S. Aboobakar, J.M. Cohen, N. Gopee, A. Bheecarry, D. Moonasar, et al. 2011. Preventing the reintroduction of malaria in Mauritius: A programmatic and financial assessment. *PLoS One* 6 (9): e23832.

Trape, J.F., G. Pison, M.P. Preziosi, C. Enel, A. Desgrees du Lou, V. Delaunay, et al. 1998. Impact of chloroquine resistance on malaria mortality. *Comptes Rendus de l'Académie des Sciences Série III* 321 (8): 689–697.

Tripura, R., T.J. Peto, C.C. Veugen, C. Nguon, C. Davoeung, N. James, et al. 2017. Submicroscopic Plasmodium prevalence in relation to malaria incidence in 20 villages in western Cambodia. *Malaria Journal* 16 (1): 56.

Tripura, R., T.J. Peto, N. Chea, D. Chan, M. Mukaka, P. Sirithiranont, et al. 2018. A controlled trial of mass drug administration to interrupt transmission of multidrug-resistant falciparum malaria in Cambodian villages. *Clinical Infectious Diseases* 67 (6): 817–826.

Tun, K.M., A. Jeeyapant, M. Imwong, M. Thein, S.S. Aung, T.M. Hlaing, et al. 2016. Parasite clearance rates in upper Myanmar indicate a distinctive artemisinin resistance phenotype: A therapeutic efficacy study. *Malaria Journal* 15: 185.

Upshur, R.E. 2002. Principles for the justification of public health intervention. *Canadian Journal of Public Health* 93 (2): 101–103.

Vandoolaeghe, P., and L. Schuerman. 2018. The RTS, S/AS01 malaria vaccine in children aged 5-17 months at first vaccination. *The Pan African Medical Journal* 30: 142.

Verdrager, J. 1986. Epidemiology of the emergence and spread of drug-resistant falciparum malaria in South-East Asia and Australasia. *The Journal of Tropical Medicine and Hygiene* 89 (6): 277–289.

von Seidlein, L. 2014. The failure of screening and treating as a malaria elimination strategy. *PLoS Medicine* 11 (1): e1001595.

von Seidlein, L., and A. Dondorp. 2015. Fighting fire with fire: Mass antimalarial drug administrations in an era of antimalarial resistance. *Expert Review of Anti-Infective Therapy* 13 (6): 715–730.

White, N.J. 2017. Does antimalarial mass drug administration increase or decrease the risk of resistance? *The Lancet Infectious Diseases* 17 (1): e15–e20.

White, N.J., S. Pukrittayakamee, T.T. Hien, M.A. Faiz, O.A. Mokuolu, and A.M. Dondorp. 2014. Malaria. *Lancet* 383 (9918): 723–735.

World Health Organization. 2011. *A global plan for artemisinin resistance containment*. Available from: http://apps.who.int/iris/bitstream/10665/44482/1/9789241500838_eng.pdf.

———. 2016a. *Guidelines for the treatment of malaria*, 3rd ed. Available from: http://apps.who.int/iris/bitstream/10665/162441/1/9789241549127_eng.pdf.

———. 2016b. *Minutes of the Evidence Review Group meeting on the emergence and spread of multidrug-resistant Plasmodium falciparum lineages in the Greater Mekong subregion 2016*. Available from: http://www.who.int/malaria/mpac/mpac-mar2017-erg-multidrug-resistance-session6.pdf?ua=1.

———. 2017. *A framework for malaria elimination 2017*. Available from: http://apps.who.int/iris/bitstream/10665/254761/1/9789241511988-eng.pdf.

World Health Organization, Global Malaria Programme. 2015a. *The role of mass drug administration, mass screening and treatment, and focal screening and treatment for malaria 2015*. Available from: http://www.who.int/malaria/publications/atoz/role-of-mda-for-malaria.pdf?ua=1.

———. 2015b. *Policy brief on single-dose primaquine as a gametocytocide in Plasmodium falciparum malaria 2015*. Available from: http://www.who.int/malaria/publications/atoz/who_htm_gmp_2015.1.pdf.

6

The Right to Refuse Treatment for Infectious Disease

Carl H. Coleman

Abstract One of the central tenets of contemporary bioethics is that mentally competent persons have a right to refuse medical treatment, even if the refusal might lead to the individual's death. Despite this principle, laws in some jurisdictions authorize the nonconsensual treatment of persons with tuberculosis (TB) or other serious infectious diseases, on the grounds that doing so is necessary to protect the safety of others. This chapter argues that, in the vast majority of situations, overriding a refusal of treatment for infectious disease is not justifiable, as the risk to third parties can be avoided by the less restrictive alternative of isolating the patient. At the same time, it rejects the extreme position that the nonconsensual treatment of infectious disease is never appropriate. Instead, it concludes that compelling an individual to undergo treatment for infectious diseases may be ethically justifiable in exceptional situations if a refusal of treatment poses a grave risk to third parties, the treatment is not overly burdensome and has been established to be safe and effective, and less restrictive alternatives, including humanely isolating the patient, are not feasible under the circumstances. The burden should be on those seeking to compel unwanted treatment to demonstrate that these requirements have been met.

Keywords Bioethics · Public Health · Infectious Diseases · Medical Law · Human Rights

The Right to Refuse Medical Treatment

If there is one unifying concept that runs through the field of bioethics, it is the doctrine of informed consent — i.e., the principle that individuals have the right to make their own decisions about medical treatment after having been informed of the risks, potential benefits, and reasonably available alternatives (Beauchamp and Childress 2013). The principle of informed consent is grounded in two interrelated

C. H. Coleman (✉)
School of Law, Seton Hall University, Newark, NJ, USA
e-mail: carl.coleman@shu.edu

justifications. First, by conditioning the imposition of medical treatment on the individual's authorization, informed consent protects persons' right to bodily integrity. Second, by requiring the provision of information needed to evaluate the desirability of proposed treatments, informed consent shows respect for individuals as autonomous decision-makers. The right to refuse medical treatment is "the logical corollary" of the informed consent doctrine: if there were no right to refuse proposed treatments, the process of soliciting consent would be a hollow charade (Cruzan v. Director 1990).

In addition to its ethical foundations, the right to refuse medical treatment is supported by internationally-recognized human rights principles. These principles include the right to security of the person (International Covenant on Civil and Political Rights 1976), the right not to be subjected to torture or to inhuman or degrading treatment (International Covenant on Civil and Political Rights 1976; European Convention on Human Rights 2010), and the right to health (International Covenant on Economic, Social and Cultural Rights 1976). The United Nations Committee on Economic, Social, and Cultural Rights has specifically recognized that the right to health includes the "right to be free from … non-consensual treatment" (United Nations Committee on Economic, Social and Cultural Rights 2000).

Courts have upheld mentally competent individuals' right to refuse medical treatment in a variety of situations, including those in which the refusal of treatment might strike some observers as irrational or unwise. For example, in the case of Fosmire v. Nicoleau, the New York Court of Appeals found that an adult Jehovah's Witness had the right to refuse blood transfusions prior to and immediately after the delivery of her baby, despite her physicians' belief that without the transfusions she was likely to die (Matter of Fosmire v. Nicoleau 1990). While some older judicial decisions in the United States suggested that the right to refuse treatment must be balanced against the state's interests in the preservation of life, the prevention of suicide, and "the maintenance of the ethical integrity of the medical profession" (Annas 1992), there are no recent cases in which any of these state interests has been deemed sufficient to override the refusal of treatment by a mentally competent adult.

However, like most individual rights, the right to refuse treatment is not absolute. First, refusals of treatment may be overridden when the patient lacks the mental capacity to provide informed consent and the imposition of treatment would be in his or her medical best interests (Steele v. Hamilton Cty. Community Mental Health Bd. 2000). This justification for compelled treatment typically arises in the psychiatric context, where a refusal of treatment may be the result of an underlying mental illness rather than the manifestation of a genuinely voluntary choice. The main issues in these situations involve the standards and procedures for determining the patient's mental incapacity (Klein 2012), as well as the appropriate role of family members and other surrogates in making decisions on the patient's behalf (Vars 2008).

Second, the nonconsensual treatment of mentally competent persons may be authorized when doing so is necessary to protect the safety of others. For example, courts have upheld the forcible medication of violent patients in emergency situations "when there is an imminent danger to a patient or others in the immediate vicinity" (Rivers v. Katz 1986). Courts have interpreted the danger-to-others rationale particularly broadly in the context of prisoners. For example, some courts have authorized the forcible feeding of prison inmates on hunger strikes on the theory that a hunger strike can threaten "institutional order and security" (Matter of Bezio v. Dorsey 2013).

Finally, competent individuals may sometimes be compelled to submit to medical interventions as part of the process of investigating or adjudicating criminal responsibility. For example, criminal suspects may be required to undergo physical examinations, which may include the collection of bodily fluids such as saliva or blood (Maryland v. King 2013; Missouri v. McNeely 2013). In addition, courts in the United States have authorized the government to administer medications to render mentally ill criminal defendants competent to stand trial, citing the governmental interest "in bringing to trial an individual accused of a serious crime." However, the forcible medication of criminal defendants is permissible only "if the treatment is medically appropriate, is substantially unlikely to have side effects that may undermine the trial's fairness, and, taking account of less intrusive alternatives, is necessary significantly to further important governmental trial-related interests" (Sell v. United States 2003).

Existing Approaches to Compelled Treatment for Infectious Diseases

Several jurisdictions have laws that authorize the nonconsensual treatment of persons with serious communicable diseases. For example, in the early 1990s, in response to a dramatic increase in TB cases, New York City amended its health code to authorize the Commissioner of Health to compel TB patients to complete treatment and, if necessary, to detain them during the process (Gasner et al. 1999). Under the law, detention can be authorized for persons with active TB "where there is a substantial likelihood, based on such person's past or present behavior, that he or she can not be relied upon to participate in and/or to complete an appropriate prescribed course of medication for tuberculosis" (N.Y.C. Health Code §11.21(d)(5)). In most cases, treatment under detention is sought only after other less restrictive alternatives, including directly-observed therapy, have already been attempted (Gasner et al. 1999). However, the Department of Health has the discretion to order treatment under detention as a first resort if it concludes attempting outpatient treatment would be futile in light of the patient's history of nonadherence.

Similar laws exist in other jurisdictions. For example, South Africa's National Health Act provides for an exception to the requirement to obtain informed consent to medical treatment in cases where "failure to treat the user ... will result in a serious risk to the public health" (Republic of South Africa National Health Act § 7(1)(d)). Relying in part on this provision, the High Court of South Africa has upheld the involuntary isolation and treatment of patients with multi-drug resistant (MDR) TB (Minister of Health v. Goliath 2008). Similarly, Canadian courts have upheld orders requiring patients with TB to submit to mandatory detention and treatment (Ries 2007), relying on provincial legislation authorizing the board of health to issue orders requiring the "care and treatment" of persons with "virulent" communicable diseases (Ontario Health Protection and Promotion Act § 22(4)(g); Silva 2011). The state of Alabama also has a law authorizing the "compulsory treatment and quarantine" of TB patients, but with an unusual exception: Confined patients are permitted to refuse treatment if they "desire treatment by prayer or spiritual means" (Ala. Code § 22-11A-10). The Alabama law does not permit patients to refuse treatment for reasons unrelated to religion.

In contrast, laws in some jurisdictions provide that patients with infectious diseases can be subject to mandatory detention but not forcible treatment. For example, the state of Minnesota authorizes the involuntary isolation of persons with diseases "that can be transmitted person to person and for which isolation or quarantine is an effective control strategy," but it specifically provides that isolated patients have "a fundamental right to refuse medical treatment" (Minn. Statutes 144.419). Similarly, Israeli law permits the involuntary isolation of persons with TB or other serious infectious diseases, but isolated patients may not be forced to undergo unwanted medical treatment (Weiler-Ravell et al. 2004). The law in Iceland appears to follow a similar approach (Eggertsson 2004).

The Model State Emergency Health Powers Act, a proposed law developed by the Center for Law and the Public's Health, initially included provisions authorizing forcible treatment of patients during an infectious disease outbreak, but after extensive criticism, those provisions were eliminated from the proposal (Annas et al. 2008). The proposed law now provides that "persons who are unable or unwilling for reasons of health, religion, or conscience to undergo treatment" may be subject to isolation (Center for Law and the Public's Health 2001). The implication is that, once isolated, infectious persons may not be subjected to treatment involuntarily.

It is unclear whether compelled treatment for infectious disease would be permitted under international human rights law. On the one hand, some human rights documents cite "the prevention and control of communicable diseases" as a situation in which "coercive medical treatments" could be justified on an "exceptional basis" (United Nations Committee on Economic, Social and Cultural Rights 2000). In addition, the European Court of Human Rights (ECHR) has found that requiring individuals to undergo TB screening by means of a tuberculin skin-reaction test or chest X-ray "can be considered necessary in a democratic society for the protection of health" (Acmanne and others v. Belgium 1984). On the other hand, no human rights tribunal has directly addressed the permissibility of compelling individuals to undergo treatment (as opposed to testing) for infectious diseases. Moreover, citing ECHR decisions condemning the force-feeding of prisoners, a World Health Organization (WHO) mission to the Ukraine concluded that "administering a TB treatment without the consent of the patient is an intrusive major intervention that constitutes a prohibited interference with a person's rights under the ECHR" (Dagron 2016).

Finally, it is worth noting that, although "compulsory vaccination" laws are sometimes cited as support for overriding the right to refuse treatment for patients with infectious diseases (Valenti 2012), those laws do not actually support the forcible imposition of medical interventions over a patient's objection. For example, in the United States, unvaccinated children who have not received an exemption from a state's vaccination requirements may be denied enrollment in the public schools (Barraza et al. 2017), but they will not be forcibly given vaccines to which their parents have objected. In a few other countries, parents can be fined for refusing to vaccinate their children (Reuters 2017), but, again, forcible vaccination does not appear to be authorized. Similarly, in the frequently-cited U.S. Supreme Court case of *Jacobson v. Massachusetts*, which upheld a Massachusetts law requiring individuals to be vaccinated for smallpox, the plaintiff was never actually required to undergo vaccination. Instead, the consequence of his refusal of the vaccine was a fine of five dollars (Jacobson v. Massachusetts 1905).

Ethical Analysis

As discussed in the preceding section, there are two dominant legal approaches to protecting third parties from the risk of serious infectious diseases: compelling such persons to undergo medical treatment, or isolating them without forcing them to accept treatments to which they object. While the latter approach does not technically override the individual's right to refuse treatment, an offer of treatment that can be refused only by submitting to isolation is inherently coercive. Because "[v]oluntary consent is usually thought incompatible with coercion" (Eyal 2012), both approaches can be seen as exceptions to the general principle that medical treatment requires the patient's voluntary informed consent.

Recognizing an exception to informed consent for patients with infectious diseases can be compared to cases authorizing nonconsensual medical treatment when necessary to protect third parties from violence. As an ethical matter, both situations implicate John Stuart Mill's "harm principle," which provides that individual liberty does not include the right to cause harm to third parties (Brink 2014). As Marcel Verweij explains, "[i]f patients with infectious diseases neglect the treatment they need, this could have harmful implications for others, and that may be reason to overrule the requirements of informed consent" (Verweij 2011).

However, even if the harm principle can justify an exception to informed consent in some situations, the mere possibility of harm, standing alone, is an insufficient basis to justify compulsion. Instead, a full analysis must consider factors such as the likelihood and magnitude of the potential harm, the burdens of compulsion on the individuals affected, the likely effectiveness of the proposed interventions, and the alternatives that are realistically available under the circumstances. This kind of fact-sensitive inquiry is an implicit requirement of consequentialist ethical theories, which require assessing the aggregate balance of potential benefits and harms of any proposed course of action (Sinnott-Armstrong 2015). It is also supported by the human rights principle of proportionality, which requires a "fair balance between the demands of the general interest of the community and the requirements of the protection of the individual's fundamental rights" (Soering v. UK 1989).

Coercive action is most justifiable in cases of highly contagious, life-threatening illnesses, such as MDR-TB. As the likelihood of transmission and/or the consequences of infection lessen, the justification for coercion diminishes as well. The precise point at which a refusal of treatment becomes sufficiently dangerous to justify coercion can be difficult to determine. For example, as Richard Coker asks, "given that the risk of relapse is higher if compliance with [TB] treatment ceases after two months of treatment compared with, say, five months (where, in most cases it is probably very small indeed), should those who fail to comply after two months face the prospect of detention if they fail to comply, whereas those who do so only after five months remain at liberty?" In answering these questions, "one is forced to question issues relating to utility, about how one measures the burden of risk, and utility gains and losses. Objective evidence to support decisions is largely lacking" (Coker 2000).

For many diseases, both the likelihood and magnitude of potential harm exist on a lengthy continuum. With respect to the likelihood of transmission, consider the case of sexually-transmitted infections (STIs). Many persons with STIs pose little or no risk to others because they are either sexually inactive or consistently use barrier protection. However, the level of risk increases if they engage in unprotected sexual encounters with multiple partners. The likelihood of transmission is particularly high for persons whose sexual partners do not recognize the need to take precautions against transmission, such as spouses who may mistakenly assume that their relationships are exclusive. In light of these uncertainties, is the likelihood of harm to unknowing third parties sufficient to justify the use of compulsion? While public health authorities generally favor a voluntary approach to STI testing and treatment (WHO Statement 2012), efforts to use compulsion sometimes occur. For example, under 2017 guidelines from the British Columbia Centre for Disease Control, public health authorities may issue orders compelling HIV-positive individuals to initiate and continue HIV treatment if they engage in high-risk sexual behavior or share needles and/or other drug paraphernalia with other persons and do not disclose their HIV status (British Columbia Centre for Disease Control 2017). Violation of such orders can result in court-ordered detention under the British Columbia Public Health Act, which allows medical health officers "to do anything that the … officer reasonably believes is necessary … to prevent the transmission of an infectious agent" (British Columbia Public Health Act). In 2018, a man from Vancouver was charged under these provisions for allegedly refusing to comply with a medical officer's order to submit to HIV treatment (Proctor). Similarly, a man in Fayetteville, Arkansas was charged in 2016 for a misdemeanor public health violation for refusing to undergo treatment for syphilis (Vendituoli 2016).

Similar uncertainties relate to the magnitude of harm resulting from an individual's refusal of treatment. For example, seasonal influenza typically resolves itself without any long-term consequences, but it can be life threatening for elderly patients or those with compromised immune systems. If a treatment were developed that quickly made patients with seasonal influenza incapable of transmitting the illness, would the magnitude of avoidable harm justify imposing this treatment over a patient's objection? Even seemingly innocuous infections diseases, such as athlete's foot, can cause severe consequences in some subgroups of patients (e.g., persons with diabetes). So far, no one has seriously proposed compelling individuals with athlete's foot to use anti-fungal medications, or to threaten infected persons with detention if they visit a public swimming pool with bare feet during an outbreak. Yet, the idea of invoking the harm principle in this situation might seem perfectly reasonable to a diabetic patient who is forced to undergo a foot amputation after being exposed to an untreated fungal infection.

In determining whether the likelihood and magnitude of harm are sufficient to justify compulsion, some commentators have suggested that the risks posed by an individual's refusal of treatment should be compared to the other risks that individuals typically confront on a day-to-day basis. For example, Mark Cherry argues that compelled treatment for infectious disease can be justified when necessary to prevent "significant and unusual risk" to "non-consenting others." He gives the example of legally-mandated treatment for patients with extensively drug-resistant TB, explaining that "[t]he risks associated with such diseases are significantly greater than the background risks that one generally assumes in daily life" (Cherry 2010).

Yet, while a comparison to the risks of daily life provides a useful framework for analysis, it does not follow that, as long as the risks of refusal are greater than the risks of daily life, the use of compulsion is necessarily warranted. Instead, the existence of a "significant and unusual risk" should be considered a necessary but insufficient criterion for justifying compulsion. In other words, if the risks of treatment refusal are less than the risks of daily life, the use of compulsion should not even be considered; if the risk are greater, compulsion *might* be justifiable, but additional considerations must also be factored into the analysis.

One of these additional considerations is the burden of compulsion on the individuals affected. For example, in upholding Belgium's policy of mandatory skin-tests and chest X-rays for TB, the ECHR pointed to the absence of evidence suggesting that those interventions involved "disadvantages comparable to the former ravages of tuberculosis" (Acmanne and others v. Belgium 1984). The implication was that more burdensome interventions would require a more compelling justification.

Some interventions might be too burdensome to be justifiable under any circumstances. By way of analogy, in refusing to authorize a Caesarean section on a dying woman who had refused the procedure, the District of Columbia Court of Appeals noted that, to perform the procedure, the patient "would have to be fastened with restraints to the operating table, or perhaps involuntarily rendered unconscious by forcibly injecting her with an anesthetic, and then subjected to unwanted major surgery." It concluded that "[s]uch actions would surely give one pause in a civilized society, especially when [the patient] had done no wrong" (In re A.C. 1990). For similar reasons, it is difficult to imagine a scenario in which it would be acceptable to force a patient with an infectious disease to submit to a major surgical procedure, even if doing so were the only way to render the patient non-infectious.

Another consideration is the likelihood that the proposed intervention will be effective in reducing the risk that the disease will be transmitted to third parties. At a minimum, as the World Health Organization emphasizes, overriding an individual's refusal of a medical intervention for the treatment of an infectious disease should not be considered unless the proposed intervention "has proven to be safe and effective and is part of the accepted medical standard of care" (World Health Organization 2016). Likewise, requiring individuals who refuse treatment to undergo isolation would not be justifiable if the disease is already so prevalent in a population that isolating untreated patients is unlikely to make a significant difference in reducing transmission.

Finally, even if an individual's refusal of treatment creates a sufficient risk of harm to others to justify the use of compulsion, the type of compulsion used should be the least restrictive option reasonably available under the circumstances. The "least restrictive alternative" requirement is a well-established principle of human rights jurisprudence. For example, the Siracusa Principles on the Limitation and Derogation Provisions in the International Covenant on Civil and Political Rights provides that any restrictions on human rights must be "strictly necessary" and that "there must be no other, less intrusive means available to reach the same objective" (American Association for the International Commission of Jurists 1985). The United States Supreme Court applies a similar standard in analyzing restrictions on fundamental constitutional rights (Chemerinsky 2015), as does the European Court of Human Rights (Brems and Lavrysen 2015).

In light of this principle, if it is possible to protect the public from harm by isolating the patient, there would be no justification for insisting that the patient, once isolated, submit to medical treatments to which he continues to object. The WHO Ethics Guidance for the Implementation of the End TB Strategy makes this point forcefully:

> While contagious persons with TB who do not adhere to treatment or who are unable or unwilling to comply with infection prevention and control measures pose significant risks to the public, those risks can be addressed by isolating the patient. Patients who are isolated should still be offered the opportunity to receive treatment, but if they do not accept it, their informed refusal should be respected. Forcing these patients to undergo treatment over their objection would require an unacceptable invasion of bodily integrity, and also could put health care providers at risk. Moreover, as a practical matter, it would likely be impossible to provide effective treatment without the patient's cooperation. Nevertheless efforts to convince the patient and re-examine his or her refusal should not be abandoned (World Health Organization 2017).

The Belgian Advisory Committee on Bioethics takes a similar position, finding that "if an MDR patient who does not have any psychiatric problems rendering him incapable of giving his consent refuses a treatment, the health authorities can hold him in isolation to avoid the spread of the disease but cannot force him to receive treatment" (Belgian Advisory Committee on Bioethics 2013).

This position is consistent with the logic of the danger-to-others exception to the informed consent requirement. In particular, cases involving the forcible medication of violent patients emphasize that the use of force is justified only as a temporary measure, "continuing only as long as the emergency persists" (Rivers v. Katz 1986). Once a violent patient has been medicated to a point that he can safely be isolated, there would be no justification for further medication unless another basis for overriding consent, such as mental incapacity, also exists.

Taken together, the considerations discussed above suggest that nonconsensual treatment for infectious disease will rarely be justifiable. Even if the magnitude and severity of harm resulting from a treatment refusal are significant, and even if the proposed treatment is not especially burdensome and is likely to work, the less restrictive alternative of isolating the patient will usually be sufficient to protect the public from harm. While involuntary isolation still involves an element of coercion, in most cases it should be up to the patient to decide whether this option is preferable to submitting to an unwanted medical intervention.

Yet, it would be a mistake to think that the option of isolation will always eliminate the need to consider the appropriateness of nonconsensual treatment. One situation in which isolation may be impractical is when individuals are already living in confined settings, such as in prisons or the military. While isolating a small number of individuals in these settings may be possible, the available space for isolation is likely to be limited. In addition, there may be other persons with a stronger case for access to these limited facilities — for example, prisoners who need to be separated from the general population because they are at heightened risk of violent attack.

Another situation in which isolation may not be a practical alternative is during an epidemic outbreak involving substantial numbers of persons with contagious infections, particularly in low-resource settings with a limited capacity to provide humane isolation facilities. In some cases, voluntary isolation at home may be a reasonable alternative, but this will work only if the patient is willing and able to follow infection control precautions (World Health Organization 2017). Otherwise, if isolation facilities are limited, protecting the public may sometimes require consideration of nonconsensual treatment. Yet, even in these scenarios, compelled treatment would be justified only if a safe and effective treatment exists that would not be unduly burdensome to the patient. If there is such a treatment, it seems unlikely that the number of people refusing it would be high enough to overwhelm available isolation facilities, particularly if public health authorities have engaged in an adequate process of community engagement (World Health Organization 2016). Thus, as a practical matter, the need to invoke this exception may be more theoretical than real.

In all cases, the burden should be on those seeking to compel unwanted treatment to demonstrate that no less restrictive alternatives, including isolation, are realistically available under the circumstances. As the World Health Organization recommends, "objections to diagnostic, therapeutic, or preventive measures should not be overridden without giving the individual notice and an opportunity to raise his or her objections before an impartial decision-maker, such as a court, interdisciplinary review panel, or other entity not involved in the initial decision" (World Health Organization 2016). Such a process provides an important check against abuse and can avoid undermining public trust in the integrity of the public health system.

References

Acmanne and others v. Belgium, No. 10435/83 (European Court of Human Rights 1984).

Ala. Code § 22-11A-10.

American Association for the International Commission of Jurists. 1985. *Siracusa principles on the limitation and derogation provisions in the International Covenant on Civil and Political Rights*. http://icj.wpengine.netdna-cdn.com/wp-content/uploads/1984/07/Siracusa-principles-ICCPR-legal-submission-1985-eng.pdf.

Annas, George J. 1992. *The rights of patients: The basic ACLU guide to patient rights*. Springer.

Annas, George J., Wendy K. Mariner, and Wendy E. Parmet. 2008. *Pandemic preparedness: The need for a public health--not a law enforcement/National Security--Approach*. ACLU. https://www.aclu.org/files/images/asset_upload_file399_33642.pdf.

Barraza, Leila, Cason Schmit, and Aila Hoss. 2017. The latest in vaccine policies: Selected issues in school vaccinations, healthcare worker vaccinations, and pharmacist vaccination authority Laws. *Journal of Law, Medicine and Ethics* 45 (S1): 16–19.

Beauchamp, Tom L., and James F. Childress. 2013. *Principles of biomedical ethics*. 7th ed. New York: Oxford University Press.

Belgian Advisory Committee on Bioethics. 2013. *Opinion No. 55 of 13 May 2013 on the Treatment of Patients with Multidrug- Resistant Tuberculosis from a Public Health Perspective*.

Brems, Eva, and Laurens Lavrysen. 2015. 'Don't use a sledgehammer to crack a nut': Less restrictive means in the case law of the European Court of Human Rights. *Human Rights Law Review* 15 (1): 139–168. https://doi.org/10.1093/hrlr/ngu040.

Brink, David. 2014. Mill's moral and political philosophy. In *The Stanford Encyclopedia of philosophy*, ed. Edward N. Zalta. Metaphysics Research Lab, Stanford University. https://plato.stanford.edu/archives/win2016/entries/mill-moral-political/.

British Columbia Centre for Disease Control. 2017. *Guidelines for medical health officers: Approach to people with HIV/AIDS who may pose a risk of harm to others*. http://www.bccdc.ca/resource-gallery/Documents/Communicable-Disease-Manual/Chapter%205%20-%20STI/MHO-guidelines-PLWH-risk-of-transmission.pdf

British Columbia Public Health Act § 27.

Center for Law and the Public's Health. 2001. *Model State Emergency Health Powers Act*. http://www.publichealthlaw.net/MSEHPA/MSEHPA.pdf.

Chemerinsky, Erwin. 2015. *Constitutional law: Principles and policies*. 5th ed. http://www.wklegaledu.com/aspen-student-treatise-series/id-9781454849476/Constitutional_Law_Principles_and_Policies_Fifth_Edition.

Cherry, Mark J. 2010. *Non-consensual treatment is (nearly always) morally impermissible*. Los Angeles, CA: SAGE Publications Sage CA.

Coker, Richard. 2000. Tuberculosis, non-compliance and detention for the public health. *Journal of Medical Ethics* 26 (3): 157–159.

Cruzan v. Director, Mo. Dept. of Health, 497 US 261 (U.S. Supreme Court 1990).

Dagron, Stéphanie. 2016. *Tuberculosis control and human rights in the National Legislation of Ukraine, report of a Mission 20–24 April 2015*.

Eggertsson, Dagur B. 2004. *Tuberculosis and human rights in Iceland*. http://lup.lub.lu.se/student-papers/record/1554865/file/1563469.pdf.

Eyal, Nir. 2012. Informed consent. In *The Stanford encyclopedia of philosophy*, ed. Edward N. Zalta. Metaphysics Research Lab, Stanford University. https://plato.stanford.edu/archives/fall2012/entries/informed-consent/.

Gasner, M. Rose, Khin Lay Maw, Gabriel E. Feldman, Paula I. Fujiwara, and Thomas R. Frieden. 1999. The Use of Legal Action in New York City to Ensure Treatment of Tuberculosis. *New England Journal of Medicine* 340 (5): 359–366.

"International Covenant on Civil and Political Rights," 1976. http://www.ohchr.org/Documents/ProfessionalInterest/ccpr.pdf.

"International Covenant on EconomicEconomics, Social and Cultural Rights," 1976. http://www.ohchr.org/EN/ProfessionalInterest/Pages/CESCR.aspx.

In re AC, 573 A. 2d 1235 (D.C. Court of Appeals 1990).

Jacobson v. Massachusetts, 197 US 11 (U.S. Supreme Court 1905).

Klein, Dora W. 2012. When coercion lacks care: Competency to make medical treatment decisions and parens patriae civil commitments. *University of Michigan Journal of Law Reform* 45 (3): 561–593.

Maryland v. King, 133 S. Ct. 1958 (U.S. Supreme Court 2013).

Matter of Bezio v. Dorsey, 21 NY.3d 93 (N.Y. Court of Appeals 2013).

Matter of Fosmire v. Nicoleau, 75 NY 2d 218 (N.Y. Court of Appeals 1990).

Minister of Health v. Goliath, No. 13741/07 (High Court of South Africa 2008).

Minn. Statutes § 144.419.

Missouri v. McNeely, 133 S. Ct. 1552 (U.S. Supreme Court 2013).

N.Y.C. Health Code § 11.21(d)(5).

Ontario Health Protection and Promotion Act § 22(4)(g).

Proctor J. Vancouver man charged with ignoring medical health officer's orders. *CBC News*, August 24, 2018.

Reuters. "Italy Passes Law Obliging Parents to Vaccinate Children." May 19, 2017. http://www.reuters.com/article/us-italy-politics-vaccines-idUSKCN18F1J7.

Republic of South Africa National Health Act § 7(1)(d).

Ries, Nola M. 2007. Legal issues in disease outbreaks: Judicial review of public health powers. *Health Law Review* 16 (1): 11–16.

Rivers v. Katz, 67 NY 2d 485 (N.Y. Court of Appeals 1986).

Sell v. United States, 539 US 166 (U.S. Supreme Court 2003).

Silva, Diego S. 2011. *Tuberculosis and persons with severe and persistent mental illnesses: When (treatment) worlds collide?* Munk School Briefings, 2010. Munk School of Global Affairs, University of Toronto.

Sinnott-Armstrong, Walter. 2015. Consequentialism. In *The Stanford encyclopedia of philosophy*, ed. Edward N. Zalta. Metaphysics Research Lab, Stanford University. https://plato.stanford.edu/archives/win2015/entries/consequentialism/.

Soering v. UK, 11 EHHR 439 (European Court of Human Rights 1989).

Steele v. Hamilton Cty. Community Mental Health Bd., 90 Ohio St. 3d 176 (Supreme Court of Ohio 2000).

United Nations Committee on EconomicEconomics, Social & Cultural Rights 2000. *General comment No. 14: The right to the highest attainable standard of health (Article 12 of the International Covenant on Economic, Social and Cultural Rights)*. http://www.nesri.org/sites/default/files/Right_to_health_Comment_14.pdf.

Valenti, Joseph Anthony. 2012. Circumstances when medical treatment may be forcibly imposed despite a patient's explicit refusal: A comprehensive analysis of Pennsylvania law. *Widener Law Review* 18: 27.

Vars, Frederick E. 2008. Illusory consent: When an incapacitated patient agrees to treatment. *Oregon Law Review* 87 (2): 353–398.

Vendituoli, Monica. 2016. Fayetteville man accused of refusing treatment for syphilis. *Fayeteville Observer* 6.

Verweij, Marcel. 2011. Infectious disease control. In *Public health ethics: Key concepts and issues in policy and practice*, ed. Angus Dawson, 100–142. Cambridge/New York: Cambridge University Press.

Weiler-Ravell, D., A. Leventhal, R.J. Coker, and D. Chemtob. 2004. Compulsory detention of recalcitrant tuberculosis patients in the context of a new tuberculosis control programme in Israel. *Public Health* 118 (5): 323–328. https://doi.org/10.1016/j.puhe.2003.10.005.

World Health Organization. 2012. *Statement on HIV testing and Counseling: WHO, UNAIDS re-affirm opposition to mandatory HIV testing*. http://www.who.int/hiv/events/2012/world_aids_day/hiv_testing_counselling/en/.

———. 2017. *Ethics guidance for the implementation of the end TB strategy*. http://apps.who.int/iris/bitstream/10665/254820/1/9789241512114-eng.pdf?ua=1.

———. 2016. *Guidance for managing ethical issues in infectious dsease outbreaks*. http://apps.who.int/iris/bitstream/10665/250580/1/9789241549837-eng.pdf.

7

Moral Responsibility and the Justification of Policies to Preserve Antimicrobial Effectiveness

Alberto Giubilini and J. Savulescu

Abstract Restrictive policies that limit antimicrobial consumption, including therapeutically justified use, might be necessary to tackle the problem of antimicrobial resistance. We argue that such policies would be ethically justified when forgoing antimicrobials constitutes a form of easy rescue for an individual. These are cases of mild and self-limiting infections in otherwise healthy patients whose overall health is not significantly compromised by the infection. In such cases, restrictive policies would be ethically justified because they would coerce individuals into fulfilling a moral obligation they independently have. However, to ensure that such justification is the strongest possible, states also have the responsibility to ensure that forgoing antimicrobials is as easy as possible for patients by implementing adequate compensation measures.

Keywords Bioethics · Public health ethics · Antimicrobial resistance · Collective responsibility · Easy rescue

---

A. Giubilini (✉)
Wellcome Centre for Ethics and Humanities, University of Oxford, Oxford, UK

Oxford Uehiro Centre for Practical Ethics, University of Oxford, Oxford, UK
e-mail: alberto.giubilini@philosophy.ox.ac.uk

J. Savulescu
Oxford Uehiro Centre for Practical Ethics, University of Oxford, Oxford, UK

Visiting Professorial Fellow in Biomedical Ethics, Murdoch Children's Research Institute, Melbourne, Australia

Distinguished Visiting Professor on Law, Melbourne Law School, University of Melbourne, Melbourne, Australia

The Problem of Antimicrobial Resistance

When Alexander Fleming was awarded the Nobel Prize for Medicine in 1945, he warned in his acceptance speech of the risk that some bacteria could develop resistance to penicillin, which he had discovered 17 years earlier. It cannot be overstated how longsighted Fleming was. Today, "bacteria are resistant to nearly all antibiotics that were earlier active against them" (Herrmann and Laxminarayan 2010, p. 4.2), and "700,000 people die of resistant infections every year" (O'Neill 2016, p. 4). As estimated by the Review on Antimicrobial Resistance commissioned by the UK government, "by 2050 10 million lives a year are at risk due to drug resistant infections, as are 100 trillion USD of economic output" (O'Neill 2016). Examples of diseases associated with antimicrobial resistance (AMR) include tuberculosis, gonorrhoea, typhoid fever, and group A streptococcus (Van der Velden et al. 2013). The problem of AMR has been framed by some in terms of a "slowly emerging disaster" (Littmann and Viens 2015) and of a "global health security issue" (Balasegaram et al. 2015).

AMR is a naturally occurring phenomenon: microbes naturally tend to adapt to antimicrobials and develop resistance. However, AMR is accelerated by human behaviour (Jamrozik and Selgelid 2019), and particularly the use and abuse of antimicrobials, both in livestock (Anomaly 2019; Giubilini et al. 2017; O'Neill 2015; Anomaly 2009) and in humans (O'Neill 2016). This paper is focussed on AMR caused by *human* consumption of antimicrobials, and therefore on the human factor in the development of AMR. There is a positive correlation between antimicrobial resistance rates and antimicrobial consumption in humans (Van der Velden et al. 2013, pp. 318–19). In fact, in the case of antibiotics, it is now widely accepted that "the use of antibiotics is the single most important factor leading to antibiotic resistance around the world: simply using antibiotics creates resistance" (CDC, About antimicrobial resistance), even when antibiotic use is medically indicated to treat infections (which is what makes AMR a particularly difficult ethical issue). Thus, the paradox of antibiotic and certain other kind of antimicrobial consumption is that while certain antimicrobials can be beneficial to individuals, their use also poses a threat to public health, to the lives of millions of people, and to the world economy. If they are not used more wisely than they currently are, i.e. if their consumption is not reduced, we might face a "post antibiotic" era (Alanis 2005; WHO 2014) characterized by two undesirable outcomes. First, we might no longer have effective means of treating severe infections. Second, medicine's achievements that require effective antibiotics, such as organ transplantation, cancer chemotherapy, and major surgery, might no longer be available (WHO, Antimicrobial resistance).

To be sure, the problem of reducing antibiotic and certain type of antimicrobial consumption mainly concerns those countries with easy access to and massive consumption of antimicrobials. These are mainly high-income countries (HICs). The consumption rate of antimicrobials in most low- and middle-income countries (LMICs), although it increased dramatically in recent years, remains much lower than that in HICs, and in many LMICs the burden of infectious disease still outweighs the burden of resistance; the increase in consumption in such countries ought to be closely monitored, but drastic measures to reduce antibiotic consumption need to be implemented *primarily* in HICs (Klein et al. 2018). Reduction of therapeutically justified antimicrobial consumption in LMICs for conservation purposes might have undesirable outcomes, especially in those countries where the level of public health is already poor. There might be exceptions, of course; for instance, India is a lower-income country and one of the major contributors to resistance through very high consumption rates (Kumar et al. 2013; WHO India 2018), so perhaps *significant* restrictions on antibiotic access – that is, restrictions that apply also to therapeutically justified use – should be implemented in such context as well. However, to make our arguments the least controversial possible, we take them to apply only to HICs where a good level of public health might allow leaving certain mild and self-limiting infections untreated without posing significant costs on patients.

This paper is focussed on two often neglected aspects of the problem of AMR, namely on the individual moral obligations with regard to antimicrobial consumption and on the type of justification that health authorities could and should offer for restricting access to antimicrobials in order to preserve antimicrobial effectiveness. As we will argue in Sect. 9.3, these two aspects are closely related: the state has an obligation to provide the strongest justification possible for restrictive interventions aimed at limiting antimicrobial consumption, and the strongest justification is one based on the existence of an individual moral obligation to forgo antimicrobials, perhaps (as we will suggest in Sect. 9.4) even in case of mild self-limiting infections that do not significantly risk worsening the individual's general health. The fact that even justified use of antimicrobials, i.e. the use that is medically necessary to treat infections (as opposed to unjustified use, e.g. when antibiotics are prescribed for viral infections, a practice that is not uncommon unfortunately), contributes to antimicrobial resistance determines a moral conflict between individual interest and collective interest that might require individuals to make sacrifices for the sake of the common good.

Such moral conflict gives rise to a "tragedy of the commons" scenario (Hollis and Maybarduk 2015), which will be presented in Sect. 9.2: we will argue, following Garrett Hardin, that the tragedy of the commons has an ethical solution, which will be presented in Sect. 9.4, where we will argue that there is a *moral* obligation to contribute to the preservation of the common good of antimicrobial effectiveness which might entail a moral obligation not to use antimicrobials in some cases of mild, self-limiting infections, provided that certain conditions obtain and that the state takes all the measures that are necessary to ensure that forgoing antimicrobials in those cases approximates a form of "easy rescue".

Thus, in Sect. 9.4 we will draw the policy implications of this ethical solution to the tragedy of the commons: the moral obligation to sometimes forgo antimicrobials, grounded in a duty of easy rescue, strengthens the justification for state interventions that prohibit or discourage the use of antimicrobials in certain cases. Since states should be able to provide the strongest justification possible for implementing restrictive policies that discourage or prohibit antimicrobial consumption, appeal to individual moral obligations to sometimes forgo antimicrobials has a political weight in terms of justification of state-imposed restrictions on antimicrobial use.

However, as we will suggest in conclusion of Sect. 9.4, the moral obligation of the state to provide the strongest justification possible for restricting access to antimicrobials implies an obligation on the state to ensure that forgoing antimicrobials does represent a form of easy rescue, i.e. that individuals bear as small a cost as possible for leaving certain infections untreated with antimicrobials (assuming this measure is necessary). This means, in practice, that the state has moral obligations towards individuals who are requested to forgo antimicrobial for the sake of the collective good, such as the obligation to provide enhanced medical follow up and to adequately compensate, financially or in other ways (e.g. higher priorities on waiting lists for other medical treatments), these individuals.

Public Goods, Tragedy of the Commons, and Policies to Address Antimicrobial Resistance

It has been claimed that "if effective antibiotics are seen as a public good, their overuse may be likened to the tragedy of the commons scenario" (Littmann and Viens 2015, p. 214). This statement is not entirely correct in the way the notion of 'public good' is applied. As we are going to see in this section, antibiotic and more generally antimicrobial effectiveness shares an essential feature with common goods or common pool resources, rather than with public goods. Let's see more in detail what this terminology means when the concepts of "public goods" and of "common goods" are applied to the case of antimicrobial effectiveness.

Some benefits associated with antimicrobial effectiveness can certainly be considered public goods. These include freedom from infectious diseases (Selgelid 2007, p. 226), the containment of infectious diseases (Woodward and Smith 2003, p. 10), or the reduced risk of infection by a resistant disease (Smith and Coast 2003, p. 78). These benefits are public goods in the technical sense of the term: they are non-excludable, in the sense that people cannot be excluded from benefitting from them; and they are non-rivalrous, in the sense that the fact that a person benefits from them does not affect the way and the extent to which others benefit as well (Cowen 2008). More precisely, freedom from infectious diseases, infectious disease containment, and the reduced risk of infection can be conceived as *global public goods*, i.e. goods "exhibiting a significant degree of publicness (i.e. non-excludability and non-rivalry) across national boundaries" (Woodward and Smith 2003, p, 8).

Effective antimicrobials are the means through which such public goods are preserved. But antimicrobial effectiveness is a common good rather than a public good because antimicrobial effectiveness is rivalrous in consumption, in virtue of what Anne Schwenkenbecher in a chapter of this volume calls "the antimicrobial footprint" of antimicrobial consumptions: "simply using antibiotics [or other antimicrobials] creates resistance" (CDC, About Antimicrobial resistance) and "more consumption of antibiotics directly leads to more resistance" (O'Neill 2016, p. 17), regardless of whether antimicrobial use is therapeutically justified or not. The use of the resource of antimicrobial effectiveness through antimicrobial consumption erodes the resource and therefore diminishes its availability. As put by Jonny Anomaly, "individually rational choices produce substantial social costs by creating reservoirs of antibiotic-resistant bacteria in human hosts and more generally in our shared microbial environment" (Anomaly 2013, p. 753). It is important to point out that, while antimicrobial use might benefit individuals in the short term, this is not necessarily the case in the long term: individuals can incur a portion of the costs associated with antimicrobial resistance (Anomaly 2013, p. 752). For example, the individual who takes antibiotics can become a carrier of resistant bacteria, which means that the individual is at greater risk in case of subsequent infections (Cars et al. 2008).

It has been observed that the effectiveness of antimicrobials can "be modelled as a natural resource in much the same way as are fish, tree, oil, and other resources" (Herrmann and Laxminarayan 2010, p. 4.3). According to John Conly, for example,

> antimicrobial resistance may be likened to [the] overfishing scenario, to cattle overgrazing the grass in the commons or to deforestation on Easter Island, which led to population dying out. Antimicrobial resistance is a consequence of continued overuse of antibiotics combined with the constant growth of resistance overtime. (WHO 2010)

Typically, consumption of natural resources determines a 'tragedy of the commons' scenario (Ostrom et al. 1999,). Garrett Hardin first described the "tragedy of the commons" in an article he published in *Science* (Hardin 1968). Hardin illustrated the problem through the example of a commons to which some herdsmen have access. The tragedy occurs when many herdsmen, acting merely out of self-interest, have their cattle overgraze the commons, thus eroding the resource (Hardin 1968, p. 1244). Particularly in a context of growing population, all herdsmen acting in the same way deplete the common good. In the context of antimicrobial effectiveness, the same problem arises (Hollis and Maybarduk 2015). As Jonny Anomaly put it, "the benefits of [antibiotic] use are borne by the individual, the costs are socialised, and the consequent harm is the product of many independent actions" (Anomaly 2013, p. 752).

According to Hardin, one characteristic of a tragedy of the commons is the fact that there is no "technical" solution to the problem, meaning that there is no solution "that requires a change only in the techniques of the natural sciences, demanding little or nothing in the way of change in human values or ideas of morality" (Hardin 1968, p. 1243). On the contrary, Hardin argued, the solution requires a "fundamental extension" of our morality (Hardin 1968, p. 1243), i.e. acting in view of protecting the public interest rather than in a merely self-interested way.

However, Hardin seemed to be sceptical about the possibility that such an extension of morality could occur, at least without some external coercive intervention (which on most accounts of morality would arguably undermine the authentically "moral" nature of the change invoked). He believed that the best way to solve a tragedy of the commons is through some degree of "mutually agreed upon" coercion (Hardin 1968, p. 1247), for example in the form of taxation that would allow to internalize the negative externalities of individual consumption.[1]

[1]Another solution Hardin proposed is the privatization of the commons (Hardin 1968, p. 1245), which in the case of antimicrobials might consist in "extending the period of exclusivity, possibly

And indeed, some have suggested that the negative externalities of antimicrobial use could be internalised through the introduction of user fees or consumption taxes (Littmann and Viens 2015; Anomaly 2013; Herrmann and Laxminarayan 2010). Internalization is typically achieved by "taxing negative externalities (...) at a rate that would offset the social cost of the activities that generate the externalities, and then (ideally) using the revenues from the tax to fund socially useful projects" (Anomaly 2009, p. 433). The idea behind the concept of internalization is that it is those who are responsible for a negative externality that should bear the cost for it.

However, it might not be possible to fully internalise the collective cost of antimicrobial consumption and to disincentivize consumers through a tax: selection for AMR will probably continue to occur in spite of the tax and in spite of the investment of the revenue in strategies to contain AMR such as research on new antimicrobials. For this reason, it has been suggested that we might need at some point to introduce policies to restrict antimicrobial use only to the most serious infections, i.e. that it might be necessary to prevent, if necessary through legal prohibition, their use in the case of milder self-limiting infections (Foster and Grundmann 2006, p. 179). We will return to this point in Sect. 9.4.

Policies might therefore aim to disincentivize individuals from using antimicrobials, in the case of taxation; or they might coercively impose restrictions on antimicrobial use, in the case of outright prohibition of antimicrobial use in certain circumstances. As said before, we are interested here not so much in determining which policies would be more effective and ethically acceptable. Thus, we do not intend to provide arguments for or against taxation of antibiotics or restrictions on their use. Rather, we are interested in what justification an authority might offer for implementing restrictive policies, whatever form they take. While such policies might be justified by considerations of public interest, it is important that the type of justification that a state can provide for interventions that limit or discourage antimicrobial use be the strongest justification possible, given that such interventions might require individuals to sacrifice some significant personal interest, such as the interest in accessing effective health care, for the sake of the common good. As we are going to argue in the next section, considerations about the morality of individual choices regarding antimicrobial consumption can strengthen the justification for such policies.

Morality and Antimicrobial Consumption

Restrictive and coercive interventions might be efficacious at protecting the common goods associated with AMR containment and in preserving the common good of antimicrobial effectiveness. However, the "tragedy of the commons" scenario

---

indefinitely" of the patents, thus giving "the patentee the ability to charge high prices and thus indirectly restrain overuse by some users" (Hollis and Maybarduk 2015, p. 33).

which preservation of antimicrobial effectiveness gives rise to suggests that there is an independent ethical dimension to the problem of AMR. In this section we will explain why discussing such an independent ethical dimension is important from a political point of view, i.e. in view of justifying coercive policies aimed at restricting antimicrobial use.

Establishing an independent *moral* responsibility to make a more appropriate use of antimicrobials would make the justification that a state could provide for policies that restrict or discourage antimicrobial use the strongest possible. And, arguably, the state does have a duty to provide individuals with the strongest justification possible for implementing policies that restrict or discourage a treatment that is in the individuals' best interest, as is often the case with antimicrobials.

Restrictive policies might be justified in light of a state's duty to protect certain common goods and public goods, such as the public goods associated with AMR containment. These possible interventions range from those that are minimally intrusive to those that more substantially infringe rights or important interests of individuals. Thus, at one end of the spectrum we find policies such as information campaigns, nudging, or incentivisation of certain pro-social behaviours; and at the other end we find more restrictive policies such as taxation and compulsion. In all such cases, the authority enforcing such policies should be able to provide the strongest justification possible for its interventions, but the more restrictive the policies become, the more difficult it is for the authority to meet such requirement. A state's duty to protect public goods and common goods by itself does not provide the strongest justification possible for interventions that sacrifice important individual interests. The justification would be stronger if, in addition to considerations of public interest, there were independent individual moral obligations to make those individual sacrifices that are required by the restrictive policy (Giubilini et al. 2018) Thus, one way to strengthen the justification for state interventions such as taxation of antimicrobials or prohibition of certain antimicrobial uses is to identify a pre-existing individual *moral* obligation not to use antimicrobials in certain cases. Such independent moral obligation to prioritize other-regarding choices over self-interested choices would make the case for introducing restrictive policies that limit or discourage antimicrobial use as compelling as possible: such policies would simply impose or encourage choices that individuals have an independent moral obligation to make anyway.

Individual Responsibility and Duty of Easy Rescue: The Ethical Solution to the Tragedy of the Commons and the Responsibilities of the State

We have noted above that, as Hardin himself acknowledged, the tragedy of the commons is first and foremost an *ethical* problem. Therefore, it has an ethical solution that is independent from the justification for legislative coercive solutions. Now, "ethical solution" means, according to Hardin's phrasing, a change in "human values" informing human behaviour. Thus, in the case of antimicrobial consumption, the ethical solution to the tragedy of the commons consists in justifying the existence of an individual *moral* obligation to act contrary to one's (short term) self interest in order to contribute to the preservation of the common good of antimicrobial effectiveness. In other words, the ethical solution consists in finding a justification for a moral duty not to use antimicrobials, if necessary even at the cost of leaving some infections untreated, in order to protect the common good of antimicrobial effectiveness. In this section we are going to provide this justification.

It is plausible to assume that individuals have what might be called a "duty of easy rescue" (Savulescu 2007). That is, if doing X (or refraining from doing Y) entails a small cost to an individual and a large benefit (or prevention of a large harm) to others, the individual has a clear prima facie moral obligation to do X (or to refrain from doing Y). Morality is essentially different from prudence, and requires the sacrifice of one's own interests for others. It is debatable what kind of individual sacrifices morality requires, but if morality requires anything, almost everyone would agree that it certainly requires at least small sacrifices for the sake of preventing great harm. This does not mean that an individual does not have a moral obligation when the cost to her is not small. However, in easy rescue case, such moral obligation seems uncontroversial. A formulation of the duty of easy rescue was famously provided by Peter Singer, according to whom "if it is in our power to prevent something bad from happening, without thereby sacrificing anything of *comparable* moral importance, we ought, morally, to do it" (Singer 1972, p. 230, emphasis added). A roughly equivalent, though way less demanding, formulation has been provided by Tim Scanlon, according to whom "[i]f we can prevent something very bad from happening to someone by making a slight or even moderate sacrifice, it would be wrong not to do so" (Scanlon 1998, p. 224). The fact that some version of a duty of easy rescue can be defended both from a utilitarian perspective- in the case of Singer – and a contractualist perspective- in the case of Scanlon – supports the idea that it is a fundamental requirement of morality on which reasonable people could agree.

The existence of a duty of easy rescue implies an individual moral obligation to forgo antimicrobials for the sake of the common good of antimicrobial effectiveness, *when forgoing antimicrobials comes at a sufficiently small cost to individuals*. This would be the case, for example, when antimicrobials are not necessary to treat an infection (for example in the case of viral infections), in which case there would be no cost at all in forgoing antimicrobials. But forgoing antimicrobials would also come at a relatively small cost to individuals when individuals have minor self-limiting infections or low risk mild infections (for example, skin infections which could be treated topically with antiseptics) that do not significantly worsen the general state of health of the individual, where the risks of complications is adequately monitored, and when the individual is adequately compensated for any financial and non-financial cost she might incur as a consequence of leaving that infection untreated. As some have suggested (Foster and Grundmann 2006) it *might* at some point be necessary to leave such self-limiting infections untreated in order to preserve antimicrobial effectiveness.

The moral duty of easy rescue represents the ethical solution to the tragedy of the commons in the context of antimicrobial consumption that Hardin advocated: individuals have a moral obligation to prioritize the public interest in the preservation of the commons of antimicrobial effectiveness over their own interest in treating with antimicrobials any type of infection (including mild and self-limiting ones), because doing so comes at a small cost to individuals, at least when all that is required of individuals is to leave self-limiting mild or minor infections untreated in circumstances in which this would not significantly worsen individual health and where adequate compensatory measures are in place.

Now, since it is necessary that a large number of individuals fulfil a duty of easy rescue in order for a public benefit to obtain, we can say that there is not only an individual, but also a *collective* responsibility to forgo antimicrobials when doing so is a way of fulfilling a duty of easy rescue. Now, in some cases of collective action, any individual contribution to a collective good, or to the prevention of a collective harm, is insignificant; for example, the contribution each individual could make to the realisation of herd immunity through individual vaccination, or the contribution each individual could make to the prevention of global warming by avoiding driving just for fun, are both negligible. However, in the case of containment of antimicrobial resistance every single individual forgoing antimicrobials could make a difference, because every single individual could become the carrier of resistant microbes that are then passed onto other people. For example, it has been shown that individuals who take antibiotics for respiratory and urinary infections might develop bacterial resistance that could last up to 12 months (Costelloe et al. 2010). Thus, the need to preserve the common good of antimicrobial effectiveness implies not only a collective responsibility, but also an individual responsibility not to use antimicrobials so as to benefit others by contributing to the preservation of antimicrobial effectiveness, at least as long as forgoing antimicrobials comes at a small enough cost to individuals.

When forgoing antimicrobials is a moral duty of easy rescue, we can claim that the state is in the position to fulfil its obligation to provide the strongest justification possible for prohibiting or at least discouraging the use of antimicrobials: as we said in Sect. 9.3, the state would be discouraging or preventing individuals from doing only what they have a moral obligation not to do anyway. Therefore, being the state in the position to fulfil its moral obligations in implementing restrictive measures, such restrictive measures regarding antimicrobial use are ethically justified. As one of us put it, "when the cost to us of forgoing some activity is small (…) and the harm to others which thereby does not occur is great (prevention of serious disease), then liberals might require that the state prevent this harm" (Savulescu 2007, p. 10).

"Duty to rescue" laws exist in many European countries; for instance, in Germany and France it is illegal not to assist a person in danger when providing assistance entails a small or no risk to the potential rescuer. From what we have said so far, laws restricting antimicrobial use could be ethically justified as special cases of "duty to rescue" laws of this kind.

The individual moral responsibility to forgo antimicrobials in certain circumstances implies that there are two other actors with specific moral responsibilities, besides patients with minor or mild self-limiting infections.

First, doctors have the responsibility to assess whether a certain infection is self-limiting and, more in general, whether leaving a certain infection untreated is compatible with a good enough level of individual health. In one important sense, the fact that the state has the strongest justification possible for imposing bans on antimicrobial use or for discouraging through taxation antimicrobial consumption takes the responsibility for decisions about antimicrobial prescription out of the hands of doctors: if a certain infection is mild and self limiting and leaving it untreated does not significantly worsen the general state of health of the patient, then the state, rather than the doctor, is justified in preventing the use of antimicrobials for the sake of the common good. However, the doctors would still have the important responsibility of determining whether the conditions specified in such laws would apply, and thus they would still be the ultimate gate-keepers of antimicrobials.

Second, but equally important, healthcare systems and states have important moral responsibilities too. We have said that having an uncontroversial individual moral obligation based on a duty of easy rescue to sometimes forgo antimicrobials strengthens the justification for state interventions that forbid or discourage antimicrobial use. Therefore, the state or the healthcare system have the responsibility to ensure that forgoing antimicrobials does represent a form of easy rescue, i.e. that it is not too burdensome for patients, so that the justification for state intervention is the strongest possible. This means, at the very least, that patients who are denied antimicrobials should be carefully monitored and provided with adequate and enhanced medical follow up to make sure that forgoing antimicrobial treatment does not significantly worsen the general state of health of the individual. It is the responsibility of states and of healthcare systems to ensure that adequate measures are in place in order to guarantee monitoring and medical supervisions of those patients who sacrifice their self-interest for the sake of the collective good, so that their sacrifice would represent a form of easy rescue.

However, we claim that the responsibility of states extends beyond the provision of medical supervision and follow up. We propose that a further measure that might be implemented in order to ensure that the rescue is an easy rescue is that of *compensating* individuals who make a sacrifice for the sake of the collective good. Compensation – financial or of other kind – would be an appropriate measure because it would provide individuals with an additional reason for forgoing antimicrobials in certain circumstances, it would be fair in consideration of the sacrifice individuals are making for the sake of the collective good, and, more importantly, if the right type of compensation is offered, it could make their condition easier to bear, thus approximating a form of easy rescue and providing a further reason for the existence of an individual ethical obligation. For example, those who forgo antimicrobials and leave infections untreated could be offered first call on future medical treatments, even for conditions that are not related to the current infection; or they might be offered discounts when they buy other medicines, such as painkillers, or discounts on future medical treatments; alternatively, they might be offered outright financial compensation, for example in the form of tax relief or by directly paying them, which would account for any financial loss that might result from enduring a prolonged infections. In this way, they would derive at least some benefit from the sacrifice they are making, which would render the sacrifice easier to bear, and at the same time society would be "making up" for the sacrifice it is imposing on these individuals.

Granted, preserving antimicrobial effectiveness by financially compensating those who forgo antimicrobials might involve a significant cost for the state. However, we saw in the introduction that there will be significant costs associated with AMR if we don't intervene now; therefore, investing money now to compensate and to guarantee adequate medical follow up to those who make sacrifices in order to contain AMR might be a good strategy also from the point of view of cost-effectiveness.

Conclusions

When is it necessary to leave infections untreated in order to preserve the common good of antimicrobial effectiveness? This is an empirical issue and the answer depends on whether and to what extent the societal optimum of antimicrobial consumption differs from the individual optimum. In other words, it concerns the issue whether and to what extent the level of individual consumption that is consistent with satisfactory AMR containment (the societal optimum) differs from the level of consumption that would effectively treat infections in any individual (the individual optimum). As Kevin Foster and Hajo Grundmann (2006, pp. 178–9) have explained, if individual and societal optima were similar, it would be sufficient to avoid inappropriate antimicrobial use, such as using antibiotics in the case of viral infections, an abuse which often occurs (Van der Velden et al. 2013). Only inappropriate use of antimicrobials would then be morally impermissible. However, if individuals and societal optimum differed significantly, in order to protect the societal interest in AMR containment individuals might be required to leave minor and mild self-limiting infections untreated in order to reserve antimicrobials for serious major infections. In such cases, coercive policies that restrict access to *some* therapeutically justified use of antimicrobials are ethically permissible, or so we have argued. However, when implementing such restrictive policies, state and health authorities have responsibilities not only towards the collective, but also towards individuals who make (small) sacrifices for the sake of the collective interested, and who should be guaranteed adequate compensation in exchange for leaving certain infections untreated.

Acknowledgment AG and JS were funded by the Wellcome Centre for Ethics and Humanities, University of Oxford, which is supported by a Wellcome Centre Grant (203132/Z/16/Z), and by the Wellcome Trust grant 104848/Z/14/Z. Through his involvement with the Murdoch Children's Research Institute, JS was supported by the Victorian Government's Operational Infrastructure Support Program. AG was also supported by the Oxford Martin School through the Oxford Martin Program on 'Collective responsibility for infectious disease'.

References

Alanis, Alfonso J. 2005. Resistance to antibiotics: Are we in the post-antibiotics era? *Archives of Medical Research* 36 (6): 597–705.

Anomaly, Jonny. 2009. Harm to others: The social cost of antibiotics in agriculture. *Journal of Agricultural and Environmental Ethics* 22: 423–435.

———. 2013. Collective action and individual choice: Rethinking how we regulate narcotics and antibiotics. *Journal of Medical Ethics* 39: 752–756.

———. 2019. Antibiotics and animal agriculture the need for global collective action. In *Ethics and drug resistance: Collective responsibility for global public health*. Cham: Springer.

Balasegaram, Manica, et al. 2015. The global innovation model for antibiotics needs reinvention. *The Journal of Law, Ethics, and Medicine* 43 (S3): 22–26.

Baquero, Fernando, and Jose Campos. 2003. The tragedy of the commons in antimicrobial chemotherapy. *Revista espanola de quimioterapia: publicacion oficial de la Sociedad Espanola de Quimioterapia* 16 (1): 11–13.

Barlam, Tamar, and Kalpana Gutpa. 2015. Antibiotic resistance spreads internationally across borders. *The Journal of Law, Medicine, and Ethics* 43 (S3): 12–16.

Cars, Otto, et al. 2008. Meeting the challenge of antibiotic resistance. *British Medical Journal* 337: 726–728.

CDC (Center for Disease Control and Prevention). About antimicrobial resistance, updated 2015. Available at: https://www.cdc.gov/drugresistance/about.html. Last access 17 Aug 2016.

CDDEP (Center for Disease Dynamics, Economics, and Policy). 2015. *The state of the world's antibiotics*. Available at: https://cddep.org/sites/default/files/swa_2015_final.pdf. Last access 15 Nov 2016.

Coast, J., R. Smith, and M.R. Millar. 1996. Superbugs: Should antimicrobial resistance be included as a cost in economic evaluation? *Health Economics* 5 (3): 217–226.

Copp, David. 2007. The collective moral autonomy thesis. *Journal of Social Philosophy* 38: 3.

Costelloe, Ceire, et al. 2010. Effect of antibiotic prescribing in primary care on antibiotic resistance in individual patients: Systematic review and meta-analysis. *British Medical Journal* 340: c2096.

Cowen, Tyler. 2008. Public goods. In *The concise encyclopedia of economics*, ed. R. Henderson. Indianapolis: Library of Economics and Liberty. Available at: http://www.econlib.org/library/Enc/PublicGoods.html. Last access 5 Aug 2016.

Daulaire, Nils, et al. 2015. Universal access to effective antibiotics is essential for tackling antibiotic resistance. *The Journal of Law, Medicine, and Ethics* 43 (S3): 17–21.

Foster, Kevin, and Hajo Grundmann. 2006. Do we need to put society first? The potential for tragedy in antimicrobial resistance. *PLoS Medicine* 3 (2): 177–180.

Giubilini, A., et al. 2017. Taxing meat: Taking responsibility for one's contribution to antibiotic resistance. *Journal of Agricultural and Environmental Ethics* 30 (2): 179–198.

Giubilini, A., T. Douglas, J. Savulescu, and Hannah Maslen. 2018. Quarantine, isolation, and the duty of easy rescue in public health. *Developing World Bioethics* 18 (2): 182–189.

Hardin, Garrett. 1968. The tragedy of the commons. *Science* 162: 1243–1248.

Held, Virginia. 1970. Can a random collection of individuals be morally responsible? *The Journal of Philosophy* 57 (14): 471–481.

Herrmann, Markus, and Ramanan Laxminarayan. 2010. Antibiotic effectiveness: New challenges in natural resource management. *The Annual Review of Resource Economics* 2 (4): 1–14.

Hoffman, Steven, and Trygve Ottersen. 2015. Addressing antibiotic resistance requires robust international accountability mechanisms. *The Journal of Law, Medicine, and Ethics* 43 (S3): 53–64.

Hoffman, Steven, et al. 2015. International law has a role to play in addressing antibiotic resistance. *The Journal of Law, Medicine, and Ethics* 43 (S3): 65–67.

Hollis, Aidan, and Peter Maybarduk. 2015. Antibiotic resistance is a tragedy of the commons that necessitates global cooperation. *The Journal of Law, Medicine, and Ethics* 43 (S3): 33–37.

Jamrozik, E., and M.J. Selgelid. Drug-resistant infection: Causes, consequences, and responses. In *Ethics and drug resistance: Collective responsibility for global public health*. Cham: Springer.

Klein, Eili, et al. 2018. *Global increase and geographic convergence in antibiotic consumption between 2000 and 2015*. In Proceedings of the National Academy of Sciences of the United States of America.

Kumar, S.G., C. Adithan, B.N. Harish, S. Sujatha, G. Roy, and A. Malini. 2013. Antimicrobial resistance in India: A review. *Journal of Natural Science, Biology, and Medicine* 4 (2): 286–291.

Lewis, H.D. 1948. Collective responsibility. *Philosophy* 23 (84): 3–18.

Littmann, J., and A.M. Viens. 2015. The ethical significance of antimicrobial resistance. *Public Health Ethics* 8 (3): 209–224.

Littmann, J., A. Buyx, and O. Cars. 2015. Antibiotic resistance: An ethical challenge. *International Journal of Antimicrobial Agents* 46: 359–361.

Miller, Seamus. 2006. Collective responsibility: An individualist account. *Midwest Studies in Philosophy* 30: 176–193.

Narveson, J. 2002. Collective responsibility. *The Journal of Ethics* 6: 179–198.

O'Neill, Jim. 2015. Antimicrobials in agriculture and the environment: Reducing unnecessary use and waste. *The Review on Antimicrobials Resistance*. Available at: https://amr-review.org/sites/default/files/Antimicrobials%20in%20agriculture%20and%20the%20environment%20-%20Reducing%20unnecessary%20use%20and%20waste.pdf. Last access 8 Oct 2016.

O'Neill. 2016. *Tackling drug resistant infections globally: Final report and recommendations*. The Review on Antimicrobial Resistance. Available at: http://amr-review.org/sites/default/files/160518_Final%20paper_with%20cover.pdf. Last access 16 Aug 2016.

Oczkowski, Simon. 2017. Antimicrobial stewardship programmes: Bedside rationing by another name? *Journal of Medical Ethics* 43 (10): 684–687.

Ostrom, E., J. Burger, C.B. Field, R.B. Norgaard, and D. Policansky. 1999. Sustainability – Revisiting the commons: Local lessons, global challenges. *Science* 284: 278–282.

Podolski, Scott, et al. 2015. History teaches us that confronting antibiotic resistance requires stronger global collective action. *The Journal of Law, Medicine, and Ethics* 43 (S3): 27–32.

Savulescu, Julian. 2007. Future people, involuntary medical treatment in pregnancy, and the duty of easy rescue. *Utilitas* 19 (1): 1–20.

Scanlon, T. 1998. *What We Owe to Each Other*. Cambridge, MA: Harvard University Press.

Schwenkenbecher, Anne. forthcoming. Antimicrobial footprints, fairness, and collective harm. In *Ethics and drug resistance: Collective responsibility for global public health*. Cham: Springer.

Selgelid, M. 2007. Ethics and drug resistance. *Bioethics* 21 (4): 218–229.

Singer, P. 1972. Famine, affluence, and morality. *Philosophy and Public Affairs* 1 (3): 229–243.

Smith, Richard, and Joanna Coast. 2002. Antimicrobial resistance: A global response. *Bulletin of the World Health Organization* 80 (2): 126–133.

———. 2003. Antimicrobial drug resistance. In *Global public goods for health*, ed. Smith et al., 73–93. New York: Oxford University Press.

Van der Velden, A., et al. 2013. Prescriber and patient responsibilities in treatment of acute respiratory tract infection – Essential for conservation of antibiotics. *Antibiotics* 2: 316–327.

WHO. 2010. Antimicrobial resistance: Revisiting the "tragedy of the commons". *Bulletin of the World Health Organization* 88: 11. Available at http://www.who.int/bulletin/volumes/88/11/10-031110/en/.

———. 2014. *Antimicrobial resistance: Global report on surveillance 2014*. Geneva: World Health Organization.

———. Antimicrobial resistance, Fact sheet n 194, updated 2015. Available at: http://www.who.int/mediacentre/factsheets/fs194/en/. Last access 17 Aug 2016.

WHO India. 2018. *Combating antimicrobial resistance in India*. Available at: http://www.searo.who.int/india/topics/antimicrobial_resistance/Combating_Antimicrobial_Resistance_in_India/en/. Last access 19 Nov 18.

Woodward, David, and Richard D. Smith. 2003. Global public goods and health: Concepts and issues. In *Global public goods for health*, ed. Smith et al., 3–29. New York: Oxford University Press.

8

Conceptualizing the Impact of MDRO Control Measures Directed at Carriers: A Capability Approach

Morten Fibieger Byskov, Babette Olga Rump, and Marcel Verweij

Abstract Many countries have implemented specific control measures directed at carriers of multidrug-resistant organisms (MDRO) in order to prevent further introduction and transmission of resistant organisms into hospitals and other healthcare related settings. These control measures may in many ways affect the lives and well-being of carriers of MDRO, resulting in complex ethical dilemmas that often remain largely implicit in practice. In this chapter, we propose to conceptualize the impact of MDRO control measures on the well-being of individual carriers in terms of capabilities and functionings. A capabilitarian framework for the ethical treatment of MDRO carriers commits us to conceptualize the harm done to carriers in terms of the impact that MDRO control measures have on what they are able to do or be. Adopting and adapting Nussbaum's list of ten central human capabilities, we present a taxonomy of capabilities and functionings that are normatively relevant for the design and evaluation of MDRO control measures.

Keywords Bioethics · Moral philosophy · Public health · Drug resistance

---

M. F. Byskov (✉) · M. Verweij
Communication, Philosophy, and Technology, Wageningen University & Research, Wageningen, Netherlands
e-mail: morten.byskov@wur.nl; Marcel.verweij@wur.nl

B. O. Rump
The Netherlands National Institute for Public Health and the Environment (RIVM), Bilthoven, Netherlands

Introduction

Antimicrobial resistance (AMR) has been described as one of the major threats to individual and public health (WHO 2014). This threat has justified extensive restrictions on the freedom of individuals (Krom 2011; Littmann 2014; Littmann and Viens 2015). Many countries have implemented control measures in order to prevent further introduction and spread of MDRO. Some more general, as addressed in Chap. 6 by Gilbert et al., and some more specific, like those targeting the individual who is found to carry an MDRO. Measures directed at MDRO carriers aim to limit the introduction and further transmission of multidrug-resistant organism (MDRO) in hospitals and other healthcare-related settings. The measures vary per microorganism and include for instance isolation and quarantine; contact precaution; eradication treatment; restrictions in the workplace; refusal of access to important activities; or contact restrictions at the one's family farm. They may in many ways affect the lives and well-being of carriers, resulting in complex ethical dilemmas that often remain largely implicit in practice.

Within the literature, little attention has been paid to how we treat carriers of MDRO, however, and Littmann et al. (2015) includes it as one of four ethical issues that needs further examination when addressing MDRO. In this chapter we aim to start filling this lacuna by proposing to conceptualize the impact of MDRO control measures on the well-being of individual carriers in terms of capabilities and functionings. A capabilitarian framework for the ethical treatment of MDRO carriers commits us to conceptualize the harm done to carriers in terms of the impact that MDRO control measures have on what they are able to do or be. Adopting and adapting Nussbaum's list of ten central human capabilities, we present a taxonomy of capabilities and functionings that are normatively relevant for the design and evaluation of MDRO control measures. Chapter 16 addresses the implications of AMR for child development and adult capabilities.

The chapter is structured as follows: In Sect. 13.2, we shortly present the issue of treating MDRO carriers as an ethical problem before we turn, in Sect. 13.3, to propose a capabilitarian framework for the conceptualization of the impact that MDRO control measures have on the well-being of carriers. In Sects. 13.4 and 13.5, we adapt Nussbaum's list of ten central human capabilities in order to develop a taxonomy of normatively relevant capabilities and functionings in the context of MDRO. In Sect. 13.4, we first present Nussbaum's list of capabilities before we argue that this list needs further specification when applied to the case of MDRO. In Sect. 13.5, we proceed to propose a taxonomy of ethical domains and normatively relevant capabilities and functionings in the context of responsible care for MDRO carriers. In Sect. 13.6, we finally argue that and show how this capabilitarian taxonomy can provide a crucial input to procedures for ethical decision-making on appropriate MDRO control measures.

The Ethical Treatment of MDRO Carriers: A Neglected Issue

Treating MDRO as an ethical issue is a double-sided coin. On the one side, it involves a concern for public health and how we can ensure that everyone, now and in the future, have access to antimicrobial treatment while minimizing the risk of further spread of MDRO. From this side of the coin, addressing MDRO is primarily an issue of global distributive justice (Littmann 2014; Littmann et al. 2015, 360): how can we distribute antimicrobials in a way that, on the one hand, adequately protects public health by ensuring that everyone has access to antibiotics while, on the other hand, ensuring that antibiotics do not become useless? In the following, however, we shall not primarily be concerned with this distributive question.[1]

The distributive focus has often been accompanied by a discussion of what kinds of control measures we can take to prevent the further spread of MDRO (Selgelid et al. 2009; Coleman et al. 2010): how can we treat carriers in a way that minimizes the risk that they contaminate other individuals? An important element in the fight against MDRO is to adequately treat infections with multi-resistant microbes in patients and to prevent that these persons are re-infected or will infect others with a resistant organism. Due to the threat that MDRO poses to individual and public health (WHO 2014), many countries have implemented specific MDRO control measures in order to prevent further introduction and spread of MDRO. Measures to prevent and control the spread of MDRO may include isolation and quarantine; eradication therapy; restrictions in the workplace; refusal of access to important activities; or contact restrictions with one's family (Verweij and Dawson 2010).

Many of these control measures threaten to seriously affect the lives of individual carriers, however, and as important as such prevention and control is, it may have burdensome implications for infected patients and healthy persons in whom a resistant organism has been colonized: they may feel stigmatized, face restrictions in their work or private life, or might be refused access to certain institutions. For example, in a healthcare context, control measures may mean that surgeons should refrain from operating due to carriership, that infected nurses should not perform patient-related activities, or that we ask infected residents of a nursing home to keep away from social activities.

In some extreme cases it is almost impossible to eradicate the resistant organism and then it may be impossible for the person to return to what used to be his/her normal life. Consider, for example, the case of a medical student who was repeatedly diagnosed as carrier of Methicillin-Resistant Staphylococcus Aureus (MRSA) (Rump 2011; Rump et al. 2016). In line with the MDRO control guidelines, the student was not allowed to be involved in patient-care, which is an implicit part of completing the internships necessary to graduate. Because of this, the student had to

---

[1] For a discussion of different approaches to the distribution of antimicrobials, see especially Anomaly (2010, 2013), Daulaire et al. (2015), Littmann (2014), and Selgelid (2007). For an introduction to and overview of distributive justice in general, see Lamont and Favor (2016).

eventually discontinue his studies. Whether this outcome was indeed necessary or not remains unclear, though, since the risk of further contamination could have been minimized through proper hygiene and guidance.

The consequences of MDRO carriership certainly have the potential to affect the lives and well-being of not only carriers themselves, but also their social connections, such as family members, friends, and colleagues. Yet, it is unclear in what ways MDRO and MDRO carriership affect these individuals. In the remainder of this chapter, we will offer a novel conceptualization of how MDRO control measures can harm carriers and other affected individuals and further reflect on how this conceptualization, and the normatively relevant issues that are thereby revealed, influences the design and evaluation of MDRO control measures. We argue that adopting a capabilitarian framework for the conceptualization of 'harm' done to (potential) carriers can help us make better and more informed decision about what control measures to implement. According to a capabilitarian framework, MDRO control measures may harm individual carriers by negatively affecting their capabilities and functionings.

A Capabilitarian Framework for Conceptualizing the Impact of MDRO Control Measures

What is the capability approach and how can it be used to conceptualize the (negative) impact that MDRO control measures have on the lives and well-being of individual carriers?[2] Originally conceived by the Indian philosopher-economist Amartya Sen (1979) and further developed by a number of theorists, such as Martha Nussbaum, David A. Crocker, and Ingrid Robeyns, the capability approach is a normative framework for the conceptualization of human well-being (Robeyns 2016a). According to this framework, human well-being should be conceptualized in terms of *capabilities* and *functionings*. Capabilities are the real freedom that people have to do or be certain things, such as falling in love, getting an education, being politically active, riding a bike, reading a book, and so on. Functionings are

[2] It is possible that the capability approach can also be used to conceptualize 'harm' within three other related domains of application, which we will not discuss in this chapter. First, we can conceptualize the risk that the spread MDRO poses to the well-being of members of the public in terms of their capabilities and functionings. For a discussion of how to conceptualize public health in terms of the capability approach, see Prah Ruger (2010), Venkatapuram (2011), and Nielsen (2014). Secondly, the capability approach can be used to conceptualize the 'harm' of control measures within infectious disease control in general. While the taxonomy that we provide in Sect. 13.5 may also apply within infectious disease control in general, more research needs to be done in this regard as different capabilities may be relevant in relation to different diseases. Thirdly, the capability approach has been used to conceptualize the idea of 'person-centered healthcare,' what it means to treat patients as persons (Entwistle and Watt 2013).

capabilities that have been realized either by choice or by chance. A person's *capability-set* refers to all the capabilities and functionings that that individual has.[3]

Real freedom in this sense means that there are no restrictions on achieving a particular functioning. Whether or not one has such real freedom crucially depends on certain *conversion factors*. Conversion factors are personal, social, and environmental circumstances that affect the extent to which one can achieve certain doings and beings. For example, whether or not one has the real freedom to be healthy – that is, whether or not one has the capability of achieving the functioning of being healthy – depends on one's physical health, for example the strength of one's immune defense system (personal conversion factors), the extent to which one can rely on family and social relations for care (social conversion factors), and where one lives and whether there are adequate infrastructures, such as accessible health care facilities (environmental conversion factors).[4]

Through the notion of conversion factors, the capability approach captures the fact that human beings are diverse: different people living in different societies would have different needs and capabilities. As we shall see in Sect. 13.5, the different conversion factors are relevant when we consider how MDRO control measures affect the lives and well-being of individual carriers.

The capability approach moves the focus from the means that people have to their ends – what they are able to do or be with these means, such as goods, resources, and formal freedoms. As Sen (1979) argues, this shift in focus is justified because resources and goods alone do not ensure that people are equally able to convert them into doings and beings. Consider, for example, two persons – one disabled, the other able-bodied – with the same amount of resources. According to Sen, the disabled person is disadvantaged relative to the able-bodied person in two regards. First, she is disadvantaged in terms of what she can do or be with her means and resources. She may, for example, be less able to move around because she is confined to a wheelchair. Secondly, she may even be doubly worse off because she only receive the same amount of resources as the able-bodied person, even though she has more expenses in order to correct for her disability, whereas the able-bodied person, *ex hypothesi*, can spend all of her resources to pursue her valued ends. Hence, when evaluating the well-being of individuals, we cannot merely compare the amount of resources that they have without also looking at what they are able to do or be with these resources.

---

[3] Capabilities and functionings can be both positive and negative, as well as neutral (Robeyns 2016b). Positive capabilities are what we consider valuable for someone to do or be. Examples of positive capabilities are good health, adequate nutrition, falling in love, and getting an education. While most applications of the capability approach are primarily concerned with positive capabilities, there are also cases where we want to consider their negative capabilities. When evaluating a person's well-being, for example, it is relevant whether her capability-set include the capabilities to be murdered or raped. Insofar as we, usually, do not consider these capabilities to be valuable, a capability-set that allows for the risks of being murdered or raped would be less valuable than a capability-set that protects the individual from these risks.

[4] This example is adapted from Crocker and Robeyns (2010).

The concepts of capabilities and functionings can help us to better understand how MDRO control measures can 'harm' (potential) carriers of MDRO in terms of how MDRO control measures influence the real freedom that MDRO carriers have to do or be certain normatively relevant things. MDRO control measures can affect the capability-sets of (potential) carriers in at least two ways. First, they may impose certain requirements on (potential) carriers. This is, for example, the case when we subject nurses to strict hygiene regimes or demand that carriers undergo mandatory screenings and eradication therapies. In terms of the capability approach, MDRO control measures thus impose certain doings and beings – that is, functionings – on carriers. Secondly, MDRO control measures can reduce the choices that carriers have to choose from (i.e., the capabilities that they can choose to turn into realized functionings). This is, for example, the case when we place carriers in isolation or ban them from social activities.[5]

Rather than merely focusing on whether or not the autonomy of carriers is being respected (Beauchamp and Childress 2001), by conceptualizing the potential impact of MDRO control measures in terms of capabilities and functionings, we get a broader picture of the many ways in which carriers are affected. In other words, it allows us to move from a singular basis for evaluation, namely in terms of their autonomy, to a multi-dimensional one. The same carrier may be impacted in many different ways by a particular control measure. For example, restricting a resident of a nursing home from participating in the weekly bingo nights not only restricts her capability for participating in social activities, but may also take away an important source of pleasure and happiness or may even lead to stigmatization. Likewise, a particular control measure may impact different carriers in different ways. For example, a child who is at a crucial stage in her social and cognitive development would arguably be negatively affected to a greater extent from being taken out of daycare (even for a short period of time) than a child who is not in this crucial stage of development (Piaget 1971).

Moreover, the capability perspective gives substance to carriers' autonomy: it allows us to identify in which ways MDRO control measures have the potential to (negatively) impact the capabilities of (potential) carriers. We are not merely concerned with the limitation of options that carriers can choose from. Rather, the capability perspective tells us that carriers are concerned with *particular* opportunities for choice (Sen 1991), such as access to day care centers, nursing homes, and physiotherapy; participation in social and leisure activities; opportunities for education and employment; freedom from stigmatization and discrimination; and possibilities

[5]That is, there might still be good normative reasons to override this concern for carriers' capabilities, for example out of a concern for the public health. While we do not engage with the discussion on how to weigh the violation of carriers' capabilities against concerns for public health in this paper, do see Sect. 13.6 for an example of how such weighing can take place within an open-ended decision-making framework. The point here is, rather, that there are certain capabilities that are so normatively relevant that we should take them into consideration when deciding on appropriate MDRO control measures – again, even if we do not consider them to have overriding normative status.

for forming and sustaining relationships to friends, family, and pets. Indeed, by employing the capability approach to conceptualize the 'harm' done by MDRO control measures to individual carriers we gain a greater, more in-depth, and more specific understanding of this impact.

As noted, this focus on particular opportunities for choice – rather than freedom or autonomy, in general – moves the discussion away from the singular dichotomy between public health versus the freedom of the individual carrier. The restriction of freedom is not necessarily a bad thing on the capabilitarian view.[6] The restriction of an individual carrier's freedom out of concern for public health is perfectly compatible with the protection of her valued capabilities. What the capability perspective does highlight, though, is that the restriction of some freedoms and opportunities, however *prima facie* insignificant, may affect capabilities that we do find normatively valuable. For example, restricting an MRSA positive child from attending kindergarten for just a few months may not seem like a big deal. However, that restriction may negatively affect a normatively crucial aspect of a person's life, namely the opportunity for a normal social, cognitive, and physical development if the MRSA positive child were, at the moment of isolation, at a crucial stage of her development.

To see how MDRO control measures can (negatively) affect the lives of MDRO carriers, it is crucial to identify what capabilities and functionings that are normatively relevant for carriers in the context of MDRO. In the following two sections, we present a taxonomy of capabilities and functionings that may be normatively relevant when deciding on appropriate control measures. This taxonomy builds on one prominent instantiation of the capability approach, namely Nussbaum's list of ten central capabilities. We first discuss Nussbaum's list in Sect. 13.4 and argue that it needs further adaptation and specification when applied to the context of deciding on appropriate MDRO control measures before we explain the taxonomy in greater detail in Sect. 13.5. In Sect. 13.6, we finally show how this capabilitarian taxonomy can help us make better and more informed decisions when deciding on appropriate MDRO control measures.

Nussbaum's Ten Central Capabilities: A Starting Point

What capabilities should we be concerned about protecting when implementing certain measures to prevent the spread of MDRO?[7] A good starting point is Nussbaum's influential list of ten central capabilities that, she argues, every

[6] See, though, Carter (2014) for a dissenting view.

[7] We have employed what Byskov (forthcoming) refers to as a *synthesizing method* to identify the relevant capabilities. Synthesizing methods compare and reconcile two or more lists of capabilities derived from different theoretical and empirical sources. We have here reconciled Nussbaum's (2000) list of central human capabilities with (i) other lists of relevant normatively domains in healthcare literature, such as Entwistle and Watt (2013) and Huber et al. (2016), (ii) empirical

government should provide for their citizens. While Nussbaum's list is thus derived from a discussion on global justice, it can nevertheless be useful for conceptualizing what kinds of capabilities that are important because it helps us to identify how well-off individuals truly are.[8] The most influential version of Nussbaum's list of capabilities can be found in her book *Women and Human Development* (Nussbaum 2000)[9]:

1. *Life:* Ability to live to the end of a normal length human life, and not to have one's life reduced to not worth living.
2. *Bodily health:* Ability to have a good life, which includes – but is not limited to – reproductive health, nourishment, and shelter.
3. *Bodily integrity:* Ability to change locations freely, in addition to having sovereignty over one's body, which includes being secure against assault (e.g., sexual assault, child abuse, and domestic violence) and the opportunity for sexual satisfaction.
4. *Senses, imagination, and thought:* Ability to use one's senses to imagine, think, and reason in a 'truly human way' informed by an adequate education. The ability to produce self-expressive works and engage in religious rituals without fear of political ramifications. The ability to have pleasurable experiences and avoid unnecessary pain. Finally, the ability to seek the meaning of life.
5. *Emotions:* Ability to have attachments of things outside of ourselves, including being able to love others, grieve at the loss of loved ones, and be angry when it is justified.
6. *Practical reason:* Ability to form a conception of the good and critically reflect on it.
7. *Affiliation:*
    (a) Ability to live with and show concern for others, empathize with and show compassion for others, and the capability of justice and friendship. Institutions help develop and protect forms of affiliation.
    (b) Ability to have self-respect and not be humiliated by others (i.e., being treated with dignity and equal worth). This entails at least protections from being discriminated on the basis of race, sex, sexuality, religion, caste, ethnicity, and nationality. In work, this means entering relationships of mutual recognition.

---

analysis of a database of ethical and practical questions concerning MDRO raised within the Dutch healthcare system as well as (iii) participatory case discussions with practitioners working with infectious disease control. For overviews of the various methods for the selection of capabilities, see Ballon (2013) and Byskov (forthcoming).

[8] Several scholars have taken build on Nussbaum's list and made changes to it, as necessary, when applied in practice (e.g., Alkire 2002). Thus, to be clear, we do not take Nussbaum's list at face value but rather hold that we can compare and specify this list to the particular case of MDRO.

[9] See also Nussbaum (1992, 2011) for similar iterations of her list, albeit based on different normative justifications.

8. *Other species:* Ability to have concern for and live with other animals, plants, and the environment at large.
9. *Play:* Ability to laugh, play, and enjoy recreational activities.
10. *Control over one's environment:*
    (a) Political: Ability to effectively participate in the political life, including having the right to free speech and association.
    (b) Material: Ability to own property, not just formally but materially. Furthermore, having the ability to seek employment on an equal basis and the freedom from unwarranted search and seizure.

Nussbaum's list of central human capabilities provides a good starting point for our attempt to identify what capabilities and functionings that are relevant for evaluating the extent to which MDRO control measures excessively interfere with the lives of MDRO carriers. However, when Nussbaum specifies a list of capabilities she is not concerned with the case of MDRO control measures and the well-being of individual carriers of MDRO but rather with setting out a partial theory of justice. For this reason, when adapting Nussbaum's list to the context of MDRO carriership, we still need to ask (a) whether all items on her list are relevant and (b) to what extent they need to be further specified and/or supplemented by additional capabilities.

First of all, while some of the items on Nussbaum's list may also be relevant for the evaluation MDRO control measures other capabilities are clearly not applicable. For example, while the capability for bodily integrity, seems to be of utmost importance for this discussion, the capability for senses, imagination and thought do not seem to be at stake here. The reason for this is not that being able to use one's senses, imagination, or thoughts are not important human characteristics. Rather, the reason that these capabilities are of little importance in the context of MDRO is that it can be argued that there are no control measures that have the potential to restrict one's use of the senses, imagination, and thoughts. Likewise, it is questionable whether the capability for practical reason – one's ability to form a conception of the good and critically reflect on it – would be thwarted or under threat by any conceivable measure we can take to control MDRO. (However, do note that we suggest to subsume (and expand) the capability for education, which is part of the capability for practical reason, under the capability for life as the capability for proper social, physical, and cognitive development.)

This leaves us the following list of capabilities that we can tentatively assume are relevant for the context of MDRO: Life, bodily health, bodily integrity, affiliation (in both senses), other species, play, and control over one's environment (in both senses). Now, we still need to ask whether these seven items are sufficient for our present purpose. This is so in two ways. We need to ask, first, whether these seven capabilities are comprehensive in the sense that we do not need to add additional capabilities and, second, whether they are sufficiently specified to capture what is at stake in the context of MDRO.

In the first case, are the seven capabilities that we retain from Nussbaum's list sufficient to capture all relevant ethical aspects of the context of MDRO? Do we need to add any further capabilities? In order to answer this, let us first distinguish between Nussbaum's *categories* of capabilities and the more *specific* capabilities that are included within the categories. Thus, for example, the category of 'bodily health' includes the more specific capabilities of adequate health, nourishment, shelter, and reproductive health. Though all of these specific capabilities support the more general categorical capability of bodily health, they can neither be reduced to each other nor to the general category. In other words, the more specific capabilities are distinct capabilities in themselves.

Are the seven categories of capabilities sufficient to capture all ethical aspects of MDRO? In general, the categories on Nussbaum's list seem comprehensive. However, it may be helpful to distinguish carriers' mental well-being from Nussbaum's category of bodily health. Many of the MDRO control measures have little impact on one's physical or bodily health. Even decreases in bodily health – for example, the displeasure caused by eradication therapies – are only temporary. The mental impact, however, may be just as profound and long lasting. Being subject to isolation measures, for instance, is known to increase the levels of perceived stress and anxiety and the stigma of having been a carrier can continue long after carriage has ceased. Thus, the mental impact of MDRO control measures can and should be seen independently from their physical impact. Let us therefore add an additional category, namely *mental health*.

How about the more specific capabilities on Nussbaum's list? Does Nussbaum identify all relevant capabilities to adequately capture what is at stake within the seven general categories in relation to the context of MDRO? Given the particular focus of her own list, Nussbaum naturally leaves off many capabilities that are relevant in the context of MDRO. For example, when deciding on how to treat children and adolescents, a major concern is how the control measure affects their physical and mental development. Prolonged isolation of children in certain age groups may cause setbacks in speech or reading that will disadvantage them later in life. Moreover, Nussbaum does not explicitly address concerns related to healthcare, such as access to timely and effective treatment and protection against intrusive and excessive examinations and therapy.

Nor are Nussbaum's capabilities sufficiently specified to the context of MDRO carriership and MDRO control measures. For example, the way Nussbaum defines sovereignty over one's body (a part of bodily integrity) seems overly abstract. In the context of MDRO, what we mean by bodily integrity and sovereignty concerns not being subjected to unnecessary, intrusive, or excessive examinations and eradication therapies. Likewise, since a large issue in relation to MDRO is how it might contribute to the stigmatization of carriers (Rump et al. 2015), we need to include protection from stigmatization along with the protection from discrimination (a part of the capability for affiliation).

Thus, we can also answer the second question that we asked above, namely whether Nussbaum's capabilities are sufficiently and adequately specified to capture the context of MDRO. There are good reasons to argue that Nussbaum's list needs to be further specified and supplemented with additional capabilities when setting out a taxonomy of normatively relevant capabilities and functionings in the context of how MDRO control measures and carriership may affect the lives and well-being of carriers.

In sum, although Nussbaum's list of ten central capabilities provides a useful starting point for identifying the normatively relevant aspects of how MDRO control measures have the potential to impact the lives of individuals, it still needs to be adapted and specified to this particular context. This is so in several ways: first, some capabilities on Nussbaum's list are irrelevant for the case of MDRO; secondly, Nussbaum's list does not distinguish all relevant capabilities, such as mental health; and, thirdly, Nussbaum's capabilities must be specified to the context of MDRO. In the following section, we proceed to present a taxonomy of normatively relevant capabilities and functionings that we need to take into consideration when deciding on and evaluating MDRO control measures.

A Taxonomy of Normatively Relevant Capabilities in the Context of Addressing MDRO Carriership

What does a taxonomy of normatively relevant capabilities and functionings look like in the context of MDRO? How can it help us understand what is at stake when deciding on measures to contain the spread of MDRO? Building on Nussbaum's list of central human capabilities, in this section we present a taxonomy that adapts and specifies Nussbaum's list to the particular context of assessing and evaluating MDRO control measures. The taxonomy supplements Nussbaum's list through an analysis of empirical literature and studies on what practitioners and MDRO carriers express as normatively relevant and divides the relevant capabilities into four ethical domains.

Table 13.1 presents a systematic overview of how MDRO control measures can potentially affect the lives and opportunities of individual carriers. The table is divided into three columns, which, from left to right, moves from four general domains of human life (the personal, the social, the institutional, and the environmental) to the more specific capabilities and functionings that are relevant in the context of MDRO.

On the right-hand side of the table, we find a list of the various capabilities and functionings that are (a) normatively relevant for living a decent or flourishing human life, as revealed by Nussbaum's list of capabilities, and (b) specifically relevant within the context of MDRO, as revealed by our empirical analyses.

In the first case, capabilities such as nourishment, shelter, the right to association, and being treated with dignity and equal worth are relevant for human life regardless of whether it involves MDRO or not. In the second case, there are capabilities that only or primarily come become relevant when combined with MDRO, such as protection against stigmatization and pathologization, protection against unnecessary or intrusive examinations and therapy, and the ability to engage in recreational activities.

Table Ethical domains and normatively relevant capabilities and functionings for the evaluation of the impact of MDRO control measures on (potential) carriers, partly adapted from Nussbaum (2000). Additional items and specifications in **bold**

Domain	Category	Specific capability
Personal	Life	Not having one's life reduced to not worth living **(especially for elderly)**
		Proper social, physical, and cognitive development (especially for children and adolescents)
	Bodily health	Adequate health **(e.g., to fight off infections)**
		Nourishment
		Shelter
		Reproductive health
	Mental health	**Happiness and peace of mind**
		Self-respect **and self-esteem (e.g., being able not to see oneself as sick or as merely a patient)**
		Protection against internalized pathologization
		Future prospects (e.g., of a speedy recovery)
	Bodily integrity	Sovereignty over one's body **(e.g., not being subjected to unnecessary, intrusive, or excessively costly examinations and intensive eradication therapy)**
		Appearance (i.e., being able to appear in public without shame)
		Freedom of choice and opportunity, both in life and in relation to one's body
		Choice in matters of reproduction
		Protection against internalized pathologization
	Play	Ability to enjoy social and recreational activities

(continued)

Table (continued)

Domain		Category		Specific capability
Social and community		Bodily integrity		Protection against assault **(e.g., not being seen as merely a threat), also in the case of relatives of carriers**
		Affiliation	A	Ability to live with others
				Friendship
				Family (incl. reproductive rights)
			B	Being treated with equal dignity and respect
				Social status and prestige
		Play		Ability to **engage and participate in** social and recreational activities
		Control over one's environment A		Right to association
				Ability to form and engage in social relations
Institutional	**(Health) care related**	Bodily health		**Access to adequate (i.e., timely and effective) health care**
		Bodily integrity		Security against assault **in the form of intrusive and excessive examinations and eradication therapy**
		Control over one's environment	A	**Access to just and fair healthcare treatment**
			B	Freedom from unwarranted search and seizure **(e.g., having to pay oneself for excessively expensive examinations)**
		Affiliation	A	Institutions help develop and protect forms of affiliation, **self-respect, and dignity**
			B	Being treated with dignity and equal worth
				Protection from discrimination **and stigmatization**
	Public life	Control over one's environment	A	Ability to effectively participate in political **and public** life (incl. free speech and association)
				Access to just and fair institutions
			B	Ability to seek employment on an equal basis
				Decent working environment (incl. protection against discrimination and abuse)
				Freedom from unwarranted search and seizure **(e.g., having to pay oneself for excessively expensive examinations)**
				Economic security

(continued)

Table (continued)

Domain	Category	Specific capability
Environmental	Bodily integrity	Ability to change locations freely/**freedom of movement (incl. the ability to live where one chooses to)**
	Other species	Ability to live with other animals **(i.e., pets and livestock)**, plants **(incl. crops)**, and the environment at large
	Control over one's environment B	Ability to own property **(e.g., livestock)**

The eight categories of capabilities can, in turn, be relevant within one or more of four domains of human life, identified on the left-hand side of the table: the personal, the social, the institutional, and the environmental. Within the personal domain, MDRO control measures influence the relationship that a carrier has to herself, her own body, and her mental satisfaction. In particular, this includes her bodily health, in the sense of being healthy, well-nourished, and having access to adequate accommodation, her mental health, including being happy, feeling dignified, and being free from stigmatization, and her bodily integrity, most importantly not being subject to excessive and intrusive examinations and eradication therapies.

The social domain concerns individual carriers' relationships to friends and family and the ability to participate in social activities. Human well-being to a large degree depends on well-functioning social relationships, both instrumentally and intrinsically. Not only do we count on friends and family to help us realize certain ends and goals in life; we also attribute intrinsic value to social relationship: we engage in and enjoy social relationships for their own sake and not because they help us fulfill personal goals.

Hence, whenever our social relationships break down it is likely to harm our well-being. Social relationships are especially vulnerable to MDRO and MDRO control measures. Stigmatization and pathologization are social mechanisms by which we respond to perceived threats. In this way, the case of MDRO has a lot in common with the plight of AIDS carriers in the 1980s. However, stigmatization and pathologization are only two ways in which MDRO measures can harm our well-being in a social context. More generally, since we derive pleasure from engaging in social relationships, MDRO measures that restrict the extent to which we can engage in social relations have the potential to lead to a decrease in our well-being.

On the institutional level, we are interested in the carriers' relationship to and standing within institutions, primarily (but not limited to) health care facilities. MDRO is primarily an issue when it comes into contact with a healthcare setting. That is, MDRO is primarily a risk when it comes into contact with already vulnerable individuals who depend on effective antimicrobial treatments for their health and survival. Such individuals are more often found within care facilities, such as hospitals, nursing homes, and rehabilitation centers. Moreover, healthcare settings also provide more fertile breeding grounds for the emergence of multidrug-resistant organism because of the increased exposure to antimicrobials and, hence, the risk that organisms will evolve resistance to these antimicrobials.

Within the environmental domain, we are primarily concerned with carriers' relations with their environments. To what extent, we ask, are carriers able to connect with their environment? Are they able to exercise any control over their environment? We can talk about a person's relationship to their environment in both literal and figurative terms. Literally, we talk about the environment as something that is *there*: a physical presence that we can interact with and influence. In this sense, our relationship with the environment concerns our ability to interact with physical entities such as plants, including flowers, trees, fungi, and so on, as well as animals, including both pets and livestock. In a figurative sense, the environment is a more abstract and indefinite entity. This is so in two ways. First, we can talk about the environment at large, including in the senses of nature and the climate without referring to specific plants or animals. This way of understanding the environment is of little relevance to the context of MDRO. However, secondly, the environment can also be understood as the indefinite but physical space that surrounds us and which we can move around within. In other words, in this sense we understand one's environment as something within which she (can) has control over herself and her choices. Given that two of the primary MDRO control measures – quarantine and isolation – aim to restrict (potential) carriers' ability to move around, this second figurative understanding of the environment is highly relevant to the context of MDRO.

Crucially, a category of capabilities can be specified differently within different domains. For example, the capability for control over one's environment in the context of the social domain concerns one's right and freedom to form social relationships, while in the institutional domain it rather concerns one's institutional status, such as the freedom to participate in political and public life and access to just and fair institutions. Thus, although the different categories of capabilities can be relevant within different domains, the more specific capabilities that they contain depend on the domain.

It is important to stress that the taxonomy here does not make any claims about which capabilities and functionings that cannot be violated by MDRO control measures. Rather, it provides a structural overview of how MDRO control measures may affect the lives and opportunities of individual carriers. We still need to engage in a weighing of the relevant capabilities and functionings in individual cases in order to determine whether they provide overriding normative reasons not to implement a particular control measure. Such weighing would take place on a case-by-case basis because each case includes contextual circumstances that influence what the best course of action would be. Hence, it is not possible to *a priori* determine what control measure (if any) to implement.

However, by offering a taxonomy of relevant domains and capabilities we do make a claim about what is normatively important and relevant when addressing MDRO. First, as argued in Sect. 13.3, MDRO control measures affect carriers in terms of their capability-sets – what they have the real freedom to do or be. Hence, it is claimed that we ought to conceptualize and describe the impact that MDRO control measures have on individual carriers in terms of capabilities and functionings.

Secondly, however incomplete and underspecified, we make a claim about the kinds of capabilities and functionings that are normatively important for (potential) carriers of MDRO and which should be taken into account when deciding on the best course of action. That is, there are good reasons to claim that *these* particular capabilities have the potential to be normatively relevant when dealing with cases of MDRO. There are both normative and empirical reasons for this claim. Normatively speaking, Nussbaum's list of capabilities provides a normative philosophical grounding of the capabilities: these are capabilities that can be subject to an overlapping consensus. Moreover, there is empirical evidence that (some or most of) these capabilities are of relevance to practitioners and carriers when dealing with cases of MDRO in a healthcare setting. The comparison with real-life queries about how to ethically address MDRO – as represented by our database and deliberations with carriers and practitioners[10] – provide empirical basis for the claim that these are the kinds of capabilities that are of concern when deciding on control measures.

How can this taxonomy be implemented in practice to analyze particular cases of MDRO and decide on appropriate control measures? In the final section, we show how our taxonomy can provide an input into ethical decision-making procedures on the appropriate measure to address MDRO carriership.

Applying the Capabilitarian Taxonomy in Practice

We have in the previous section repeatedly argued that the more general categories of capabilities that Nussbaum identifies – life, bodily health, mental health, bodily integrity, play, affiliation, control over one's environment, and other species – can and should be specified to the particular context of how MDRO control measures impact the lives and freedoms of individual carriers. We further argued that we can and should specify these categories of capabilities differently according to whether they relate to either of four domains of human life, namely the personal, the social, the institutional, and the environmental. While the taxonomy that we have presented in Table 13.1 provides an overview of how the different categories of capabilities can be specified in relation to the different domains, how it contributes to the practice of implementing appropriate MDRO control measures is still unclear.

The above taxonomy can provide a useful input to ethical decision-making procedures on the implementation of MDRO control measures, such as the frameworks developed by Verweij et al. (2012; Krom 2014) or Grill and Dawson (2015). How does the capabilitarian framework help us make decisions about how to address MDRO? How can our taxonomy help us make better and more informed decisions about what kinds of MDRO control measures that are preferable, acceptable, or justifiable? In this section, we briefly consider how the capabilitarian taxonomy can be applied in practice to ethical deliberations on MDRO and what issues that are left unaddressed.

[10] See footnote 7.

The capabilitarian taxonomy presented in this chapter is especially useful in two regards. First, it can help professionals better describe cases of MDRO by making explicit what is at stake for the individual carriers and relevant stakeholders. Secondly, it can help us to identify and evaluate possible courses of action by showing how various MDRO control measures may impact the capabilities and functionings of affected carriers and stakeholders. Let us, by way of a case study, briefly show how the taxonomy of normatively relevant capabilities can be put into practice in these two ways.

To illustrate how the capabilitarian taxonomy can be applied in practice, consider, for example, the case of a young, 19-year-old mother with no income or higher education who shares a household with her own mother. The father of her newborn child is unknown or absent and the woman therefore relies on her own mother for economic assistance and care help. However, the grandmother of the child turns out to be MDRO positive and there are concerns that she is a threat to the health of the newborn child. If there is close contact, it is very likely that the grandmother would transmit the resistant organism to the newborn. To make matters worse, the child in case has a heart valve condition and needs to go to the hospital for regular check-ups. Because of the likelihood that the child will become an MDRO carrier if the grandmother is involved in the post-partum care of the child, the hospital insists that the grandmother cannot provide this care or that she should take far-reaching protection measures, such as wearing gowns and masks, that would interfere with the bond between child and grandmother.

How can our taxonomy contribute to the understanding and resolution of this case? What capabilities are at stake in this case? While this case involves a lot of different capabilities within several domains, the primary concern here is the ability to live with others, including family (part 'affiliation A' within the social domain). This capability is restricted not only for the young mother but also for the newborn child as well as the grandmother. However, although we can assume that they value this relationship intrinsically – and hence contributes to the capability of happiness and peace of mind (a part of the capability for 'mental health' within the personal domain) – in this case there are at least two instrumental reasons why this capability is important.

First of all, bonding with relatives may be considered an important part of a child's development (a part of the capability for 'life') and restricting the newborn child's relationship to the grandmother risks harming this development. Secondly, in this case, the social relationship between the young mother and her own mother can also be seen as a proxy for more formal institutional care-relationships. That is, not allowing the grandmother to care for the newborn child is mainly problematic insofar as the mother does not have alternative opportunities for care assistance. Within the taxonomy this is represented by the institutional capabilities for 'bodily health' (access to timely and effective healthcare) and 'affiliation A' (institutions help develop and protect forms of affiliation).

In the described case we have multiple courses of action, which can be employed either independently or in conjunction. How can the capabilitarian taxonomy help us identify and evaluate possible measures? Some of the measures would be directed solely or primarily at the grandmother. First of all, in order to minimize contamination, we could demand that the grandmother undergoes eradication therapy and subsequently attends regular screenings. Secondly, we could demand that the grandmother adhere to a strict hygiene regiment, including the donning of a gown, mask, and gloves when tending to the child. Other measures would be directed at the other stakeholders, in particular the newborn child. For example, thirdly, we could subject the newborn to regular screenings to test for MDRO and, when positive, to eradication therapy.

However, as the case describes, these measures have potentially negative consequences for not only the mother's abilities to engage in social relations and to care for her child, but also the child's well-being, especially in relation to her early childhood development as well as her capability to form an affiliation with her grandmother. From a capability perspective, then, we would do well to look for alternative courses of action that provide better protection of these normatively valuable capabilities.

The analysis of the case from the capability perspective shows that a major issue is that the mother is reliant on *informal care* for her child. Informal care is – usually unpaid – care that is provided by family members or social relations. In contrast, formal care is institutionalized and usually performed by trained professionals. By applying the taxonomy, our analysis shows that the case extends beyond the personal and social domains to reveal a lack of normatively relevant capabilities and functionings at within institutional domain. In the present case, then, a possible solution to the issue could be to increase the access to *formal institutional* healthcare for the young mother and her infant, so that she does not have to rely so much on informal care, thereby avoiding many of the negative consequences that follow from limiting the analysis to focus solely on the informal care-relation between the child, the mother, and the grandmother.[11]

While the proposed course of action in this case might be intuitively clear, in general, a major issue of applying the capabilitarian taxonomy in practice, especially when evaluating the various MDRO control measures, concerns the question of how to weigh different capabilities against each other. That is, we need to ask, when does the reduction of a carrier's capability-set provide an overriding reason to dismiss or provide compensation for a particular control measure? When applying the capabilitarian taxonomy in practice to evaluate different control measures, we should weigh capabilities on at least three levels, namely the intrapersonal, the interpersonal, and the public health level.

The first level at which we need to weight the importance or value of different capabilities against each other when evaluating potential MDRO control measures is at the intrapersonal level. At the intrapersonal level, we ask whether a person is better off within one scenario *as compared to other scenarios*. That is, we can ask, is the person's capability-set more valuable as a result of a particular control

[11] A possible objection, also based on the capabilitarian taxonomy, to the proposed solution is that it would negatively affect the grandmother's capability for affiliation with her grandchild.

measure (or combination of control measures) than it would be if we implement another (combination of) control measure(s)?

At the interpersonal level, second, we are concerned with comparing the capability-sets of different stakeholders *within one particular scenario*. Here we should ask: does a particular control measure diminish the value of the capability sets of one or more of the relevant stakeholders to the extent that it outweighs the positive impact on the value of the capability sets of other relevant stakeholders?[12] Finally, thirdly, we should weigh the positive or negative impact to the value of the capability-sets of individual stakeholders against the estimated benefit to public health that the implementation of a particular MDRO control measure has.

It is beyond the scope of this chapter to consider how such a weighing may be done. Since this decision must eventually be made on a case-by-case basis, it must be a subject for further research to set out normative (or pragmatic) principles for the weighing of capabilities. Such principles might include a threshold level of capabilities and functionings: do we really need to compensate someone for a lost job-opportunity if she already has ample opportunity to find alternative employment? Other principles are principles of proportionality and acceptable risk, that can help us determine when a particular MDRO control measure is (dis)proportionate to the harm, conceptualized in terms of capabilities and functionings, that it does to the individual carrier. In this regard, possible connections could, for example, be made between our capabilitarian taxonomy and the approaches of Viens et al. (2009), who set out a principle of reciprocity, Krom (2011), who discusses the shortcomings of the harm principle in infectious disease control, and Grill and Dawson (2015) who propose a value-based approach.

Moreover, the weighing of capabilities and capability-sets should be done in consultation with the relevant stakeholders in order to identify relevant capabilities and their normative weight. This leaves quite a bit of space for professional autonomy in ethical decision-making. It is simply quite impossible *a priori* to determine the normatively relevant capabilities and their relative, normative weight. In this regard, the taxonomy of normatively relevant capabilities and functionings presented in this chapter should be taken as an open-ended and underspecified basis for further deliberation between the various stakeholders (carriers, relatives, professionals, and possibly policy-makers) on a case-by-case basis. Again, how much room to leave for professional autonomy and how exactly to conduct such deliberative exercises must be subject to further research. We have here proposed two promising frameworks for ethical decision-making, namely Verweij et al. (2012; Krom 2014) or Grill and Dawson (2015).

Finally, it might be objected that, while intuitively attractive, the capabilitarian taxonomy presented in this chapter does not add to professional practice on MDRO. That is, it is not clear that the capability perspective would change what professionals already do when addressing cases of MDRO. This objection holds

[12] Conversely, this could also be framed as: does a particular control measure increase the value of the capability sets of one or more of the relevant stakeholders to the extent that it outweighs the negative impact on the value of the capability sets of other relevant stakeholders?

that one of the supposed advantages of adopting the taxonomy of capabilities, namely its intuitive appeal, at the same time makes the contribution of this chapter trivial. However, even if the taxonomy largely corresponds to existing practice, there are at least four benefits to making the tacit or implicit assumptions of professional practice explicit through the language of the capability approach and the taxonomy that has been presented in this chapter.

First of all, the taxonomy provides a substantive – yet underspecified and open-ended – view of carriers' well-being. Rather than a person's autonomy, generally speaking, we are, on this view, concerned with protecting carriers' normatively relevant or valuable capabilities and functionings. This allows us, secondly, to provide a structured way of discussing how MDRO control measures impact the lives and well-being of carriers, namely by influencing their normatively relevant or valuable doings and beings. In this sense, the proposed taxonomy could serve as a basis for consultation among professionals and with relevant stakeholders. Third, the capability view presents a multi-dimensional view of the impact that MDRO control measures can have. Different individuals might be impacted in different ways by similar control measures and one individual might be affected in many different ways by a particular control measure. Fourth, by conceptualizing the impact of MDRO control measures in terms of people's capabilities and functionings, it possible to see how affecting one aspect of an individual's life may affect other, less immediately obvious, capabilities and functionings.

In sum, the capability framework to MDRO and the accompanying taxonomy of normatively relevant capabilities does contribute to both the literature on the ethical aspects of MDRO as well as, potentially, to real practice of addressing cases of MDRO.

Concluding Remarks

In this chapter, we have presented and discussed a capabilitarian conceptualization of how MDRO control measures can (negatively) impact the lives and well-being of individual MDRO carriers. According to the capability approach, we should measure and evaluate this impact in terms of how MDRO control measures (negatively) influence what they are able to do or be. Building on Nussbaum list of central human capabilities, we introduced a taxonomy of normatively relevant capabilities and functionings in the context of MDRO. This taxonomy proposes that measures to contain the spread of MDRO may potentially affect carriers in one or more of four domains human life, namely the personal, social, institutional, and environmental domains. We identified eight categories of capabilities – life, bodily health, mental health, bodily integrity, affiliation, other species, play, and control over one's environment – that can and should be specified differently within the four domains of human life when applied to the context of analyzing how MDRO control measures impact the lives of individual carriers. An overview of this taxonomy can be found in Table 13.1.

The taxonomy, we finally argued, should be used as an ethical input to a decision-making framework when deciding on the best measures to take when dealing with cases of MDRO. As such, the taxonomy is both underspecified and open-ended: it still needs to be expanded and adapted when applied to particular, individual cases of MDRO. It does not, by itself, determine when the infringement of a particular capability or range of capabilities is unjust and should be supplemented with a notion of when the reduction of a carrier's capability-set provides an overriding reason to dismiss a particular control measure.

References

Alkire, S. 2002. *Valuing Freedoms*. Oxford: Oxford University Press.

Anomaly, J. 2010. Combating resistance: The case for a global antibiotics treaty. *Public Health Ethics* 3: 13–22.

———. 2013. Collective action and individual choice: Rethinking how we regulate narcotics and antibiotics. *Journal of Medical Ethics* 39: 752–756.

Ballon, P. 2013. The selection of functionings and capabilities: A survey of empirical studies. *Partnership for Economic Policy (PEP)*.

Beauchamp, T.L., and J.F. Childress. 2001. *Principles of biomedical ethics*. Oxford: Oxford University Press.

Byskov, M.F. forthcoming. Methods for the selection of capabilities and functionings. In *New frontiers of the capability approach*, ed. F. Comim, S. Fennell, and P.B. Anand. Cambridge: Cambridge University Press.

Carter, I. 2014. Is the capability approach paternalist? *Economics and Philosophy* 30: 75–98.

Coleman, C.H., Organization WH, E. Jaramillo, et al. 2010. *Guidance on ethics of tuberculosis prevention, care and control*. Geneva: World Health Organization.

Crocker, D.A., and I. Robeyns. 2010. Capability and agency. In *Amartya Sen*, ed. C. Morris, 60–90. Cambridge: Cambridge University Press.

Daulaire, N., A. Bang, G. Tomson, et al. 2015. Universal access to effective antibiotics is essential for tackling antibiotic resistance. *The Journal of Law, Medicine & Ethics* 43: 17–21.

Entwistle, V.A., and I.S. Watt. 2013. Treating patients as persons: A capabilities approach to support delivery of person-centered care. *The American Journal of Bioethics* 13: 29–39.

Grill, K., and A. Dawson. 2015. Ethical frameworks in public health decision-making: Defending a value-based and pluralist approach. *Health Care Analysis*: 1–17.

Huber, M., M. van Vliet, M. Giezenberg, et al. 2016. Towards a "patient-centred" operationalisation of the new dynamic concept of health: A mixed methods study. *BMJ Open* 6: 1–11.

Krom, A. 2011. The harm principle as a mid-level principle? Three problems from the context of infectious disease control. *Bioethics* 25: 437–444.

———. 2014. *Not to be sneezed at. On the possibility of justifying infectious disease control by appealing to a mid-level harm principle*. Utrecht University.

Lamont, J., and C. Favor. 2016, Winter. Distributive justice. In *The stanford encyclopedia of philosophy*, ed. E.N. Zalta.

Littmann, J. 2014. *Antimicrobial resistance and distributive justice*. Doctoral, UCL (University College London).

Littmann, J., and A.M. Viens. 2015. The ethical significance of antimicrobial resistance. *Public Health Ethics*: phv025.

Littmann, J., A. Buyx, and O. Cars. 2015. Antibiotic resistance: An ethical challenge. *International Journal of Antimicrobial Agents* 46: 359–361.

Nielsen, L. 2014. Why health matters to justice: A capability theory perspective. *Ethical Theory and Moral Practice*: 1–13.

Nussbaum, M. 1992. Human functioning and social justice: In defence of Aristotelian essentialism. *Polit Theory* 20: 202–246.

———. 2000. *Women and human development. The capabilities approach*. Cambridge: Cambridge University Press.

———. 2011. *Creating capabilities. The human development approach*. Cambridge, MA: Belknap Press of Harvard University Press.

Piaget, J. 1971. The theory of stages in cognitive development. In *Measurement and Piaget*, ix, 283. New York: McGraw-Hill.

Prah Ruger, J. 2010. Health capability: Conceptualization and operationalization. *American Journal of Public Health* 100: 41–49.

Robeyns, I. 2016a, Winter. The capability approach. In *The Stanford Encyclopedia of philosophy*, ed. E.N. Zalta. Metaphysics Research Lab, Stanford University.

———. 2016b. Capabilitarianism. *Journal of Human Development and Capabilities* 17: 397–414.

Rump, B. 2011. Stoppen met de studie geneeskunde omwille van MRSA-dragerschap? *Ethiek Infect 19*.

Rump B., M. De Boer, R. Reis, et al. 2015. *Signs of stigma and poor mental health among carriers of MRSA*.

Rump, B., C. Kessler, E. Fanoy, et al. 2016. Case 2: Exceptions to national MRSA prevention policy for a medical resident with untreatable MRSA colonization. In *Public health ethics: Cases spanning the globe*, ed. D.H. Barrett, L.W. Ortmann, A. Dawson, et al., 191–194. Berlin: Springer.

Selgelid, M.J. 2007. Ethics and drug resistance. *Bioethics* 21: 218–229.

Selgelid, M.J., A.R. McLean, N. Arinaminpathy, and J. Savulescu. 2009. Infectious disease ethics: Limiting liberty in contexts of contagion. *Journal of Bioethical Inquiry* 6: 149–152.

Sen, A. 1979. Equality of what? *Tann Lect Hum Values*: 197–220.

———. 1991. Welfare, preference and freedom. *Journal of Econometrics* 50: 15–29.

Venkatapuram, S. 2011. *Health justice. An argument from the capability approach*. Cambridge: Polity Press.

Verweij, M., and A. Dawson. 2010. Shutting up infected houses: Infectious disease control, past and present. *Public Health Ethics*: 1–3.

Verweij, M., A. Krom, and J. Van Steenbergen. 2012. Ethische kwesties in de infectieziektebestrijding. Rijksinstituut voor Volksgezondheid and Milieu.

Viens, A.M., C.M. Bensimon, and R.E.G. Upshur. 2009. Your liberty or your life: Reciprocity in the use of restrictive measures in contexts of contagion. *Journal of Bioethical Inquiry* 6: 207–217.

WHO. 2014. *Antimicrobial resistance global report on surveillance: 2014 summary*. Geneva: World Health Organization.

9

Epidemiology and Ethics of Antimicrobial Resistance in Animals

Lisa Boden and Dominic Mellor

Abstract Despite a large and rapidly growing volume of research activity and output, primarily on the biological bases of antimicrobial resistance (AMR), epidemiological understanding of the causal mechanisms at play behind the apparent recent global rise in prevalence of AMR has, arguably, progressed very little. Despite this inconvenient fact, political imperative and expedience, among other drivers, have given substantial impetus to an interventionist approach against what are considered to be the culprits for the apparent growing prevalence of AMR and its impacts. Concern about the rise in prevalence of microbial infections that are resistant to therapeutic agents designed to kill them has arisen almost exclusively in relation to human health. (Public awareness and concern about antihelmintic resistance, for which the impacts are much more substantial for animal health, at least in developed temperate countries, are trivial by comparison). Nevertheless, antimicrobial drugs have been, and are, widely used in animal health and production throughout the world, and the contribution of this diverse usage to the 'global AMR problem' has historically been controversial. There is growing acceptance, notwithstanding the limitations in causal understanding noted previously, of AMR as an ecological problem of competing populations of microorganisms experiencing both natural and anthropogenic selection pressures in compartments that transcend species and other boundaries. Typifying what is described as a 'One Health' problem, AMR is therefore considered to be most amenable to conjoint mitigation efforts in all compartments: i.e. interventions in human health, animal health, food and the environment in a coherent manner.

In animals, this calls into question the motivations and practices for antimicrobial drug usage, the majority of which are justified on the basis of promoting animal

L. Boden
Global Academy of Agriculture and Food Security, The Royal (Dick) School of Veterinary Studies and The Roslin Institute, University of Edinburgh, Edinburgh, UK
e-mail: lisa.boden@ed.ac.uk

D. Mellor (✉)
School of Veterinary Medicine, College of Medical, Veterinary and Life Sciences, University of Glasgow, Glasgow, UK
e-mail: dominic.mellor@glasgow.ac.uk

health and welfare and securing a food supply for a growing human population. Not surprisingly, there are great differences in animal husbandry and food demand, and in availability, access and regulation of antimicrobial usage in animals, and in surveillance of AMR, which are likely to be starkest between developed and developing countries. Thus, it is unlikely that the impacts of AMR, and the impacts of efforts to mitigate AMR that are directed to the 'animal compartment' of the ecosystem, will be felt equally across the world.

Keywords AMR · Ethics · One Health · Veterinary · Animal · Causality

Introduction: Evolutionary History of Antimicrobial Resistance as a Natural Phenomenon

Antimicrobial resistance has occurred as a natural phenomenon for millennia, as a response to inhibitory substances produced by microbial populations competing for resources in different ecosystems (Hall and Barlow 2004). Human discovery of the existence of these substances was exploited in the early twentieth century leading to the development of the first antibacterial drugs for therapeutic use. The rapid discovery and development of both natural and synthetic antimicrobial drugs (active against bacteria, fungi, viruses, and protozoa), and their widespread use to treat and prevent human and animal infectious diseases, took place throughout the latter half of the twentieth century. As predicted by Alexander Fleming himself, as therapeutic use of antibiotics grew there closely followed the emergence of untreatable strains of organisms that had hitherto responded to treatment.

Any microorganism that isn't inhibited or killed by appropriate, effective antimicrobials is classified as resistant (Ridge et al. 2011). This phenomenon is now widely explained in terms of a 'selection pressure' being exerted on the populations of microorganisms which are exposed to antimicrobial agents. Such microbial populations are usually comprised of an almost unimaginable number and diversity of individual organisms, amongst which the target 'pathogen' population for antimicrobial therapy may constitute only a fraction of those exposed to the agent. Under these circumstances, those organisms susceptible to the agent are inactivated, and cease to compete for resources, and those that are equipped with mechanism(s) to resist the effects of the agent thrive through access to the resources no longer consumed by the inactivated organisms (Levin et al. 2000). In the case of therapeutic use of antimicrobial agents, if the organisms equipped with mechanism(s) to resist the effects of the agent are members of the 'pathogen' population, the result is likely to be treatment failure and prolonged clinical disease for the patient. If the organisms equipped with mechanism(s) to resist the effects of the agent are members of the non-pathogen population (usually referred to as commensals), the effect is to select for populations that carry resistance mechanisms, but is unlikely to result in treatment failure at that time. Nevertheless, and especially for bacteria, many of the mechanisms to resist the effects of antimicrobial agents are coded for by genes carried on transmissible genetic elements which can be passed between organisms of the same or different species or genera. Thus, selection for resistance in members of the non-pathogen population could subsequently lead to transfer to 'pathogen' populations and increased likelihood of subsequent treatment failure.

Drug Resistance as an Animal or Public Health Concern

Treatment failure and prolonged and/or more serious clinical disease for the patient are probably much more widely recognized consequences of drug resistance in human than in veterinary medicine. In efforts to mitigate these principally public health effects of antimicrobial resistance in the developed world, much attention has been focussed on human healthcare settings, particularly hospitals and care homes (Edwards et al. 2012). Efforts to improve infection prevention and control (IPC) in these settings are paramount, because they are needed not only to reduce the transmission between people of infectious agents likely to require drug therapy, but also the transmission of antimicrobial resistance genes. Principles of IPC form the mainstays of current strategies to combat antimicrobial resistance and are coupled with measures to promote 'better' prescribing of antimicrobial agents through guidelines and audit, and initiatives to educate the healthcare profession and the public. Judicial antimicrobial use (i.e. "better prescribing") is based on evidence which supports using a particular agent against a particular organism in a particular patient for a particular reason and period of time (e.g. British Veterinary Association 2015).

The contribution and nature of veterinary use of antimicrobial agents to the problem of antimicrobial resistance on a global scale has been a controversial issue for many years, with conflicting, polarized views espoused by different respected research groups (Aarestrup et al. 2000; Collignon 2013; Mather et al. 2013; van Bunnik and Woolhouse 2017). Much has been made of the widespread and varied use of antimicrobial agents in veterinary medicine and the potential for this to contribute to the (largely) public health problem posed by antimicrobial resistance. In this, it is noteworthy that, with few exceptions, relatively little is made of treatment failure and prolonged and/or more serious clinical disease for animal patients. The use of the broad term 'antimicrobial' has been unhelpful in this regard as it is inclusive of agents such as anti-coccidials, which are important for animal health and food security, but have no effect on other organisms (such as bacteria or fungi) which drive resistance in humans (Mendelson et al. 2017). Mendelson et al. (2017) argue for more precision in the language around drug-resistant infections, and for more specific terms such as "antibiotic" or "antifungal" to be used in preference to '"antimicrobials" when referring to medicines against a specific type of organism.

There is a growing acceptance that drug-resistant infections are a 'One Health' problem that transcends species (and other) barriers (Karesh et al. 2012). Expanding on this, it is obvious that agents that carry resistance determinants exist very well and evolve outside animal or human hosts. There is increasing recognition of the need to consider environmental reservoirs, and inanimate vehicles of transmission, not least among which are foods of animal origin – home produced and imported – and integrate these into thinking about the ecology and epidemiology of resistance (Wellington et al. 2013). Resistance genes may spread directly from people to animals and from animals to people through food-borne and environmental contamination (via wastewater, soil and the spread of contaminated manure from livestock and wild animals) (Casey et al. 2013; Kim et al. 2013; Davis and Rutkow 2012; Johnson and Becker 2010; Cantas et al. 2013; Roe and Pillai 2003; Soonthornchaikul and Garelick 2009; Levy et al. 1976; Thanner et al. 2016; Literak et al. 2011). However, the relative importance of these routes of transmission is uncertain; exposure is complex and not unequivocally in one direction (Carlet et al. 2011; Mather et al. 2013; Zhu et al. 2013). Additionally, there are other epidemiological pathways (such as transmission of resistance via irrigation and waste-water, plant production and the disposal or presence of disinfectants and heavy metals in the environment) that have been shown to be associated with the emergence of drug resistance. These are not well researched due to the lack of analytical methods to monitor contaminants in waste, surface and drinking water and soil (Thanner et al. 2016). Thus, the epidemiological drivers associated with the selection for and against resistant organisms in animals are unlikely to be different to the causal mechanisms believed to exist in humans or the environment. There are important caveats to this assertion: (1) many parts of the relevant ecosystem are ignored by surveillance approaches adopted to date, notably the environment and food (home produced and imported), (2) it is difficult to partition antibiotic resistance into that which arises naturally from bacterial competition in various ecological niches and that which is selected for anthropogenically through therapeutic or other use of drugs and/or biocides. Of course, the relative intensity of the various selection pressures for the emergence of drug-resistant infections is itself driven in part by broader socio-economic issues (e.g. poverty, sanitation, hygiene and public health resources) which are harder to quantify and even more difficult for governments to address. These caveats arise due to the limitations of the evidence provided by surveillance for drug-resistant infections, which has largely focused on trying to compare observations of antibiotic resistance in bacterial isolates from human patients to those of antibiotic resistance in animal populations (often using different methods of antimicrobial resistance determination) in developed countries.

High rates of drug-resistant infections are found in densely populated, developing countries where there is corruption and unreliable enforcement of laws and regulations pertaining to the practice of human and veterinary medicine (Collignon et al. 2015). Individuals who are exposed to resistant bacteria or fungi in these hotspots through international travel and medical tourism can subsequently import resistance into other countries, resulting in rapid global spread (World Health Assembly Resolution 51.9 1998).

There is still a need to convince some sectors that this is a shared problem with shared accountability and shared responsibility, but that principle is pretty much implicit in nationally and internationally agreed accords (e.g. Department of Health 2013; O'Neill 2016). Based on experience from the UK, plans to implement the recommendations of such accords, whilst all claiming to be taking a 'One Health' approach, can vary even among devolved administrations. In this sense, creation of a bespoke 'One Health' agency, with appropriately balanced multidisciplinary representation (and buy-in and trust), acting in a collegiate manner to coordinate a collective and coherent response seems intuitively more likely to succeed than simply hoping that separate agencies will be able to work in parallel towards a common aim without 'funding the arrows' (Campbell 2006).

In conclusion, considering the epidemiology of drug-resistance in animals in isolation is missing the point.

Antimicrobial Use in Animals

Similar to antimicrobial use in humans, there is substantial variation throughout the world in the availability, regulation, control and administration of antimicrobials to animals. Whilst these factors themselves are not expected to alter the postulated causal mechanisms by which drug use affects drug resistance in microorganisms, they are likely to modify the extent to which these mechanisms have the opportunity to act. Simply put, it appears that greater usage of particular antimicrobial drugs, in a relevant time and place, is positively correlated with greater proportions of isolates tested for susceptibility in that time and place being designated as resistant. Thus, greater control over the quality and supply of antimicrobial drugs and greater regulation and professionalism over their administration should correlate with reduced proportions of resistant isolates.

It is worthy of note that this general observation appears also to be true of anthelmintic drugs, although the ecology of macroparasites is of course different to microbes. However, in the developed world, the problem of anthelmintic resistance is more of an immediate issue for animals than humans, which means that it has received much less attention from a public health point of view. Nevertheless, sophisticated guidance on control of parasitic infestations, based on understanding their ecology, and seeking to preserve the efficacy of anthelmintic drugs, are seen as critical to future food security (e.g. see Sustainable Control of Parasites in Sheep (http://www.scops.org.uk/)).

A range of antimicrobial drugs is used widely to treat disease in domestic animals through a large and internationally varying number of preparations and through a number of different routes of administration. In most developed countries of the world, the classes of antimicrobial drug available for animal administration, and the preparations and routes by which they can be administered, have to be specifically licensed for animal use and are highly regulated, especially for animal species likely to enter the human food chain. In these countries, there are also strictly enforced 'withdrawal periods' which define for how long an animal must be 'off' treatment before products form that animal can be used for human consumption. In some parts of the world, so-called 'off-label' use (i.e. an unlicensed product and/or an unlicensed route of administration) is sometimes permitted under derogation for the treatment of companion animals. Lists of critically important antimicrobials (CIAs) in humans and animals have been agreed, and are periodically updated, by the OIE and WHO and others, and the use of these drugs should be restricted to treating infections that have been demonstrated to be susceptible (and resistant to less important, so-called first-line, drugs) (OIE list of antimicrobials of veterinary importance 2007; WHO list of Critically Important Antimicrobials (CIA) 2017). In developing countries, due to limitations in infrastructure, such regulations, where they exist, are much more difficult to make effective. Coupled with a very high demand due to a high disease burden and often high population densities, and issues such as uncontrolled, unauthorized markets and counterfeit drugs, the conditions appear likely to favour intense selection for antimicrobial resistance and subsequent dissemination, though there are few reliable data to provide firm evidence of this.

Much of the controversy around use of antimicrobials in animals has concentrated on their use as growth promoters. It has been considered that routine addition of some antimicrobial compounds (usually antibacterial drugs and often at sub-therapeutic concentrations) to livestock feed increases food conversion efficiency by more than enough to outweigh the cost of adding the drugs, though this is disputed (Graham et al. 2007). However, other agents, such as anti-coccidials used by the poultry sector, are also included in this broad classification (Mendelson et al. 2017). Use of antibiotic growth promoters is considered by many to be particularly undesirable due to the selection pressure being applied in an almost unrelenting way to the populations of microorganisms colonizing these animals, especially in instances in which drugs are used at sub-therapeutic concentrations, as this is thought to select more strongly for antimicrobial resistance. Much research has sought to investigate the impact of the use of antimicrobials for growth promotion and has been interpreted by most as demonstrating a positive association with increased prevalence of resistant organisms in exposed microbial populations (O'Neill (2015)). On the basis of this evidence, their use as growth promoters has been banned in many parts of the world, notably Europe, yet still persists in others.

In the EU, "the use of agents from classes which are or may be used in human or veterinary medicine (i.e. where there is a risk of selecting for cross-resistance to drugs used to treat bacterial infections)" as growth promoters has not been permitted since 2006 (Regulation (EC) No 1831/2003/EC) and withdrawal periods for antimicrobial use prior to animal slaughter are designed to ensure that there are no antimicrobial residues in food. In the USA, non-therapeutic use is still widespread in industrial farming. The USA FDA has historically been slow to respond to calls to reduce antimicrobial use and unwilling to exert its authority over the antimicrobial approval process (see Natural Resources Defense Council, et al. v. United States Food and Drug Administration, et al.). Until recently, the FDA implemented a voluntary approach to antimicrobial conservation that encouraged drug companies to withdraw approvals for antimicrobials for non-therapeutic use and replace them with approvals for other uses such as chemoprophylaxis (USDA 2012a, b). However, this policy has had little real effect on antimicrobial usage because, in many cases, the doses and durations of drug use for chemoprophylaxis and growth promotion are the same (Outterson 2014).

In emerging economies, such as the BRICS and MINT countries, it is anticipated that non-therapeutic use of antibiotics in animals may exponentially increase because of increasing intensification of agriculture/aquaculture, high prevalences of production and endemic diseases (which are likely to be better controlled in other countries) and lack of resources to ensure appropriate governance over antimicrobial use (Carlet et al. 2011; Van Boeckel 2015). In some of these countries, AMR and antimicrobial conservation aren't on the "political agenda" at all (Grace 2015 at p 11–12) because addressing other issues such as poverty, starvation, malnutrition through (un)sustainable livestock and farmed fish production are more urgent for the current population. The impact of antimicrobial use on accessibility of animal food sources hasn't been quantified for most countries, partly due to the variability and uncertainty regarding the quantities of antimicrobials used even in similarly intensive systems elsewhere (Rushton et al. 2014), and there is no agreement on the desired levels of antimicrobial consumption. Even if an enforced ban on the non-therapeutic use of antimicrobials were to be introduced, in some places, the absence of national R&D investment means that there are few alternative mechanisms (such as vaccines) to concurrently improve animal husbandry and avoid production losses which could paradoxically increase AMR prevalence through off-label or unprescribed use of poor quality or counterfeit antimicrobials. The relative costs of not using antimicrobials on the security of the global food supply and the success of the Sustainable Development Goals (in eradicating poverty and hunger in the current generation) have not been compared to AMR treatment failure in people (in future generations). Although developed countries arguably have sufficient means to assist developing countries address some of these issues, they have so far focussed on their own national priorities in order to achieve wider international societal benefits (Clift 2013).

Distinction is made in veterinary medicine (at least in the developed world) between prophylactic (administering antimicrobial drugs to prevent anticipated infection) and metaphylactic use of antimicrobials (administering antimicrobial drugs to clinically well members of a population in contact with an index case of infectious disease to prevent anticipated infection), which is not recognized in human medicine. Prophylaxis in veterinary medicine is criticized by many as an excuse for poor infection prevention and control (often referred to as 'biosecurity' in animal production) in a particular animal husbandry system, but presents ethical dilemmas to veterinarians who struggle with the notion of withholding treatment in the face of what is considered to be almost inevitable disease and associated welfare compromise. In many instances, the clinical use of antimicrobials in animals is empirical and sensitivity testing of an isolate of the putative causative agent of infection is not carried out. The reasons for this are largely to do with cost and expediency in starting treatment to improve the clinical condition of the patient. Thus, data that characterize the resistance profiles of clinical isolates from animals represent a very small proportion of the putative infections treated by veterinarians, and their use for epidemiological purposes often appears to overlook this fact. However, this is also true of human medicine.

The notion that antimicrobial resistant organisms somehow 'arise' in animals, driven by selection pressures applied by veterinary use of antimicrobials, and pass to humans, principally through the food chain, has been a popular model of antimicrobial resistance 'acquisition' for some time. However, some recent research shows that transmission is likely to occur in both directions between animals and people directly and indirectly through the environment and various fomites (Mather et al. 2013). As discussed in the introduction, it is probably more reasonable to think of animals and people as inextricably linked 'samplers' of a shared environmental pool of organisms subject to different selection pressures in different compartments.

Surveillance for Antimicrobial Resistance in Animals

'Better' surveillance for antimicrobial resistance in animals is a more or less universal feature of international concordats, calls to action and other declarations on antimicrobial resistance (Department of Health 2013; O'Neill 2016). As the bedrock of epidemiology, surveillance activity, and the intelligence generated by it, offers the greatest potential to understand fully the causal relationships at play within the complex landscape ecology underlying the antimicrobial resistance 'phenomenon' (Singer et al. 2006). Nevertheless, there are a great many limitations, often overlooked, that can apply to data derived from surveillance of infections in animals (and people) for the purposes of exploring causal relationships of relevance to the emergence and spread of antimicrobial resistance. Chief among these is the question of how well the isolate(s) derived from the sample(s) collected from the individual(s) and/or their environment(s) under study represent the actual nature and dynamics of the interactions between host and microbial populations and the selection pressures experienced by them. Confounding this, in many instances, is a lack of standardization of the microbiological methods applied and inconsistent definitions of how antimicrobial sensitivity or lack of it is defined for individual drug/bug combinations derived from different species (animals and humans).

The World Health Organization (WHO) has led international efforts to develop action plans to monitor and reduce drug-resistant infections (WHO Strategy 2001). However, without a legally-binding mandate, it has been difficult implement this strategy within Member States. Indeed, between 1998 and 2015 (when the WHO first published its global action plan), there have been at least seven World Health Assembly (WHA) Resolutions promoting surveillance of drug-resistant infections, but still no internationally coordinated or standardized AMR surveillance strategy within either the human or veterinary sectors. Although collaboration between the WHO, Food and Agricultural Organization of the United Nations (FAO) and World Organization of Animal Health (OIE) is improving coordination between human and animal surveillance, within individual Member States the two sectors remain distinct and regulated independently of one another. Surveillance, if undertaken at all, has hitherto been implemented separately by each sector, without harmonization or standardization of approach.

Existing national action plans within Member States describe broad strategic aims to mitigate, and reduce current rates of drug-resistant infections and resultant treatment failures. These include: improvements in infection prevention and control, education and training initiatives, optimization of prescribing practices (particularly in animals with respect to critically important antimicrobials) and incentives to innovate new, effective therapies. For the most part, these aims have not been translated yet into specific actions with explicit timescales for delivery or agreed outcome metrics. In some countries, technical and financial constraints, such as lack of existing public health infrastructure, access to diagnostic technologies and changing public attitudes towards public health mean that surveillance is poor (STAG-AMR 2013; WHO 2011). Accurate inferences (and/or between-country comparisons) about antibiotic or antifungal consumption rates aren't always possible because of the scarcity and variability of available information on consumption, species treated, routes of administration, dose rate, and pharmaceutical costs (Rushton et al. 2014 at p 11). Other important differences, such as husbandry practices, diversity of available drugs and prescribing habits of veterinarians, mean that comparisons of antimicrobial use based on animal demographics are potentially misleading. For example, Chile is the second largest producer of farmed salmon and the only important developing country producer. However, it uses around 300 times more antibiotics than the largest salmon producer, Norway because Norway has the resources to access and implement vaccination and alternative husbandry measures instead of antimicrobials to control diseases (Grace 2015 at page 11). Thus, it is currently not possible to accurately chart progress towards AMR reduction or identify early-warning performance indicators for actions that aren't effective in achieving these aims.

Despite these limitations, surveillance and research data generated, principally in the developed world, are subject to ever more sophisticated epidemiological analyses to infer risk factors and causal relationships for resistance emergence, persistence and spread. Entrenched in this aim is the notion that population patterns of drug-resistant infections can be explained by a complex web of multiple interconnected factors, which if identified, can be used to inform and target interventions to improve public health (Krieger 1994). Increasingly, these analyses seek to be comparative and inferential about the impacts of antimicrobial use in one species (animals or man) on antimicrobial resistance in the other, as the 'One Health' construct of drug resistance becomes more widely accepted. However, caution is required in the interpretation of these findings. 'Causal webs' are not unbiased; they are necessarily hierarchical, focusing "attention on risk factors closest to the outcome under inspection", inevitably prioritizing biological factors (amenable to medical or veterinary intervention) over other broader social or environmental determinants which could be addressed through social action (Krieger 1994; Thanner et al. 2016). For example, addressing a lack of access to education, sanitation and adequate healthcare (including infection prevention and control, scarcity of new antibiotics, poor prescribing practices and absence of concurrent diagnostic tools to ensure appropriate treatment) will affect rates of disease, which will influence subsequent amounts of antimicrobial used (Buckland Merrett 2013). Reduction of antimicrobial use may reduce selection pressure for resistance, but at the same reduces the numbers of antimicrobial 'customers' and thus incentives to innovate new drugs. Equally, economic strategies that are driven by sales rewards will inevitably conflict with principles of conservation and IPC. Understanding of the epidemiology of AMR (and this broader socio-economic and ecological 'web of causation') and an appreciation for the gaps in communication and coordination between stakeholders and regulators involved across multiple sectors and disciplines at each of these foci is therefore necessary to ensure policy decisions are robust and ethical.

Summary and Conclusion

The epidemiology of antimicrobial resistance in animals seems very unlikely to be extricable or distinct from that in people. A powerful epidemiological model of the causation and dissemination of antimicrobial resistance as a feature of microbiological ecology among a very complex web of interconnected host and environmental compartments has emerged and gained widespread acceptance under the construct of 'One Health'. However, the limitations in the quality of the data that have been used to build this model leave room for uncertainty about its validity. In addition, there needs to be 'thinking time and space' to consider and account for cognitive biases in such models and to incorporate socio-economic modifiers of such biological models in order to inform efficient and effective measured interventions. As rapidly developing scientific advances offer the potential to improve the quality (e.g. WGS) and representativeness (e.g. through properly and purposively designed comparative surveillance programmes) of data, it is to be hoped that epidemiological inference will be able to keep pace and offer better, and what yet may be surprising, insights into the problem of antimicrobial resistance and ways in which it might be tackled.

References

Aarestrup, F.M., Y. Agerso, P. Gerner-Schmidt, M. Madsen, and L.B. Jense. 2000. Comparison of antimicrobial resistance phenotypes and resistance genes in *Enterococcus faecalis* and *Enterococcus faecium* from humans in the community, broilers and pigs in Denmark. *Diagnostic Microbiology and Infectious Disease* 27: 127–137.

British Veterinary Association. 2015. *Responsible use of antimicrobials in veterinary practice*. Available from: https://www.bva.co.uk/uploadedFiles/Content/News,_campaigns_and_policies/Policies/Medicines/responsible-use-of-antimicrobials-in-veterinary-practice.pdf.

Buckland Merrett, G.L. 2013. *Tackling antibiotic resistance for greater global health security*. Centre on Global Health Security. Available from: http://www.chathamhouse.org/sites/files/chathamhouse/public/Research/Global%20Health/1013bp_antibioticresistance.pdf.

Campbell, A. 2006. *The Australian natural resource management knowledge system*. Available from: http://lwa.gov.au/products/pr061081.

Cantas, L., S.Q.A. Shah, L.M. Cavaco, C.M. Manaia, F. Walsh, M. Popowska, H. Garelick, H. Bürgmann, and H. Sørum. 2013. A brief multi-disciplinary review on antimicrobial resistance in medicine and its linkage to the global environmental microbiota. *Frontiers in Microbiology* 4: 96. https://doi.org/10.3389/fmicb.2013.00096.

Carlet, J., P. Collignon, D. Goldmann, H. Goossens, Gyssens ICJ, S. Harbarth, V. Jarlier, S.B. Levy, B. N'Doye, D. Pittet, R. Richtmann, W.H. Seto, J.W.M. van der Meer, and A. Voss. 2011. Society's failure to protect A precious resource: Antibiotics. *The Lancet* 378 (9788): 369–371.

Casey, J.A., F.C. Curriero, F.C. Cosgrove, K.E. Nachman, and B.S. Schwartz. 2013. High-density livestock operations, crop field application of manure, and risk of community-associated methicillin-resistant Staphylococcus Aureus infection. *Journal of the American Medical Association of Internal Medicine* 173 (21): 1980–1990. https://doi.org/10.1001/jamainternmed.2013.10408.

Clift, C. 2013. The UK's new antimicrobial resistance strategy. Available at https://www.chathamhouse.org/media/comment/clift/amr (last accessed 31 July 2015).

Collignon, P. 2013. Superbugs in food: A severe public health concern. *The Lancet Infectious Disease* 13 (8): 641–643.

Collignon, P., A. Prema-chandra, S. Senanayake, and F. Khan. 2015. Antimicrobial resistance: The major contribution of poor governance and corruption to this growing problem. *PLoS One* 10 (3): e0116746. https://doi.org/10.1371/journal.pone.0116746.

Davis, M.F., and L. Rutkow. 2012. Regulatory strategies to combat antimicrobial resistance of animal origin: Recommendations for a science-based US approach. *Tulane Environmental Law Journal* 25: 327–387.

Department of Health. 2013. *UK five year antimicrobial resistance strategy 2013 to 2018*. Available from: https://www.gov.uk/government/uploads/system/uploads/attachment_data/file/244058/20130902_UK_5_year_AMR_strategy.pdf.

Edwards, R., E. Charani, N. Sevdalis, B. Alexandrou, E. Sibley, D. Mullett, H.P. Loveday, L.N. Drumright, and A. Holmes. 2012. Optimisation of infection prevention and control in acute health care by use of behaviour change: A systematic review. *Lancet Infectious Diseases* 12: 318–329. https://doi.org/10.1016/S1473-3099(11)70283-3.

Grace, D. 2015. *Review of evidence on antimicrobial resistance and animal agriculture in developing countries*. ILRI Available from: http://www.evidenceondemand.info/review-of-evidence-on-antimicrobial-resistance-and-animal-agriculture-in-developing-countries.

Graham, J.P., J.J. Boland, and E. Silbergeld. 2007. Growth promoting antibiotics in food animal production: An economic analysis. *Public Health Reports* 122: 79–87.

Hall, B.G., and M. Barlow. 2004. Evolution of the serine beta-lactamases: Past, present and future. *Drug Resistance Updates* 7: 111–123. https://doi.org/10.1016/j.drup.2004.02.003.

Johnson, R., and G. Becker. 2010. *US-Russia meat and poultry trade issues*. Washington, DC: Congressional Research Service for Congress. Available from: http://nationalaglawcenter.org/wp-content/uploads/assets/crs/RS22948.pdf.

Karesh, W.B., A. Dobson, J.O. Lloyd-Smith, J. Lubroth, M.A. Dixon, M. Bennett, S. Aldrich, T. Harrington, P. Formenty, E.H. Loh, C.C. Machalaba, M.J. Thomas, and D.L. Heymann. 2012. Ecology of zoonoses: Natural and unnatural histories. *The Lancet* 380: 1936–1945.

Kim, B.F., L.I. Laestadius, R.S. Lawrence, R.P. Martin, S.E. Mckenzie, K.E. Nachman, T.J.S. Smith, and P. Truant. (2013). *Industrial food animal production in America: Examining the impact of the Pew Commission's Priority Recommendations*. John's Hopkins Centre for a Liveable Future. Available at http://www.jhsph.edu/research/centers-and-institutes/johns-hopkins-center-for-a-livable-future/_pdf/research/clf_reports/CLF-PEW-for%20Web.pdf.

Krieger, N. 1994. Epidemiology and the web of causation: Has anyone seen the spider? *Social Science Medicine* 39 (7): 887–903.

Levin, B.R., V. Perrot, and N. Walker. 2000. Compensatory mutations, antibiotic resistance and population genetics of adaptive evolution in bacteria. *Genetics* 154: 985–997.

Levy, S.B., G.B. FitzGerald, and A.B. Macone. 1976. Changes in intestinal flora of farm personnel after introduction of a tetracycline-supplemented feed on a farm. *New England Journal of Medicine* 295: 583–588. https://doi.org/10.1056/NEJM197609092951103.

Literak, I., R. Petro, M. Dolejska, E. Gruberova, H. Dobiasova, J. Petr, et al. 2011. Antimicrobial resistance in fecal *Escherichia coli* isolates from healthy urban children of two age groups in relation to their antibiotic therapy. *Antimicrobial Agents and Chemotherapy* 55: 3005–3007. https://doi.org/10.1128/AAC.01724-10.

Mather, A.E., S.W.J. Reid, D.J. Maskell, J. Parkhill, M.C. Fookes, S.R. Harris, D.J. Brown, J.E. Coia, M.R. Mulvey, M.W. Gilmour, L. Petrovska, E. de Pinna, M. Kuroda, M. Akiba, H. Izumiya, T.R. Connor, M.A. Suchard, P. Lemey, D.J. Mellor, D.T. Haydon, and N.R. Thomson. 2013. Distinguishable epidemics of multidrug-resistant Salmonella Typhimurium DT104 in different hosts. *Science* 341: 1514–1517. https://doi.org/10.1126/science.1240578.

Mendelson, M., M. Balasegaram, T. Jinks, C. Pulcini, and T. Sharland. 2017. Antibiotic resistance has a language problem. *Nature* 545 (7652): 23–25.

Natural Resources Defense Council. et al. 2012a. v. United States Food and Drug Administration, et al. 884 F.Supp.2d 127 (S.D.N.Y.).

Natural Resources Defense Council. et al. 2012b. v. United States Food and Drug Administration, 872 F.Supp.2d 318 (S.D.N.Y.).

O'Neill, J. 2015. *Antimicrobials in agriculture and the environment: Reducing unnecessary use and waste*. Available from: https://amr-review.org/sites/default/files/160525_Final%20paper_with%20cover.pdf.

———. 2016. *Tackling drug-resistant infections globally: Final report and recommendations*. Available from: https://amr-review.org/sites/default/files/160525_Final%20paper_with%20cover.pdf.

OIE list of antimicrobials of veterinary importance. 2007. Available from: https://www.oie.int/fileadmin/Home/eng/Our_scientific_expertise/docs/pdf/AMR/A_OIE_List_antimicrobials_July2019.pdf

Outterson, K. 2014. *New business models for sustainable antibiotics*. Centre on global health security working group papers 1–31. Available from: http://www.chathamhouse.org/sites/files/chathamhouse/public/Research/Global%20Health/0214SustainableAntibiotics.pdf.

Regulation (EC) No 1831/2003/EC Of The European Parliament and of the Council of 22 September 2003 On additives for use in animal nutrition, replacing directive 70/524/EEC on additives in feeding-stuffs. 2003. Official Journal of the European Union L 268: 0029–0043.

Ridge, K.W., K. Hand, M. Sharland, I. Abubakar, and D.M. Livermore. 2011. Antimicrobial resistance. In *The annual report of the chief medical officer volume 2, Infections and the rise of antimicrobial resistance*. Available at https://www.gov.uk/government/uploads/system/uploads/attachment_data/file/138331/CMO_Annual_Report_Volume_2_2011.pdf

Roe, M.T., and S.D. Pillai. 2003. Monitoring and identifying antibiotic resistance mechanisms in bacteria. *Poultry Science* 82: 622–626.

Rushton, J., J. Pinto Ferreira, and K.D. Stärk. 2014. *Antimicrobial resistance: The use of antimicrobials in the livestock sector*, OECD Food, Agriculture and Fisheries Papers No. 68. Paris: OECD Publishing. https://doi.org/10.1787/5jxvl3dwk3f0-en.

Singer, R.S., M.P. Ward, and G. Maldonado. 2006. Can landscape ecology untangle the complexity of antimicrobial resistance? *Nature Reviews Microbiology* 4: 943–952.

Soonthornchaikul, N., and H. Garelick. 2009. Antimicrobial resistance of campylobacter species isolated from edible bivalve molluscs purchased from Bangkok markets, Thailand. *Foodborne Pathogens and Disease* 6: 947–951. https://doi.org/10.1089/fpd.2008.0236.

Strategic and Technical Advisory Group on Antimicrobial Resistance (STAG-AMR). Report of the first meeting Geneva, 19–20 September 2013. Available from: http://www.who.int/drugresistance/stag/amr_stag_meetingreport0913.pdf.

Sustainable Control of Parasites in Sheep. Available from: http://www.scops.org.uk/.

Thanner, S., D. Drissner, and F. Walsh. 2016. Antimicrobial resistance in agriculture. *MBio* 7 (2): e02227–e02215. https://doi.org/10.1128/mBio.02227-15.

Van Boeckel, T.P. 2015. Global Trends In Antimicrobial Use In Food Animals. *Proceedings of the National Academy of Science* 112 (18): 649–5654. https://doi.org/10.1073/pnas.1503141112.

van Bunnik, B.A.D., and M.E.J. Woolhouse. 2017. Modelling the impact of curtailing antibiotic usage in food animals on antibiotic resistance in humans. *Royal Society Open Science* 4: 161067. https://doi.org/10.1098/rsos.161067.

Wellington, E.M.H., A.B.A. Boxall, P. Cross, E.J. Feil, W.H. Gaze, P.M. Hawkey, A.S. Johnson-Rollings, D.L. Jones, N.M. Lee, W. Otten, C.M. Thomas, and A.P. Williams. 2013. The role of the natural environment in the emergence of antibiotic resistance in Gram-negative bacteria. *Lancet Infectious Diseases* 13: 155–165.

World Health Assembly Resolution 51.9. 1998. Emerging and other communicable diseases: Antimicrobial resistance. In *51st world health assembly*. Available from: http://apps.who.int/medicinedocs/index/assoc/s16335e/s16335e.pdf?ua=1.

World Health Organisation. 2001. *WHO global strategy for containment of antimicrobial resistance*. Available from: http://www.who.int/drugresistance/WHO_Global_Strategy_English.pdf.

———. 2011. *Tackling antibiotic resistance from a food safety perspective in Europe*. Available from: http://www.euro.who.int/__data/assets/pdf_file/0005/136454/e94889.pdf at page 9.

World Health Organisation List of Critically Important Antimicrobials (CIA). 2017. Available from: https://www.who.int/foodsafety/publications/antimicrobials-sixth/en/

Zhu, Y.-G., T.A. Johnson, J.-Q. Su, M. Qiao, G.-X. Guo, R.D. Stedtfield, S.A. Hashsham, and J.M. Tiedje. 2013. Diverse and abundant antibiotic resistance genes in Chinese swine farms. *Proceedings of the National Academy of Science* 110 (9): 3435–3440.

10

Antimicrobial Resistance and the Private Sector in Southeast Asia

Marco Liverani, Lauren Oliveira Hashiguchi, Mishal Khan, and Richard Coker

Abstract Southeast Asia is considered a regional hotspot for the emergence and spread of antimicrobial resistance (AMR). A commonality across countries in the region, particularly those with lower incomes such as Cambodia, Myanmar, Lao PDR and Vietnam, is the high utilisation of private healthcare providers, often unregulated, which may play a role in driving AMR. In this chapter we discuss challenges to the control of AMR in Southeast Asia, with a focus on the role of the private sector. After providing an overview of the problem and current policy responses, we consider ethical issues of equity and fairness that may arise from the implementation of established and proposed interventions.

Keywords Drug resistance · Ethics · Medicine & Pubic Health · Private sector · Southeast Asia.

M. Liverani (✉)
Department of Global Health and Development, London School of Hygiene and Tropical Medicine, London, UK

Faculty of Public Health, Mahidol University, Bangkok, Thailand

School of Tropical Medicine and Global Health, Nagasaki University, Nagasaki, Japan
e-mail: Marco.Liverani@lshtm.ac.uk

L. Oliveira Hashiguchi
Department of Global Health and Development, London School of Hygiene and Tropical Medicine, London, UK

School of Tropical Medicine and Global Health, Nagasaki University, Nagasaki, Japan
e-mail: Lauren.Hashiguchi@lshtm.ac.uk

M. Khan · R. Coker
Department of Global Health and Development, London School of Hygiene and Tropical Medicine, London, UK

Faculty of Public Health, Mahidol University, Bangkok, Thailand
e-mail: Mishal.Khan@lshtm.ac.uk; richard.coker@lshtm.ac.uk

Diversity, Epidemiology and Surveillance Capacity

Southeast Asia is a loosely defined geographic region, whose configuration is variable and depends on different political, institutional, and cultural perspectives. For the purpose of this chapter, we refer to Southeast Asia as the ten member countries of the Association of Southeast Asian Nations (ASEAN), that is, Brunei, Cambodia, Indonesia, Lao PDR, Malaysia, Myanmar, the Philippines, Singapore, Thailand, and Vietnam. As such, this region includes small, wealthy countries such as Singapore (5.6 million population, US$ 52,960 per capita) and populous, lower middle-income countries such as Indonesia (261.2 million population, 3570 US per capita) (The World Bank 2017). It is also characterised by socio-cultural differences and vast diversity in ecosystems including farming, natural habitats, and urbanisation. Although gaps remain in our understanding of AMR in Southeast Asia, available evidence indicates that this is an important and growing challenge (Cherau et al. 2017). For example, studies have identified a high prevalence of antimicrobial resistant infections in hospitalized paediatric populations in several regional countries (Al-Taiar et al. 2013; Stoesser et al. 2013; Turner et al. 2016). The Asian Network for Surveillance of Resistant Pathogens (ANSORP) reported rates of pneumococcal resistance to penicillin exceeding 50% in some contexts (Song et al. 1999) and that resistance had spread across the region. Resistance to enteric pathogens is becoming increasingly prominent (Coker et al. 2017), with studies in Thailand and Cambodia identifying high *Campylobacter coli* and *Campylobacter jejuni* rates of resistance to ciprofloxacin among isolate samples from children hospitalized with acute diarrhoea (Bodhidatta et al. 2002; Meng et al. 2011). In terms of respiratory infections, the World Health Organization (WHO) 2016 Global Tuberculosis Report lists Myanmar, Indonesia, Thailand, Philippines, and Vietnam among the 27 countries bearing the highest burden of multidrug resistant tuberculosis in the world (WHO 2015). Drug-resistant malaria is also prevalent across the region, including resistance of the malaria parasite *P. falciparum* to chloroquine, sulfadoxine–pyrimethamine, and most recently, and of considerable concern, artemisinin (WHO 2017). It is well documented that Western Cambodia, near the border with Thailand, has been an epicentre of antimalarial resistance since the 1950s (Dondorp et al. 2010; Alam et al. 2011; Vinayak et al. 2010). Despite much documentation of resistance throughout the region (Ashley et al. 2014; Imwong et al. 2017), the full epidemiological profile of resistance to antimalarials in Southeast Asia, as with AMR more broadly, is not known.

Fragmented surveillance systems and weak laboratory capacity remain major barriers to acquiring quality surveillance data and information for AMR in the region, especially in LMICs (Lee and Wakabayashi 2013). These barriers were echoed in the findings of the Joint External Evaluation (JEE) (WHO 2016), a WHO-led process to assess country capacity to prevent, detect, and respond to public health threats. In Southeast Asia, JEEs have been conducted in Lao PDR, Vietnam, and Cambodia. Vietnam and Cambodia, the only countries with public JEE reports at present (Joint External Evaluation of the IHR Core Capacities of the Kingdom of

Table Joint external evaluation scoring for AMR Technical Area Indicator, Cambodia and Vietnam (Joint External Evaluation Tool and Process Overview 2016; Joint External Evaluation of the IHR Core Capacities of the Kingdom of Cambodia 2017; Joint External Evaluation of IHR Core Capacities of Viet Nam 2017)

	AMR detection	Surveillance of infections caused by AMR pathogens	Healthcare associated infection prevention and control programs	Antimicrobial stewardship activities
Cambodia	3	2	2	2
	Developed capacity	Limited capacity	Limited capacity	Limited capacity
Vietnam	2	2	3	2
	Limited capacity	Limited capacity	Developed capacity	Limited capacity

Cambodia 2017; Joint External Evaluation of IHR Core Capacities of Viet Nam 2017), reported limited capacity for surveillance of infections caused by AMR pathogens and advocated improved stewardship to prevent inappropriate use of antimicrobials (Table 5.1) (see also Chap. 23 in this book).

Private Health Services and AMR

The private sector is the dominant health care provider in many countries in the region. For example, about 70% of Cambodian patients first seek treatment from the private sector and private drug sellers are the preferred healthcare providers for the majority of those who are ill (NIS Cambodia 2014). Across the region, out-of-pocket payment is a common method to finance health care, despite good progress toward universal health coverage in Thailand, Malaysia, Singapore, and Indonesia (Van Minh et al. 2014). Out-of-pocket health expenditure as a percentage of total health expenditure is more than 50% in Cambodia, Singapore, the Philippines, and Myanmar (Table 5.2) (The World Bank 2017). A study including data from 47 countries indicated that out-of-pocket health expenditure was strongly correlated with AMR in low-income countries, with the authors concluding that high demand for the private sector may be related to higher AMR owing to heightened incentives among private providers to overprescribe and less standardized quality assurance of antimicrobials (Alsan et al. 2015).

Prior to discussing the role of private providers in AMR, it is important to briefly describe the diversity of the private health sector in Southeast Asia and reasons for its popularity. Broadly, private providers include persons operating outside of the government-financed system, alone or in groups, to provide diagnosis, treatment or advice to individuals for health-related concerns. In Southeast Asia, as in other regions, the private sector includes a variety of providers, ranging from large private hospitals, small clinics and pharmacies to road-side informal drug vendors and traditional healers (Khan 2016). The level of training varies greatly. Some private

Table Health sector expenditure indicators in ASEAN (The World Bank 2017)

	Population (thousands), 2016	GDP (billions) 2016	Health expenditure as proportion of the GDP, 2014	Public health expenditure as % of total health expenditure, 2014	Out-of-pocket health expenditure as % of total expenditure on health, 2014
Brunei	423,196	11.4	2.7%	93.9%	6.0%
Cambodia	15,762,370	20.0	5.6%	22.0%	95.2%
Indonesia	261,115,456	932.3	2.9%	37.8%	46.9%
Lao PDR	6,758,353	15.9	1.9%	50.5%	38.9%
Malaysia	31,187,265	296.4	4.1%	55.2%	35.3%
Myanmar	52,885,223	67.4	2.3%	45.9%	50.7%
Philippines	103,320,222	304.9	4.7%	32.3%	53.7%
Singapore	5,607,283	297.0	4.9%	41.7%	54.8%
Thailand	68,863,514	406.8	4.1%	77.8%	11.9%
Vietnam	92,701,100	202.6	7.1%	54.1%	36.8%

practitioners have no training or claim to have qualifications that they do not have, while others have several years of specialist training. In addition to allopathic healthcare providers, there are alternative therapeutic approaches, which include homeopathy and traditional healing. Private providers also vary in terms of the fees charged. Some are highly priced and accessible only to a fraction of the population while others are more accessible and may offer flexible payment arrangements.

Why do patients use the private sector? A recent systematic review comparing the performance of private and public health-care systems in LMICs found that patients' preferences for private providers were related to shorter waiting times, better hospitality, increased time spent with doctors, cleanliness of facilities, longer and flexible opening times, personal attitude, and better availability of staff (Basu et al. 2012). However, quality of care in terms of competence and adherence to guidelines is often low (Morgan et al. 2017).

In terms of AMR specifically, over-prescribing or over-selling of antimicrobial drugs by for-profit healthcare providers appears to be fairly common, although inappropriate prescribing practices have also been reported in public hospitals and health centres (Apisarnthanarak et al. 2008; Om et al. 2017; Yeung et al. 2011). A large study of over 400 healthcare providers including drug shops, private clinics and hospitals in Vietnam found that 79% would dispense antibiotics for common colds with fever and only 19% had knowledge of antibiotic prescribing according to national guidelines (Hoa et al. 2009). Drug sellers were more likely to dispense antibiotics inappropriately than other types of healthcare providers in this study. Other studies in the region have shown that, among drugs sold, antimicrobials are very common as they are reported to be the most profit-generating (Gollogly 2002; Chuc and Tomson 1999).

Drug quality is also a problem in the region. There is evidence from Cambodia, particularly on antimalarial drugs (Novotny et al. 2016), and from neighbouring countries such as Vietnam, that unregulated drug shops often sell poor-quality medications. According to the WHO, substandard drugs are products whose composition and ingredients do not meet the correct scientific specifications (WHO 2003). This could be due to inappropriate storage at high temperature and humidity or poor quality assurance during the manufacturing process. Both of these conditions are more likely to occur in less-developed countries. Counterfeit drugs are considered a subset of substandard drugs that are deliberately and fraudulently mislabelled with respect to identity and/or source. Antibiotics and antimalarials are at particular risk of targeting by counterfeiters and drug manufacturers that use poor practices owing to large volumes of sales, their relatively low production cost, and the challenges met by regulatory mechanisms and their enforcement. In 2013, a multi-governmental investigation across Cambodia, Indonesia, Lao PDR, Myanmar, Thailand, and Vietnam found that nearly one third of both antimalarials and antibiotics were of poor quality and potentially counterfeited (Weraphong et al. 2013). Similarly, a 2004 cross-sectional survey of pharmacies and drug shops in Myanmar found an "alarming high proportion" of counterfeit artesunate (Dondorp et al. 2004), although a recent survey provides encouraging evidence that the quality of artemisinin-based combination therapies has improved (Yeung et al. 2015).

As noted earlier, this chapter focuses on the use of antimicrobials in human health. But the use in animals is also important, and is a major contributor to AMR globally (Nhung et al. 2015), as further discussed in Chaps. 7 and 18. Subtherapeutic use of antibiotics in livestock for growth promotion or prophylaxis is of particular concern, as the low doses used can lead to the emergence of drug resistance (Van Boeckel et al. 2015). While there are regulations around the use of growth promoters in Europe and America, the use of antibiotics by unregulated veterinarians and drug sellers in Southeast Asia is poorly understood. Multiple studies in the region do, however, indicate a high prevalence of confirmed resistance to ciprofloxacin, and gentamicin, and of particular concern, colistin among *E. coli* isolates in pig and chicken farms (Nhung et al. 2015, 2016; Nguyen et al. 2015, 2016). Colistin is one of the last line of drugs available for treating multidrug resistant Gram-negative pathogens in humans.

Policy Challenges in Tackling AMR

Most governments in Southeast Asia have recognised the dangers of AMR and taken action to control the use of antimicrobials through policy making, legal provisions, and program implementation. Legal frameworks to regulate the pharmaceutical supply chain have been improved in many countries, providing stronger legal bases to counter the problem of substandard medicines and poor management practices (Lamy and Liverani 2015). Operational capacities of drug regulatory authorities have also increased, leading to more effective quality control, closure of unlicensed businesses and a crackdown of the trade in counterfeit medicines, with major enforcement operations being conducted throughout the Mekong region (Interpol 2015). Further, new laws have been introduced to regulate drug sellers, particularly for antimalarial medications, although provisions are variable across regional countries. In Thailand, for example, the sale of antimalarial medications in the private sector is banned since 1995, but in other countries regulations are less stringent. In Myanmar, there is no prohibition, while in Lao PDR, the ban applies only to grocery stores, general retailers and itinerant vendors (Akulayi et al. 2017).

Despite increasing commitment, the control of AMR remains a major policy challenge in Southeast Asia, particularly in relation to the sale and use of antibiotics. In Thailand, for example, pharmacists can dispense antibiotics without prescription, leaving more room to profit-motivated sale (Apisarnthanarak et al. 2008; Saengcharoen and Lerkiatbundit 2010). In 2007, the "Antibiotic Smart Use" programme was piloted in community health centres and hospitals to reduce unnecessary prescription of antibiotics for respiratory infections, diarrhoea, and simple wounds. Based on promotional material and performance-based incentives, this programme was subsequently scaled up nationwide and described as a workable model to improve the rational use of antibiotics in Thailand (Akulayi et al. 2017). However, efforts to engage private pharmacies have been less effective (Chalker et al. 2005). In other countries, such as Vietnam and Indonesia, regulations on prescribing and dispensing of antibiotics are more restrictive, but enforcement has been difficult to achieve due to either lack of resources, weak sanctions, or challenges in monitoring compliance in highly diversified markets (Nga et al. 2014; Widayati et al. 2011; Mao et al. 2015). Antimicrobial use is particularly difficult to control in remote rural areas, where access to public health services is more limited, patients tend to self-medicate, and medicines of dubious origin are more likely to be available in road stalls and other informal outlets (Lon et al. 2006; Hadi et al. 2010; Om et al. 2017).

In general, AMR is a complex, multi-dimensional health issue which requires a comprehensive multi-sector policy approach, able to tackle structural drivers and determinants across human and animal health sectors. However, policy development and program implementation have often targeted particular diseases, especially in LMICs where donors have prioritised vertical health programmes. In Cambodia, for example, innovative social marketing schemes have been introduced to improve access to good-quality antimalarials in the private sector and control of pharmaceutical drivers of drug resistance, such as the use of artemisinin monotherapies (Yeung et al. 2011; Yamey et al. 2012). As in other countries, however, no comprehensive policy response to promote the responsible use of medicines has been developed to date. Professional development, supervision, and behaviour change activities are driven by vertical disease programmes as well as the systems for the collection, analysis, and dissemination of surveillance data on antimicrobial resistance. Engagement with the agricultural sector has also been relatively weak in many countries, with gaps in legal provisions and operational capacities to regulate and monitor antibiotic use for animal health prophylaxis and growth promotion (Archawakulathep et al. 2014). Further challenges result from the diversity of the livestock sector in Southeast Asia. While supervision is more feasible in large production units, there is less or no control of antibiotic use in smallholders and contracted farmers (Om and McLaws 2016).

In recognition of these challenges and the need for a more comprehensive policy approach, action plans on AMR have been adopted in Cambodia, Indonesia, the Philippines, Thailand, and Vietnam, while the Lao PDR, Malaysia and Singapore are currently developing their national plans (Cheng 2016). In line with WHO global guidelines (WHO 2015), these plans have been informed by One Health approaches and a commitment to strengthening cooperative arrangements across sectors and national authorities. To this end, inter-ministerial and inter-agency committees have been established to guide policy implementation and monitor progress. Since these plans have been adopted only recently, it is too early to assess outcomes and their value in promoting more effective responses to AMR. However, it is expected that the achievement of the stated policy and governance goals will require a significant increase in resource allocation, which may be challenging to achieve in LMICs. Further, as in other contexts, the divisive forces of institutional mandates and professional interests are likely to counteract the imperative of multi-sectoral cooperation, requiring political will at the highest level of policymaking. Finally, as we will see below, achieving a good balance between *access* to antimicrobials, as well as other vital resources for human and animal health, and curbing inappropriate use and *excess* is arguably one the most important challenges ahead (Das and Horton 2017), posing key ethical questions about policy choices in the short and the long term.

Ethical Issues

The challenges to controlling the emergence of AMR in Southeast Asia are multi-sectoral and complex, requiring policies that can address the diverse range of contributing factors, including behaviour and practices, gaps in health service provision and regulations, and macro- and micro-economic drivers in the antimicrobial supply chain and market at the national, regional, and global level. In the process, particular attention should be given to the private health sector and food production systems, as these are arguably the largest channels for the distribution, sale, and use of a wide range of antimicrobials in many regional countries. Yet policy and planning in this area is problematic. In addition to governance challenges noted above, policy options to control AMR in the private sector raise ethical issues of equity and fairness, which have been recognised only recently in research and policy communities (Heyman et al. 2014; Littmann and Viens 2015). While a reduction of antibiotics use is necessary to avert the potentially disastrous impact of future drug-resistant pandemics, a single focus on this policy goal may result in undesirable consequences in the short term, particularly in relation to equitable access to essential goods and services, as we discuss below.

Access to Health Services Informal providers account for a significant fraction of diagnosis and treatment services in parts of Southeast Asia, raising concerns about the quality of care and their role in driving AMR. Efforts are being made in some countries to ban unlicensed practitioners. However, "village doctors" and other informal providers may be the only accessible source of primary care in some areas, particularly in remote rural communities where public health facilities are hard to reach and other options are not available. In such contexts, regulatory enforcement may be necessary to control potentially harmful practices and key drivers of AMR, but may also reduce access to care where it is needed most. Engagement with the informal sector, including training and supervision programmes, might be a solution to this problem. Yet informal providers have weak legitimacy in relation to the formal health system. The implicit recognition of unqualified providers as legitimate health workers might be challenging if conducted or sanctioned by government agencies and is likely to face strong opposition from established professional categories. On the other hand, informal providers may be reluctant to participate in projects with public health authorities for fear of being exposed (Khan et al. 2015).

Access to Medicines Policy and regulations on prescription and dispensing of antimicrobials raise similar concerns (see also Chap. 24 in this book). Since 1998, the WHO has urged Member States to "prohibit the dispensing of antimicrobials without the prescription of a qualified health care professional" and to strengthen legislation "to prevent the sale of antibiotics on the informal market" (WHO 1998). In many countries, however, the government health system or other authorised suppliers might not be able to reach all population groups or gaps may exist in their ability to meet the demand for antimicrobials. In Cambodia and Lao PDR, for example, health volunteers have been appointed in remote communities to diagnose suspected malaria cases by using rapid diagnostic tests, administer subsidised artemisinin-based combination therapy (ACT), and refer severe patients to the nearest public health facility (Liverani et al. 2017; Alum et al. 2017). These programmes have been successful in improving adherence to malaria policy and treatment where other health services are either lacking or inadequate. However, informal drug outlets and grocery stores remain the only accessible and affordable suppliers of medicines in some areas or for some hard-to-reach groups such as mobile and migrant workers. In addition, stronger quality control and higher standards are likely to increase the cost of medicines, making them less affordable to the poor. While subsidization of particular categories of antimicrobials, such as anti-malarial and anti-tuberculosis treatments, has been implemented with good results (Novotny et al. 2016; Hill and Mao 2007), this approach might not be feasible for mass-market drugs such as antibiotics.

Access to Food As noted earlier, evidence indicates that the use of antibiotics in the livestock sector is an important driver of AMR (Witte 1998). Thus, it is suggested that this practice should be reduced or banned outright. However, it is also known that regulatory restrictions may have significant economic effects on farmers, as the use of antibiotics allows larger numbers of healthy animals to be maintained with lower cost to the producer (National Research Council 1999). Further, the effects of restrictions or bans are likely to be unequally distributed across livestock production systems. While large companies and production units may replace antibiotics with other disease prevention practices and veterinary services, smallholders may not be able to do so, bearing higher cost of regulatory change. Finally, more stringent regulations raise concerns of fairness and equity in access to food. Low and sub-therapeutic use of antibiotics contributes to growth promotion and improved feed efficiency, resulting in lower costs of meat and eggs (National Research Council 1999). While the effect of reduced antibiotics use on the price of meat products is difficult to gauge with precision, organic foods are generally more expensive and therefore less affordable to lower income groups (Chander et al. 2011). As Littman (Littmann and Viens 2015) pointed out, "these considerations do not appear to weigh heavily enough to justify the continuation of current practices"; however, we should recognise, "who will be disadvantaged by proposed policy changes, and discuss what kind of subsidy or compensation may be warranted".

Conclusion

In conclusion, AMR is a complex problem that extends far beyond the technical challenge of reducing or improving the use of antimicrobials, as interventions are likely to have externalities on other important issues for human well-being and livelihood. Thus, in Southeast Asia as in other contexts, policy and planning in this area, and modelling and pilot exercises that provide evidence, will need to incorporate a wide range of issues and a calculation of costs and benefits to individuals, enterprises, and across the whole of society. This will likely require us to find a difficult balance between the urgent need to address the rising challenge of AMR while addressing the moral obligations to broad public health benefits and limiting economic hardship. And all of this within complex social and political environments. Simple solutions are likely to induce undesirable, and perhaps unforeseen, consequences.

References

Alum, A., A. Andrada, J. Archer, E. Auko, K. Bates, P. Bouanchaud, et al. 2017. The malaria testing and treatment landscape in the southern Lao People's Democratic Republic (PDR). *Malaria Journal* 16 (1): 169.

Akulayi, L., A. Alum, A. Andrada, J. Archer, E. D. Arogundade, E. Auko, et al. 2017. Private sector opportunities and threats to achieving malaria elimination in the Greater Mekong Subregion: Results from malaria outlet surveys in Cambodia, the Lao PDR, Myanmar, and Thailand. *Malaria Journal* 16: 180.

Alam, M.T., S. Vinayak, K. Congpuong, C. Wongsrichanalai, W. Satimai, L. Slutsker, et al. 2011. Tracking origins and spread of sulfadoxine-resistant Plasmodium falciparum dhps alleles in Thailand. *Antimicrobial Agents and Chemotherapy* 55 (1): 155–164.

Alsan, M., L. Schoemaker, K. Eggleston, N. Kammili, P. Kolli, and J. Bhattacharya. 2015. Out-of-pocket health expenditures and antimicrobial resistance in low- and middle-income countries. *The Lancet Infectious Diseases* 15 (10): 1203–1210.

Al-Taiar A, M.S. Hammoud, L. Cuiqing, J.K.F. Lee, K.-M. Lui, N. Nakwan, et al. 2013. Neonatal infections in China, Malaysia, Hong Kong and Thailand. *Archives of Disease in Childhood – Fetal and Neonatal Edition* 98 (3): F249–F255.

Anomaly, Jonathan. this volume. Antibiotics and animal agriculture: The need for global collective action. In *Ethics and drug resistance: Collective responsibility for Global Public Health*, 299–310. Cham: Springer.

Apisarnthanarak, A., J. Tunpornchai, K. Tanawitt, and L.M. Mundy. 2008. Nonjudicious dispensing of antibiotics by drug stores in Pratumthani, Thailand. *Infection Control and Hospital Epidemiology* 29 (6): 572–575.

Archawakulathep, A., C.T. Thi Kim, D. Meunsene, D. Handijatno, H.A. Hassim, H.R.G. Rovira, et al. 2014. Perspectives on antimicrobial resistance in livestock and livestock products in ASEAN countries. *Thai Journal of Veterinary Medicine* 44: 5–13.

Ashley, E.A., M. Dhorda, R.M. Fairhurst, C. Amaratunga, P. Lim, S. Suon, et al. 2014. Spread of artemisinin resistance in Plasmodium falciparum malaria. *The New England Journal of Medicine* 371 (5): 411–423.

Basu, S., J. Andrews, S. Kishore, R. Panjabi, and D. Stuckler. 2012. Comparative performance of private and public healthcare systems in low- and middle-income countries: A systematic review. *PLoS Medicine* 9 (6): e1001244.

Boden, Lisa and Dominic Mellor. this volume. Epidemiology and ethics of antimicrobial resistance in animals. In Ethics and drug resistance: *Collective responsibility for Global Public Health*, 109–121. Cham: Springer.

Bodhidatta, L., N. Vithayasai, B. Eimpokalarp, C. Pitarangsi, O. Serichantalergs, and D.W. Isenbarger. 2002. Bacterial enteric pathogens in children with acute dysentery in Thailand: Increasing importance of quinolone-resistant Campylobacter. *The Southeast Asian Journal of Tropical Medicine and Public Health* 33 (4): 752–757.

Chalker, J., S. Ratanawijitrasin, N.T.K. Chuc, M. Petzold, and G. Tomson. 2005. Effectiveness of a multi-component intervention on dispensing practices at private pharmacies in Vietnam and Thailand – A randomized controlled trial. *Social Science and Medicine* 60: 131–141.

Chander, M., B. Subrahmanyeswari, R. Mukherjee, and S. Kumar. 2011. Organic livestock production: An emerging opportunity with new challenges for producers in tropical countries. *Revue Scientifique et Technique* (International Office of Epizootics) 30 (3): 969–983.

Cheng, L. 2016. *State of play of antimicrobial resistance research and surveillance in Southeast Asia*. Bonn, Germany: SEA-EU-NET II. Available from: https://sea-eu.net/object/document/274/attach/20161201_State_of_Play_on_AMR_Research__Surveillance_-_FINAL.pdf[Accessed May 2020]

Chereau, F., L. Opatowski, M. Tourdjman, and S. Vong. 2017. Risk assessment for antibiotic resistance in South East Asia. *BMJ* 358: j3393. https://doi.org/10.1136/bmj.j3393

Chuc, N.T., and G. Tomson. 1999. "Doi moi" and private pharmacies: A case study on dispensing and financial issues in Hanoi, Vietnam. *European Journal of Clinical Pharmacology* 55 (4): 325–332.

Coker, R.J., B.M. Hunter, J.W. Rudge, M. Liverani, and P. Hanvoravongchai. 2017. Emerging infectious diseases in southeast Asia: Regional challenges to control. *Lancet* 377 (9765): 599–609.

Das, P., and R. Horton. 2017. Antibiotics: Achieving the balance between access and excess. *Lancet* 387 (10014): 102–104.

Dondorp, A.M., P.N. Newton, M. Mayxay, W. Van Damme, F.M. Smithuis, S. Yeung, et al. 2004. Fake antimalarials in Southeast Asia are a major impediment to malaria control: Multinational cross-sectional survey on the prevalence of fake antimalarials. *Tropical Medicine & International Health* 9 (12): 1241–1246.

Dondorp, A.M., S. Yeung, L. White, C. Nguon, N.P.J. Day, D. Socheat, et al. 2010. Artemisinin resistance: Current status and scenarios for containment. *Nature Reviews in Microbiology* 8 (4): 272–280.

Gollogly, L. 2002. The dilemmas of aid: Cambodia 1992–2002. *Lancet* 360 (9335): 793–798.

Hadi, U., P. van den Broek, E.P. Kolopaking, N. Zairina, W. Gardjito, I.C. Gyssens, et al. 2010. Cross-sectional study of availability and pharmaceutical quality of antibiotics requested with or without prescription (over the counter) in Surabaya, Indonesia. *BMC Infectious Diseases* 10: 203.

Heyman, G., O. Cars, M.-T. Bejarano, and S. Peterson. 2014. Access, excess, and ethics – Towards a sustainable distribution model for antibiotics. *Upsala Journal of Medical Sciences* 119 (2): 134–141.

Hill, P.S., and T.E. Mao. 2007. Resistance and renewal: Health sector reform and Cambodia's national tuberculosis programme. *Bulletin of the World Health Organization* 85: 631–636.

Hoa, N.Q., M. Larson, N.T. Kim Chuc, B. Eriksson, N.V. Trung, and C.L. Stalsby. 2009. Antibiotics and paediatric acute respiratory infections in rural Vietnam: Health-care providers' knowledge, practical competence and reported practice. *Tropical Medicine & International Health* 14 (5): 546–555.

Imwong, M., K. Suwannasin, C. Kunasol, K. Sutawong, M. Mayxay, H. Rekol, et al. 2017. The spread of artemisinin-resistant Plasmodium falciparum in the Greater Mekong subregion: A molecular epidemiology observational study. *The Lancet Infectious Diseases* 17 (5): 491–497.

Interpol. 2015. Falsified and illicit medicines worth USD 7 million seized across Asia in INTERPOL-led operation. Available from: https://www.interpol.int/en/News-and-Events/News/2015/Falsified-and-illicit-medicines-worth-USD-7-million-seized-across-Asia-in-INTERPOL-led-operation [Accessed May 2020].

WHO. 2017a. Joint External Evaluation of IHR Core Capacities of Viet Nam. Geneva: World Health Organization.

WHO. 2017b. Joint External Evaluation of the IHR Core Capacities of the Kingdom of Cambodia. Geneva: World Health Organization.

WHO. 2016. Joint External Evaluation Tool and Process Overview. Geneva: World Health Organization.

Khan, M. 2016. *Health markets and antibiotics: Unlikely places you can buy them.* Health Policy and Planning Debated Blog, London School of Hygiene and Tropical Medicine. Available from: http://blogs.lshtm.ac.uk/hppdebated/2016/11/29/health-markets-and-antibiotics/#respond [Accessed May 2020].

Khan, M.S., S. Salve, and J.D.H. Porter. 2015. Engaging for-profit providers in TB control: Lessons learnt from initiatives in South Asia. *Health Policy and Planning* 30 (10): 1289–1295.

Lamy, M., and M. Liverani. 2015. Tackling substandard and falsified medicines in the Mekong: National responses and regional prospects. *Asia & the Pacific Policy Studies* 2 (2): 245–254.

Lee, Y., and M. Wakabayashi. 2013. Key informant interview on antimicrobial resistance (AMR) in some countries in the western pacific region. *Global Health* 9: 34.

Littmann, J., and A.M. Viens. 2015. The ethical significance of antimicrobial resistance. *Public Health Ethics* 8 (3): 209–224.

Liverani, M., C. Nguon, R. Sok, D. Kim, P. Nou, S. Nguon, et al. 2017. Improving access to health care amongst vulnerable populations: A qualitative study of village malaria workers in Kampot, Cambodia. *BMC Health Services Research* 17 (1): 335.

Lon, C.T., R. Tsuyuoka, S. Phanouvong, N. Nivanna, D. Socheat, C. Sokhan, et al. 2006. Counterfeit and substandard antimalarial drugs in Cambodia. *Transactions of the Royal Society of Tropical Medicine and Hygiene* 100 (11): 1019–1024.

Mao, W., H. Vu, Z. Xie, W. Chen, and S. Tang. 2015. Systematic review on irrational use of medicines in China and Vietnam. *PLoS ONE* 10: e0117710.

Meng, C.Y., B.L. Smith, L. Bodhidatta, S.A. Richard, K. Vansith, B. Thy, et al. 2011. Etiology of diarrhea in young children and patterns of antibiotic resistance in Cambodia. *The Pediatric Infectious Disease Journal* 30 (4): 331-335.

Morgan, R., T. Ensor, and H. Waters. 2017. Performance of private sector health care: Implications for universal health coverage. *Lancet* 388 (10044): 606–612.

NIS Cambodia. 2014. Cambodia Demographic and Health Survey 2014. Phnom Penh, Cambodia: National Institute of Statistics.

National Research Council. 1999. *The use of drugs in food animals: Benefits and risks.* Washington, DC: The National Academies Press.

Nga, D.T.T., N.T.K. Chuc, N.P. Hoa, N.Q. Hoa, N.T.T. Nguyen, H.T. Loan, et al. 2014. Antibiotic sales in rural and urban pharmacies in northern Vietnam: an observational study. *BMC Pharmacology and Toxicology* 15 (1): 6.

Nguyen, V.T., J.J. Carrique-Mas, T.H. Ngo, H.M. Ho, T.T. Ha, J.I. Campbell, et al. 2015. Prevalence and risk factors for carriage of antimicrobial-resistant Escherichia coli on household and small-scale chicken farms in the Mekong Delta of Vietnam. *The Journal of Antimicrobial Chemotherapy* 70 (7): 2144–2152.

Nguyen, N.T., H.M. Nguyen, C.V. Nguyen, T.V. Nguyen, M.T. Nguyen, H.Q. Thai, et al. 2016. Use of colistin and other critical antimicrobials on pig and chicken farms in Southern Vietnam and its association with resistance in commensal Escherichia coli bacteria. *Applied and Environmental Microbiology* 82 (13): 3727–3735. http://www.ncbi.nlm.nih.gov/pmc/articles/PMC4907207/

Nhung, N.T., N.V. Cuong, J. Campbell, N.T. Hoa, J.E. Bryant, V.N.T. Truc, et al. 2015. High levels of antimicrobial resistance among Escherichia coli isolates from livestock farms and synanthropic rats and shrews in the Mekong Delta of Vietnam. *Applied and Environmental Microbiology* [Internet] 81 (3): 812–820.

Nhung, N.T., N.V. Cuong, G. Thwaites, J. Carrique-Mas. 2016. Antimicrobial usage and antimicrobial resistance in animal production in Southeast Asia: A review. *Antibiotics* 5 (4). pii: E37.

Novotny, J., A. Singh, L. Dysoley, S. Sovannaroth, and H. Rekol. 2016. Evidence of successful malaria case management policy implementation in Cambodia: Results from national ACTwatch outlet surveys. *Malaria Journal* 15 (1): 194.

Om, C., and M.-L. McLaws. 2016. Antibiotics: Practice and opinions of Cambodian commercial farmers, animal feed retailers and veterinarians. *Antimicrobial Resistance and Infection Control* 5: 42.

Om, C., F. Daily, E. Vlieghe, J.C. Mclaughlin, M.-L. Mclaws. 2017. Pervasive antibiotic misuse in the Cambodian community: antibiotic-seeking behaviour with unrestricted access. *Antimicrobial Resistance and Infection Control* [Internet] 6: 30. Available from: https://doi.org/10.1186/s13756-017-0187-y

Saengcharoen, W., and S. Lerkiatbundit. 2010. Practice and attitudes regarding the management of childhood diarrhoea among pharmacies in Thailand. *The International Journal of Pharmacy Practice* 18 (6): 323–331.

Song, J.-H., N.Y. Lee, S. Ichiyama, R. Yoshida, Y. Hirakata, W. Fu, et al. 1999. Spread of drug-resistant Streptococcus pneumoniae in Asian Countries: Asian Network for Surveillance of Resistant Pathogens (ANSORP) study. *Clinical Infectious Diseases* 28 (6): 1206–1211.

Stoesser, N., C.E. Moore, J.M. Pocock, K.P. An, K. Emary, M. Carter, et al. 2013. Pediatric bloodstream infections in Cambodia, 2007 to 2011. *The Pediatric Infectious Disease Journal* 32 (7): e272–e276.

The World Bank. 2017. *World Bank Data Bank* Available from: http://data.worldbank.org.

Turner, P., S. Pol, S. Soeng, P. Sar, L. Neou, P. Chea, et al. 2016 Aug. High prevalence of antimicrobial-resistant gram-negative colonization in hospitalized Cambodian infants. *The Pediatric Infectious Disease Journal* 35 (8): 856–861.

Van Boeckel, T.P., C. Brower, M. Gilbert, B.T. Grenfell, S.A. Levin, T.P. Robinson, et al. 2015. Global trends in antimicrobial use in food animals. *Proceedings of the National Academy of Sciences of the United States of America* 16: 1–6.

Van Minh, H., N.S. Pocock, N. Chaiyakunapruk, C. Chhorvann, H.A. Duc, P. Hanvoravongchai, et al. 2014. Progress toward universal health coverage in ASEAN. *Global Health Action* 7. https://doi.org/10.3402/gha.v7.25856.

Vinayak, S., M.T. Alam, T. Mixson-Hayden, A.M. McCollum, R. Sem, N.K. Shah, et al. 2010. Origin and evolution of sulfadoxine resistant Plasmodium falciparum. *PLOS Patho*gens 6 (3):e 1000830.

Weraphong, J., S. Pannarunothai, T. Luxananun, N. Junsri, and S. Deesawatsripetch. 2013. Catastrophic health expenditure in an urban city: Seven years after universal coverage policy in Thailand. *The Southeast Asian Journal of Tropical Medicine and Public Health* 44 (1): 124–136.

WHO. 2015. *Use of high burden countries for TB by WHO in the post-2015 era*. Geneva, Switzerland: World Health Organization.

Widayati, A., S. Suryawati, C. de Crespigny, and J.E. Hiller. 2011. Knowledge and beliefs about antibiotics among people in Yogyakarta City Indonesia: A cross sectional population-based survey. *BMC Research Notes* 4 (1): 491.

Witte, W. 1998. Medical consequences of antibiotic use in agriculture. *Science* 279: 996–997.

WHO 1998. *Emerging and other communicable diseases: Antimicrobial resistance*. World Health Assembly (WHA5117). Geneva, Switzerland: World Health Organization.

———. 2003. *Fact sheet 275: Substandard and counterfeit medicines*. Geneva: World Health Organization.

———. 2015. *Global action plan on antimicrobial resistance*. WHO Press, 1–28. Geneva, Switzerland: World Health Organization. Available from: http://www.who.int/drugresistance/global_action_plan/en/ [Accessed May 2020].

———. 2017. *Global database on antimalarial drug efficacy and resistance*. Geneva, Switzerland: World Health Organization.

Yamey, G., D. Montagu, and M. Schäferhoff. 2012. Piloting the affordable medicines facility-malaria: What will success look like? *Bulletin of the World Health Organization* 90 (6): 452–460.

Yeung, S., E. Patouillard, H. Allen, and D. Socheat. 2011. Socially-marketed rapid diagnostic tests and ACT in the private sector: Ten years of experience in Cambodia. *Malaria Journal* 10 (1): 243.

Yeung, S., H.L.S. Lawford, P. Tabernero, C. Nguon, A. van Wyk, N. Malik, et al. 2015. Quality of antimalarials at the epicenter of antimalarial drug resistance: Results from an overt and mystery client survey in Cambodia. *The American Journal of Tropical Medicine and Hygiene* 92 (Suppl 6): 39–50.

11

Access to Effective Diagnosis and Treatment for Drug-Resistant Tuberculosis: Deepening the Human Rights-Based Approach

Remmy Shawa, Fons Coomans, Helen Cox, and Leslie London

Abstract The lack of access to effective diagnosis and treatment for drug-resistant tuberculosis (DR-TB) remains a persistent ethical, human rights and public health challenge globally. In addressing this challenge, arguments based on a Human Rights-Based Approach (HRBA) to health have most often been focused on the Right to Health. However, a key challenge in multidrug-resistant (MDR-) and extensively drug-resistant (XDR-) TB is the glaring absence of scientific research; ranging from basic science and drug discovery through to implementation science once new tools have been developed. Although the Right to Enjoy the Benefits of Scientific Progress and its Applications (REBSP) is a little theorised human right, it has the potential to enrich our understanding and use of the Rights-Based Approach to health. In this chapter, we argue that States' duties to *respect, protect* and *fulfil* the REBSP within and outside their borders is an important vehicle that can be drawn on to redress the lack of research into new drug development and appropriate use of existing drugs for DR-TB in high burden settings. We call for urgent attention to minimum core obligations for the REBSP and the need for a General Comment by a UN human rights monitoring body to provide for its interpretation. We also note that conceptualization of the REBSP has the potential to complement Right to Health claims intended to enhance access to treatment for DR-TB on a global scale.

R. Shawa (✉)
School of Public Health and Family Medicine, University of Cape Town, Cape Town, South Africa

F. Coomans
Department of International and European Law, Maastricht University, Maastricht, The Netherlands

H. Cox
Division of Medical Microbiology and Institute of Infectious Disease and Molecular Medicine, University of Cape Town, Cape Town, South Africa

L. London
Division of Public Health Medicine, University of Cape Town, Cape Town, South Africa

Keywords Drug resistance · Human rights · Tuberculosis · Scientific progress · Rights-based approach

Introduction

In this chapter we explore how the Right to Enjoy the Benefits of Scientific Progress and its Applications (REBSP), a little theorized human right found in both the Universal Declaration of Human Rights (UDHR) and the International Covenant on Economic, Social and Cultural Rights (ICESCR), can deepen our understanding of a Human Rights Based Approach (HRBA) to health, taking access to effective treatment for drug-resistant tuberculosis (DR-TB) as an example. We bring attention to the slow progress in research, development and implementation of new and repurposing of existing drugs for treating DR-TB. Further, we attempt to frame poor access to effective diagnosis and treatment as a human rights problem, not only with respect to the right to health, but also with respect to the REBSP. In locating DR-TB within this right, we articulate what we mean by scientific progress, or lack of, in DR-TB, and discuss the broad context in which scientific progress must occur. Finally, we highlight some of the challenges in the conceptualization and realization of the REBSP, and make recommendations calling for urgent attention to minimum core obligations for the right and the need for a General Comment by a UN human rights monitoring body to provide for its interpretation.

Tuberculosis remains the world's deadliest communicable disease, responsible for more than 1.6 million deaths in 2017 alone (WHO 2018). More than a century after the bacterium causing TB was first identified, it continues to kill millions of people because diagnostic tools remain poor and current life-saving, essential medicines require a minimum of 6 months to effect cure. TB is particularly difficult to both diagnose and treat when TB bacteria have become resistant to available drugs. While standard care for drug-sensitive TB requires 6 months of treatment, DR-TB treatment may take up to 2 years. Access to diagnostic tools for DR-TB remains limited with currently available technology, despite some progress such as the GeneXpert MTB/RIF (a relatively rapid test that can, in some cases, quickly diagnose TB and some types of resistance) (Evans 2011), for which accessibility is limited due to the slow pace of implementation and high costs. In 2016, only 25% of the estimated number of multidrug-resistant (MDR-) or rifampicin-resistant (RR-) TB patients emerging that year were diagnosed, and even fewer started on treatment(WHO 2017). Of those who received treatment, only 54% of MDR/RR-TB patients are successfully treated and only 26% of those treated for extensively drug-resistant (XDR-) TB were successfully treated(WHO 2017). Current treatments for RR-TB (which includes MDR- and XDR-TB) are long, and have debilitating and often severe side effects, including irreversible hearing loss in more than a third of patients (Seddon et al. 2012). Other drugs included in the currently recommended

MDR/RR-TB regimen have been known to cause renal failure, cardiac arrhythmias, and psychiatric disturbances (Skrahina et al. 2016).

As much as DR-TB is a public health problem, it is also a human rights problem because it compromises the rights and dignity of the individuals who get infected. DR-TB highlights the glaring divide that exists between high-income countries (HICs) and low-middle income countries (LMICs), as well as the divide between the rich and the poor within countries. The majority of those who get TB and DR-TB reside in LMICs (WHO 2016). In HICs, TB and DR-TB are predominantly among the vulnerable and marginalized such as migrants and refugees (Figueroa-Munoz and Ramon-Pardo 2008). This skewed burden of TB disease effectively makes it a disease of the poor, who have little capacity to pay for medical care. Eliminating TB will require special attention to these marginalized populations as part of the moral duty of HICs and LMICs alike. Therefore, framing poor access to effective treatment for DR-TB as both a public health and human rights issue calls for solutions beyond public health, into the sphere of human rights. Moreover, human rights and public health are irrevocably inter-related; the promotion of one significantly contributes to the realization of the other, while, conversely, the infringement of human rights has negative effects on public health (Mann et al. 1994).

Access to Effective DR-TB Diagnosis and Treatment

Access to effective diagnosis and treatment for DR-TB is constrained by multiple problems; three of which are discussed in this chapter. The first problem is slow, or lack of progress and innovation in TB with regard to the development of new drugs or diagnostic technology. For example, since the introduction of the inexpensive and effective four-drug (isoniazid, rifampicin, pyrazinamide and ethambutol) treatment regimen, in the 1970s (Zumla et al. 2013), there were no novel drugs developed until the appearance of bedaquiline in 2012 (Cox et al. 2015); this is in spite of TB being one of the oldest diseases, spanning centuries (Daniel 2006). The current vaccine for TB, BCG, is almost 100 years old, and is considered effective in reducing severe and disseminated TB in young children but is not effective in adults (Kernodle 2010).

In most high TB burden settings the mainstay of TB diagnosis remains sputum smear microscopy, a test essentially unchanged in a century (Steingart et al. 2006). The slow or absent innovation in TB diagnosis and treatment arises from major challenges at different stages of the research continuum from basic science through to product availability. TB drug research is hugely underfunded, and key players in the pharmaceutical industry have been withdrawing from or cutting down on their investment in TB research and drug development, predominantly due to the real or perceived lack of a profitable market (Frick 2016). While treatment of drug sensitive TB still relies on the four drug combination developed more than 40 years ago, treatment of DR-TB has utilized both older drugs previously replaced in TB treatment due to lower efficacy and/or high side effects, along with drugs that were originally meant to treat other illnesses, repurposed for TB (Zumla et al. 2013). Currently, these repurposed drugs, together with some of the new drugs on the market are being used to improve treatment success rates for MDR-TB (Ndjeka et al. 2015).

The second problem is inadequate evidence-based guidance on effective use of new or repurposed drugs. New drugs need to be registered through clinical trials, which are often lengthy and costly; and guidance on use of new drugs is restricted until further clinical trials are conducted. For example, bedaquiline is not registered for use by the FDA and other agencies in pregnant women, children or people living with HIV who are co-infected with MDR-TB (Mase et al. 2013) because there were no clinical trials on its use in these populations. Yet, in many high burden countries, co-infection with HIV and TB is very common, and in reality bedaquiline is being used in these populations (Ndjeka et al. 2015). Similarly, for repurposed medicines, the evidence base to inform guidelines for their use is inadequate (London et al. 2016; Mafukidze et al. 2016). The third problem, which is often a result of the first two, is the high cost and complexity of diagnostics and treatment, and the lack of feasible models of care for scale-up in high burden settings.

Rights Based Approach to DR-TB

To appreciate a rights-based approach to DR-TB, one needs to have an appreciation for human rights in general. Human rights are entitlements and freedoms that people have simply because they are human. They refer to moral principles or norms, which describe certain standards and moral beliefs that people have. For example, the right to food was a result of the moral belief that people should not die of starvation. Similarly, moral beliefs have been significant in defining human rights, "from resisting torture and arbitrary incarceration to demanding the end of hunger and of medical neglect" (Sen 2005). This view of human rights as morally justifiable claims entails that, if a moral claim is that no person should be enslaved to another, then the claim not to be enslaved is, by a matter of law, a human right (McFarland 2015). Likewise, the moral belief that everyone deserves equal opportunities to be in a state of mental, physical and emotional wellbeing, gives credence to the right to health. But the right to health alone is not adequate to fulfill this moral belief. Without scientific progress in prevention, treatment, or in addressing determinants of ill-health, the aspiration of good health cannot be realized. Similarly, without good trade policies, proper housing adequate food or adequate infrastructure, securing good health becomes an unrealistic aspiration.

A human rights-based approach (HRBA) to health is a way of analysing health through the framework of human rights. It entails examining the impact of health policies and programmes on human rights, and likewise, how promotion or violation of human rights impact public health. A rights-based approach to health focuses on equity of health outcomes by analyzing and addressing the inequalities, discriminatory practices (*de jure* and *de facto*) and unjust power relations which are often at the center of health problems. Under a rights-based approach, health is anchored in a system of the recognition of individuals as right-holders and states as duty-bearers. A State has obligations to realize the human rights of its people, governed by international law. Perhaps, even more importantly, a rights-based approach to health means that citizens have the power and means to hold their governments accountable to their duties and responsibilities, and in turn, governments account to their citizens in a just and transparent manner.

The right to health is included in the ICESCR, which is a legally binding treaty. Article 12(2d) provides for an obligation for States to take steps for the creation of conditions which would assure medical services and medical attention to all in the event of sickness. The United Nations Committee on Economic, Social and Cultural Rights summed up the obligations of the State as the obligation to respect, protect and fulfill. Each treaty body adopts its interpretation of the provisions of its respective treaty in the form of "general comments" or "general recommendations". The Committee's guidance on the right to health in General Comment no. 14 provides an authoritative interpretation of the right to health), and unpacks state obligations and what this right looks like in real terms.

The emergence of the rights-based approach to health in recent years brought with it a paradigm shift in the fields of public health and human rights, owing, in part, to the HIV epidemic, but also to stronger civil society movements working on both health and human rights. But what does a rights-based approach to health mean for access to effective treatment of drug-resistant tuberculosis? And what human rights, other than the right to health can this approach be anchored in? Previously, public health concerns focused on the epidemiology of diseases, analysis of risk factors and interventions to control morbidity and prevent mortality. Particularly for TB, a communicable disease, the concern was around infection control and protecting the health of the public rather than those affected (London 2008). In this "public health view" of the TB disease, the State embarks on efforts to respond to TB because it is a public health threat, and not because the State is obligated to provide for the right to health of its citizens.

The Right to Enjoy the Benefits of Scientific Progress

The REBSP is proclaimed in article 15 paragraph 1(b) of the ICESCR; that [everyone has the right] to enjoy the benefits of scientific progress and its applications. This right is closely related to other rights contained in article 15; namely, the right to take part in cultural life (article 15, paragraph 1(a); the right of everyone to benefit from the protection of moral and material interests resulting from any scientific, literary or artistic production of which they are the author (article 15, paragraph 1(c)); and the right to freedom indispensable for scientific research and creative activity (article 15, paragraph 3).

Although it is proclaimed in these two important human rights documents, the REBSP is one of the least theorised human rights, and consequently, one of the least realized. Despite its textual existence dating back to the 1940s, in the UDHR, this right is relatively new in terms of its conceptualisation (Shaver 2015). Even human rights activists and lawyers are all too often unaware of the existence of the REBSP, much less of its meaning (Chapman 2009). As such, the REBSP is one right whose conceptual content needs to be interrogated and further developed (Shaver 2015). Despite its lack of clarity, the REBSP cannot be isolated from other human rights; because of the interdependent nature of human rights (United Nations 2005), but also because science is a vehicle that is used in almost every sphere of human development (UNDP 2012). This interrelation is best exemplified in debates about unequal access to the benefits of scientific progress – not only in relation to access to essential medicines (the right to health) (FM't Hoen 2002) but also in access to seed technology (the right to food) (Dommen 2002) to scientific discoveries that can improve environmental protection (the right to a safe environment) (Maskus 2002) and to information and communication technologies (right to privacy and access to information).

Three types of obligations result from the right to enjoy the benefits of scientific progress.

The Obligation to Respect

For the REBSP, the State's obligation to respect this right means that the State must desist from curtailing, or interfering with people's ability to access the benefits of scientific progress. In relation to access to treatmemt for DR-TB, the state must therefore not interfere with the production of medicines and technology necessary for treatment and prevention of DR-TB. Such interference can take many forms, from having overly bureaucratic procedures for acquiring ethical clearance for research in drug development to unnecessary delay in approval of new drugs that have already been approved in other countries. Another interference might be in the form of patent protection laws and policies that prioritise protection of patents resulting from research and development ahead of access to treatment. The World Trade Organization adopted rules on intellectual property rights, which impose obligations on states to protect patents on new and existing medicines. Such rules often act as obstacles to making medicines available and accessible to all.

The Obligation to Protect

While a State may not engage in deliberate efforts to violate the REBSP, a failure to protect people from third parties constitutes a potential infringement on the right, and a violation of its obligation to protect. High pricing of life-saving medicines by private corporations through, for example, anti-competitive protectionism, requires the State to act in defence of people's REBSP. For example, where a pharmaceutical company holds a patent of essential TB drugs, the State can incorporate into its laws, some of the TRIPS[1] flexibilities, such as compulsory licensing. In both South Africa and Kenya, the States compelled pharmaceutical companies holding patents to Antiretroviral drugs (ARVs), to enter into "voluntary" licencing agreements with local producers (Musungu et al. 2006).

Obligation to Fulfill

The obligation to fulfill is the third obligation. It speaks to the State's duty to adopt positive measures, and create an enabling environment for human rights to be realised. These measures may include "legislative, administrative, judicial, promotional and other measures" (CESCR 2006). Some of the challenges in drug development, or in research and development in general, are lack of infrastructure and unfriendly regulatory policies. For the state to fulfill the REBSP for TB patients, therefore, it has to take deliberate steps, within its means, to create an environment for science to thrive. These steps do not necessarily require financial expenditure, but would entail mobilising political will for agenda setting and intentional policies to encourage the sharing of scientific knowledge.

For DR-TB, the State's duty to respect, protect and fulfil, does not solely apply to the state with the burden of the disease; countries with a low DR-TB burden, but whose multinational corporations manufacture drugs for use in high burden countries, have an ethical obligation to protect citizens of in other countries from exploitation by their multinational corporations. This speaks to what others have termed 'extraterritorial obligations'- human rights obligations that a state has beyond its borders (Coomans and Kamminga 2004). And in the context of extraterritorial obligations, states that have the skills and resources to develop better and effective medicines, need to also put in place deliberate measures that would make access to such drugs possible outside their jurisdiction.

Realising the REBSP

Crucial to the realisation of the REBSP is the understanding of who the right holders and duty bearers of the right are. Primary duty bearers of any given right are the States, but also the International community (other States and international agencies); they have the duty to respect, protect and fulfil rights. The people, as individuals and as a collective, are therefore rights holders, in that they have individual and collective rights, and hold claims to entitlements provided for in a particular right. One of the most important issues in human rights is to understand different actors and the relationship between rights holders and duty bearers. A distinction should

[1] Trade-Related Aspects of Intellectual Property Rights.

be made between duties and responsibilities. For example, under the right to health, the state has the duty to provide health care to the people, and may do so through private and public health providers; in that case, health providers assume the responsibility to provide health care, but the State still holds the duty under international law. Similarly, under the REBSP, the state has a series of obligations such as creating an enabling environment for scientific progress to thrive, ensuring that people benefit from such scientific progress; non-state actors, such us the private sector (corporations), and academic institutions, have the responsibility to meaningfully contribute to scientific progress through their work. Under international law non-state actors, such as companies or private health providers, do not have legal obligations, only responsibilities. The legal nature of the latter is much weaker.

Minimum Core Obligations

Core obligations are important in realising human rights as they provide a frame of reference in determining what the State needs to do, at the bare minimum (and not subject to progressive realisation[2]). Minimum core obligations require the State to demonstrate that it has made every effort to use all available resources to satisfy, as a matter of priority, those core obligations. In the General Comment on the interpretation of the nature of ICECR obligations, General Comment No. 3 (1990), the Committee on Economic, Social and Cultural Rights stated that "States parties have a core obligation to ensure the satisfaction of minimum essential levels of each of the rights enunciated in the Covenant." Core obligations should be framed as both positive steps to be taken by the State, and actions that the state will need to refrain from.

Unfortunately, for the REBSP, there are, as yet, no defined core obligations, making the application of the right difficult. As a result, there is no standard or benchmark against which people and Civil Society can compel the State's immediate efforts to realize the right. Secondly, the State lacks guidance on what it has to prioritise within its minimal resources. There is therefore an urgent need for agreed minimum core obligations under the REBSP, which would also apply to scientific progress in DR-TB.

For example, minimum core obligations in REBSP could be used to prevent harmful effects of science, to promote access to benefits and to encourage international cooperation:

(a) To monitor the potential harmful effects of science and technology, to effectively react to the findings and inform the public in a transparent way; for

[2] Given the resource and knowledge restraints faced by many countries, the CESCR recognizes that the fulfillment of economic and social rights can only be achieved over time, and calls for the *progressive realization* of ESCR.

instance, where drug development for TB poses threats to the people, the state does not need to wait before it intervenes and prevents such harm.

(b) To promote access to the benefits of science and its applications on a non-discriminatory basis including measures necessary to address the needs of disadvantaged and marginalized groups. This includes ensuring that TB patients, especially the poor and marginalized, benefit from scientific progress that informs the development of new drugs, the use of repurposed drugs as well as the application of such drugs in high burden settings;

(c) To take measures to encourage and strengthen international cooperation and assistance in science and technology to the benefit of all people and to comply in this regard with the States' obligations under international law. This includes, inter-alia, the state entering into international agreements that fosters exchange of knowledge and products of such knowledge. It also implies that states push for better patent laws, which promote access to scientific knowledge even for those in LMICs.

Lack of Scientific Progress in DR-TB

A critical element of scientific progress is research and development (R&D), which is key to ensuring access to effective medicines, especially when coupled with deliberate policies to address access-related challenges for the poor and the marginalized. In the current environment, research can either be for-profit or not, regardless of whether it is meant to add value to people's health. Unfortunately, investments in not-for-profit research tend to be significantly lower than investments in for-profit research. Modern research is largely driven by funding external to the researchers/ scientists and that how research is financed will determine how the knowledge arising from it will be used (Yamey 2008).

While not being the only element of the right, access to the benefits of scientific progress is one that is most controversial as it involves navigating the political landscapes in the production of science itself (Besson 2015a, b) and foregrounds the need for universal agreement on what defines scientific progress (Donders 2015). Moreover, the context in which the production of science takes place, often stretches beyond national jurisdictions (Besson 2015a, b). For example, for pharmaceutical companies based in HICs to test the effectiveness of new and repurposed drugs for TB, they need to conduct clinical trials in high burden settings like South Africa. Therefore, defining scientific progress is not the responsibility of one state, but requires a shared understanding by both those on the giving and receiving end of scientific development. Progress in TB is not just about the development of new drugs. It is also about the discovery and sharing of knowledge; and ensuring that such knowledge is accessible to those who need it the most.

Nevertheless, one of the main barriers is that countries from the North and the pharmaceutical companies domiciled there are reluctant to share and transfer knowledge with and to the South because of economic competition and return upon investment reasons. To counter the current static positions, the WHO, in partnership with United Nations Conference on Trade and Development (UNCTAD) and the International Centre for Trade and Sustainable Development, initiated a project on Improving Access to Medicines in Developing Countries through Technology Transfer and Local Production. One of the findings of the project has been that local production has the potential to enhance access to affordable medicines if supported by appropriate and accessible technology (WHO 2011).

Furthermore, the benefits of scientific progress, as opposed to the protection of scientific discoveries and production have not been well explored. The latter has been a topic of thorough discussion and debate under intellectual property rights and law (Besson 2015a, b). This has arguably led to a situation where attention (and legal protection) is typically given to creation of scientific knowledge most likely to benefit the innovators (Yamey and Torreele 2002), while knowledge to address key public health problems of significant magnitude, particularly for poor populations unable to purchase the applications of scientific progress, have been neglected. Or if pursued, the scientific discoveries have been too costly to benefit the majority in need (Yamey 2008). International treaties and agreements on the development, sharing and use of science need to account for the fact that, although the capacity of most LMICs to contribute to scientific progress is more limited than for high income countries, their need to benefit is far greater than that of high-income countries. This imbalance in need versus capacity should be factored into the discourse on intellectual property rights, particularly in terms of impact on access to essential life-saving medicines.

Intellectual Property Rights and Access to Essential Medicines

The dominant paradigm in scientific development favours the strengthening and protection of Intellectual Property Rights (IPRs) in efforts to encourage and reward innovation. This paradigm was institutionalised after the introduction of patents, which in turn made scientific research more lucrative (Timmermann 2014). A patent is a "government-granted limited property right to exclude others from making, using or selling the patented invention" (Clark et al. 2000).

Patents can have a dramatic impact on access to medicines when they are used to prevent competition. A drug company that holds patents on a medicine has the right to prevent others from manufacturing it and therefore can charge an artificially high price. When a company is selling commodities such as computer components, for example, this might be of no great significance. But when life-saving treatments for diseases such as HIV or cancer become unaffordable to those that need them, the consequences can be – and are – devastating. In many LMICs, where people pay for drugs out of their own pockets and very seldom have health insurance, the high price of medicines becomes a question of life and death.

To advance the protection of intellectual property rights, the Member States of the World Trade Organization (WTO) agreed on the Trade-Related Aspects of Intellectual Property Rights (TRIPS) legal regime that progressively became effective from 1994 onwards (Correa 2007). TRIPS elicited a challenge from developing countries and from Civil Society across the globe, who saw them as an impediment to access to essential medicines. Prior to TRIPS, patent protection on pharmaceuticals was almost non-existent in developing countries and the absence of patents led to the flourishing of generic medicine production in these countries, which significantly lowered the cost of essential medicines. While rewarding innovation is important, it should not occur at the expense of access to the benefits. What is needed is a system for balancing promotion of innovation and access to benefits, which is what the REBSP potentially provides.

For example, in 2001, developing countries initiated negotiations on the interpretations of TRIPS Agreement because they restricted access to drugs for patients with HIV infection, the majority of whom live in developing countries (Correa and WHO 2002). Although the TRIPS agreement itself did not change, a compromise was reached in Doha[3] in the form of a Declaration that clarified that TRIPS should not prevent developing states from dealing with public health crises, that they should not restrict universal access to essential medicines and provided for mechanisms to bypass potential IP obstacles when public health was at stake. This is a case where the right to health was used as a basis to facilitate international trade agreements that would favour access to life-saving medicines, thereby also opening opportunities for realising the benefits of scientific progress.

Creating an Enabling Environment

In order for scientific progress in TB to thrive, states need to create an enabling environment for research. State duties to meet this right might include those proposed by London, Cox and Coomans (2016): – (i) measures to ensure that researchers have access to infrastructure and equipment to conduct research such as drug development; (ii) adoption of research policies and strategies that foreground research to develop applications for neglected diseases of the poor; (iii) shaping of research funding opportunities to make more attractive research that has lower commercial opportunity; (iv) capacity building of researchers; but also, (v) Public-Private Partnerships to encourage the public sector to contribute to access to treatment; (vi) strengthening collaboration with other countries, especially those contributing to R&D; (vii) reprioritising resources from other sectors such as military to health; and (vi) putting in place more efficient regulatory laws and policies, for providing approval for both research and new drugs.

[3] Declaration on the TRIPS Agreement and Public Health, adopted 14 November 2001 by the Ministerial Conference of the World Trade Organisation.

However, for the realisation of the REBSP, there has to be a vehicle or pathways for benefits to be derived from this progress and its applications. Put simply, such a system needs to ensure access to effective treatments for people needing treatment. Where appropriate, the State should make use of the TRIPS flexibilities to develop domestic policies that foster scientific progress in TB as a neglected disease. The case of South Africa and Kenya, which made use of TRIPS flexibilities to enforce compulsory licencing of patents to local producers (Musungu et al. 2006) is an example of the State ensuring access to ARVs. Others efforts can take the form of subsidies for researchers, and tax benefits to encourage research in DR-TB.

International Cooperation to Improve Access to DR-TB Drugs

International cooperation is integral to the international human rights framework, requiring states to recognise the role of international cooperation in realising human rights globally.. Article 2 of the ICESCR sets out that governments are obligated to "[…] take steps, individually and through international assistance and co-operation, […] to the maximum of its available resources, with a view to achieving progressively the full realization of the rights recognized in the present Covenant […]. The REBSP is not exempted from the international cooperation. Science is too broad to be pursued within the confines of one country, and its benefits, particularly in TB, are far reaching. The new drugs bedaquiline and delamanid have a larger market in LMICs than in high-income countries in which they were developed. Similarly, with ARVs, the market is larger in less-developed countries hit by the HIV epidemic, than it is in the high-income countries, where most R&D takes place. The REBSP, like other social and economic rights, has collective dimensions, in that its realization requires functioning social systems involving population-wide application rather than being a right exercised for any particular individual. This is further underscored by the international dimensions of cooperation across communities and territories. Furthermore, while the REBSP can benefit from international cooperation, it can also be a vehicle to promote such cooperation through the sharing of knowledge and its application.

Some initiatives have been established, proposing how this global ethical responsibility might actually be operationalised in the DR-TB response. One of such initiatives is the 3P project,[4] which seeks to encourage the development of affordable, effective new drugs to treat TB. It makes use of an open collaborative approach to conduct drug research and development (R&D), and recommends some new ways of funding and coordinating the drug research and development process. The

[4] https://www.msfaccess.org/sites/default/files/MSF_assets/TB/Docs/TB_briefing_3P-2016_EN.pdf.

process has identified significant weaknesses in the process that hamper development of new regimens and proposes three interventions to address the weakness, these are

- Push funding to finance R&D activities upfront (i.e. through grants);
- Pull funding to incentivise R&D activities through the promise of financial rewards on the achievement of certain R&D objectives (i.e. through milestone prizes)
- Pooling of data and intellectual property to ensure open collaborative research and to ensure fair licensing for competitive production of the final products.

Conclusion

In conclusion, the REBSP offers great potential for deepening the rights-based approach to health, as well as for enhancing access to effective diagnosis and treatment of DR-TB, and by extension other neglected diseases of the poor, by promoting the development of new drugs, and research in the use of existing regimens in high burden settings. However, the right needs clarity and a universal understanding of the entitlements it confers on right-holders and corresponding obligations of duty bearers. There is also need for clarity on the application of the right beyond national borders, to account for the broad scope of science or global trade-related policies. A thorough conceptualisation of the REBSP will require more than the attention of human rights experts, but also trade experts as well as research and development practitioners.

Despite progress made to advance the right to health, health inequality continues to undermine human rights. For DR-TB, health inequality is apparent at multiple levels; the burden of disease is higher in poorer countries, while access to effective treatment is lower. The moral belief that every human being has the right to health entails a collective global responsibility to those people or countries with poor health outcomes. Therefore, "Everyone with TB should have access to the innovative tools and services they need for rapid diagnosis, treatment and care" (WHO 2015) particularly with DR-TB, ensuring access to products and services will not only benefit patients of TB, but will also benefit global health security. This requires a closer look at how other human rights can, together with the right to health, advance health for all. The REBSP is such a right.

The responsibility to ensure scientific progress in DR-TB and access to such progress cannot lie on most affected countries alone. DR-TB will require a global response and a collective responsibility in an effort to advance the right to health. States' duties to respect, protect and fulfill the REBSP within and beyond their borders is an important vehicle to redress the lack of research into new drug development and repurposing existing drugs for DR-TB and their use in high burden settings. REBSP provides some practical ways in which countries can strengthen their rights based approaches to DR-TB. This includes creating an enabling environment for R&D, promoting public-private partnerships, strengthening international cooperation, prioritizing resources to DR-TB, and implementing more efficient regulatory process for new drugs.

References

Besson, S. 2015a. Mapping the issues. *European Journal of Human Rights* 2015: 403–411.

———. 2015b. Science without borders and the boundaries of human rights: Who owes the human right to science ? *European Journal of Human Rights* 2015: 462–486.

CESCR. 2006. *General comment 17: The right of everyone to benefit from the protection of the moral and material interests resulting from any scientific, literary or artistic production of which he or she is the author*. New York: United Nations Economic and Social Council.

Chapman, A.R. 2009. Towards an understanding of the right to enjoy the benefits of scientific progress and its applications. *Journal of Human Rights* 8: 1–36.

Clark, J., et al. 2000. *Patent pools: A solution to the problem of access in biotechnology patents?* Washington, DC: United States Patent and Trademark Office.

Coomans, F., and M.T. Kamminga. 2004. *Extraterritorial application of human rights treaties*. Antwerp: Intersentia.

Correa, C. 2007. *Trade related aspects of intellectual property rights: A commentary on the TRIPS Agreement*. Oxford: Oxford University Press.

Correa, C.M., and WHO. 2002. *Implications of the Doha Declaration on the TRIPS Agreement and public health*. Geneva: World Health Organisation.

Cox, H.S., et al. 2015. The need to accelerate access to new drugs for multidrug-resistant tuberculosis. *Bulletin of the World Health Organization* 93: 491–497.

Daniel, T.M. 2006. The history of tuberculosis. *Respiratory Medicine* 100 (11): 1862–1870.

Dommen, C. 2002. Raising human rights concerns in the World Trade Organization actors, processes and possible strategies. *Human Rights Quarterly* 24 (1): 1–50.

Donders, Y. 2015. Balancing interests: Limitations to the right to enjoy the benefits of scientific progress and its applications. *European Journal of Human Rights* 2015: 486–504.

Evans, C.A. 2011. GeneXpert – A game-changer for tuberculosis control? *PLoS Medicine* 8 (7): e1001064.

Figueroa-Munoz, J.I., and P. Ramon-Pardo. 2008. Tuberculosis control in vulnerable groups. *Bulletin of the World Health Organization* 86 (9): 733–735.

FM't Hoen, E. 2002. TRIPS, pharmaceutical patents and access to essential medicines: Seattle, Doha and beyond. *Journal of International Law* 3: 39–68.

Frick, M. 2016. *2016 report on tuberculosis research funding trends, 2005–2015: No time to lose*. New York: Treatment Action Group.

Kernodle, D.S. 2010. Decrease in the effectiveness of Bacille Calmette-Guérin vaccine against pulmonary tuberculosis: A consequence of increased immune suppression by microbial antioxidants, not over attenuation. *Clinical Infectious Diseases* 51 (2): 177–184.

London, L. 2008. What is a human-rights based approach to health and does it matter? *Health and Human Rights* 10: 65–80.

London, L., et al. 2016. Multidrug-resistant TB: Implementing the right to health through the right to enjoy the benefits of scientific progress. *Health & Human Rights: An International Journal* 18 (1).

Mafukidze, A., et al. 2016. An update on repurposed medications for the treatment of drug-resistant tuberculosis. *Expert Review of Clinical Pharmacology* 9 (10): 1331–1340.

Mann, J., L. Gostin, S. Gruskin, T. Brennan, Z. Lazzarini, and H.V. Fineberg. 1994. Health and human rights. *Health and Human Rights* 1 (1): 6–24.

Mase, S., et al. 2013. Provisional CDC guidelines for the use and safety monitoring of bedaquiline fumarate (Sirturo) for the treatment of multidrug-resistant tuberculosis. *Morbidity and Mortality Weekly Report: Recommendations and Reports* 62 (9): 1–12.

Maskus, K.E. 2002. Regulatory standards in the WTO: Comparing intellectual property rights with competition policy, environmental protection, and core labor standards. *World Trade Review* 1 (2): 135–152.

McFarland, S. 2015. Culture, individual differences, and support for human rights: A general review. *Peace and Conflict: Journal of Peace Psychology* 21 (1): 10.

Musungu, S.F., et al. 2006. *The use of flexibilities in TRIPS by developing countries: Can they promote access to medicines?* Geneva: World Health Organisation.

Ndjeka, N., et al. 2015. Treatment of drug-resistant tuberculosis with bedaquiline in a high HIV prevalence setting: An interim cohort analysis. *The International Journal of Tuberculosis and Lung Disease* 19 (8): 979–985.

Seddon, J.A., et al. 2012. Hearing loss in patients on treatment for drug-resistant tuberculosis. *European Respiratory Journal* 40 (5): 1277.

Sen, A. 2005. Human rights and capabilities. *Journal of Human Development* 6 (2): 151–166.

Shaver, L. 2015. The right to science: Ensuring that everyone benefits from scientific and technological progress. *European Journal of Human Rights* 2015: 411–431.

Skrahina, A., et al. 2016. Bedaquiline in the multidrug-resistant tuberculosis treatment: Belarus experience. *International Journal of Mycobacteriology* 5: S62–S63.

Steingart, K.R., et al. 2006. Sputum processing methods to improve the sensitivity of smear microscopy for tuberculosis: A systematic review. *The Lancet Infectious Diseases* 6 (10): 664–674.

Timmermann, C. 2014. Sharing in or benefiting from scientific advancement? *Science and Engineering Ethics* 20: 111–133.

UNDP. 2012. *MDG report 2012: Assessing progress in Africa toward the Millennium Development Goals*. Addis Ababa: Economic Commission for Africa.

United Nations. 2005. *Economic, social and cultural rights: Handbook for national human rights institutions*. New York: United Nations.

WHO. 2011. *Local production for access to medical products: Developing a framework to improve public health*, 32–36. Geneva: World Health Organisation.

———. 2015. *The end TB strategy*. Geneva: World Health Organisation.

———. 2016. *Global tuberculosis report*. Geneva: World Health Organisation.

———. 2017. *Multidrug- resistant tuberculosis (MDR) TB 2017 update*. Geneva: World Health Organisation.

———. 2018. *Global tuberculosis report*. Geneva: World Health Organisation.

Yamey, G. 2008. Excluding the poor from accessing biomedical literature: A rights violation that impedes global health. *Health and Human Rights* 10: 21–42.

Yamey, G., and E. Torreele. 2002. The world's most neglected diseases. *The British Medical Journal* 325: 176–177.

Zumla, A., et al. 2013. Advances in the development of new tuberculosis drugs and treatment regimens. *Nature Reviews Drug Discovery* 12 (5): 388–404.

12

Drug-Resistant Infection: Causes, Consequences, and Responses

Euzebiusz Jamrozik and Michael J. Selgelid

Abstract This chapter provides an overview of the causes and consequences of, and possible policy responses to, the problem of drug resistance. Throughout, we highlight the ways that ethical and conceptual analyses can help to clarify relevant issues and improve policy, especially in public health, broadly conceived. Drug resistant pathogens arise, persist, spread, and produce harm due to a complex set of causes: biological processes (e.g., related to microbial evolution, the transmission of genetic determinants of resistance between microbes, and human host immunity) as well as human behaviors (e.g., antimicrobial use and hygiene practices) and other social factors (e.g., access to clean water, sanitation, healthcare, and antimicrobials). Furthermore, the ethically salient consequences of drug resistance include not only morbidity and mortality from untreatable infections (that are often inequitably distributed), but also broader effects on human freedom, privacy, and well-being. Public health ethicists are ideally placed to identify and weigh the values that might be promoted or compromised by potential policies and/or interventions that aim to address the problem of drug resistance. This chapter concludes by discussing potential policy responses, including those related to surveillance, research, animal and human antimicrobial use, the broader social determinants of health, infection control practices, and vaccination.

Keywords Antimicrobial resistance · Drug resistance · Drug resistant infection · Ethics · Bioethics · Public health ethics

---

E. Jamrozik (✉)
Monash Bioethics Centre, Monash University, Melbourne, VIC, Australia

Department of Medicine, Royal Melbourne Hospital, University of Melbourne, Melbourne, VIC, Australia

Wellcome Centre for Ethics and the Humanities and The Ethox Centre, Nuffield Department of Population Health, University of Oxford, Oxford, UK
e-mail: zeb.jamrozik@gmail.com

M. J. Selgelid
Monash Bioethics Centre, Monash University, Melbourne, VIC, Australia
e-mail: michael.selgelid@monash.edu

Introduction

It is widely acknowledged that drug resistance poses one of the greatest threats to global public health during the coming decades. Drug resistance compromises the treatment of infections (that were commonly debilitating and/or fatal before the development of antimicrobial drugs), and thereby undermines many advances in surgery, cancer treatment, and immunosuppression that depend on our ability to treat infections effectively. Microbes – bacteria, mycobacteria, parasites, fungi, and viruses – have, over billions of years and untold numbers of microbial generations, developed mechanisms (via evolutionary processes) to protect themselves from harm and transmit such portective mechanisms to other microbes (of the same or different species) (Holmes et al. 2016). The rapid increase in antimicrobial drug resistance in the twentieth and twenty-first centuries is a result of these powerful evolutionary mechanisms combined with human activities that affect the microbial world, including the widespread production and use of antimicrobial drugs. Resistance is a matter of degree (for example, low levels of resistance can be overcome with a higher dose or longer course of antimicrobials) and its impact is also relative to the availability of alternative treatments (where second line drugs are readily available, resistance to first line agents may initially be less of a concern). Thus, the recent emergence of strains of clinically important pathogens that are highly resistant to all, or nearly all, available therapies (e.g. extensively drug-resistant tuberculosis (TB) and pan-resistant gram negative bacteria) is an urgent challenge for public health (Schwaber et al. 2011; Birgand et al. 2016; World Health Organisation 2017a).

Drug resistance is an important topic for ethical analysis since (i) human actions and inactions are major contributors to the problem, (ii) the consequences for human health and well-being are highly significant and inequitably distributed, and (iii) policies aiming to reduce the rates of resistant pathogens may involve balancing this reduction in risk with other morally salient risks, burdens, and benefits. Thus, this volume aims to provide a timely exploration of many of the ethical aspects of the phenomenon of drug resistance. This first chapter highlights the complex causes and significant consequences of drug resistance, and the ways in which ethical and conceptual analysis can inform and improve relevant policy responses. We link these discussions with other chapters in this volume, as well as gesturing towards future directions for ethicists, empirical scientists, and public health policymakers.

Causes

Evolution and Transmission of Resistance Genes

The microbial world is ancient, abundant, ubiquitous, and complex. As a result of random mutation over trillions of microbial generations, bacteria have adapted to their environments, in part by developing genes that code for mechanisms of resistance to various threats – including, for example, heavy metals, naturally occurring antibacterial compounds (including beta-lactams such as penicillins and carbapenems) and synthetic antimicrobials (e.g. fluroquinolones and sulphonamides) (Holmes et al. 2016; D'Costa et al. 2011). Certain microbes are also able to horizontally transfer genes coding for resistance mechanisms to other microbes (Holmes et al. 2016; Chang et al. 2015). With the dramatic, unprecedented increase in human interventions in the microbial world (especially the widespread use and overuse of antimicrobial agents), strong evolutionary selection pressures have been applied to microbes leading to the emergence, increasing frequency, and persistence of resistant microbes in humans, animals and the environment (Holmes et al. 2016).

Antimicrobial Use in Humans

In his 1945 Nobel Prize speech, Alexander Fleming (who first discovered the antibiotic properties of penicillin) famously noted that 'the ignorant man may easily underdose himself and by exposing his microbes to non-lethal quantities of the drug make them resistant' (Fleming 1945). If antimicrobial treatment is inadequate, that is, then resistant strains of microbes that otherwise would have been killed off may survive and become more strongly established in the absence of microbal competitors, in the environment of a person's body. Resistant pathogen strains thus selected can then be transmitted to other persons. For pathogens like tuberculosis (TB) and HIV, requiring months (or, for HIV and extensively drug-resistant TB, years) of multi-drug therapy, undertreatment (e.g. due to 'noncompliance' of patients, or inadequate access to medicine, etc.) has played a central role in the emergence and persistence of highly resistant strains (see Chaps. 2, 3, 5, 10 and 26). In the case of malaria – where, for various reasons, parasites may be exposed (in human patients) to sporadic and/or sub-therapeutic concentrations of antimalarials, sometimes as a result of partial treatment – underuse of drugs likewise plays a role in the emergence of antimalarial resistance (White 2017) (See Chap. 4).

In the case of antibiotic resistance in common bacterial pathogens, however, *overuse* of antibiotics is far more important than undertreatment. Despite years of rhetoric regarding the need to 'complete the prescribed course' for common uncomplicated bacterial infections, this now appears, except among a subset of pathogens and specific sites of infection, to have been ill-founded[1] and, on balance (when generalised to all infections), harmful advice (Llewelyn et al. 2017). Overuse and 'appropriate' use are much more dominant causes of resistance. This is because the human body (particularly in the digestive and respiratory tracts, and on the skin) contains billions of bacteria, many of which are indiscriminately exposed to an antibiotic used either appropriately to treat one particular pathogen (e.g. bacterial pneumonia) or inappropriately (e.g. a viral infection mistaken for a bacterial

[1] In part because, until recently, few trials had addressed the question of whether shorter courses for common infections may be just as effective, with less development of resistance (and less side effects) – the few trials that have now been done generally support the use of shorter courses in uncomplicated infections.

infection) (Llewelyn et al. 2017; Carlet 2012). Exposure to more antibiotics in a given individual is predictive of a higher rate of asymptomatic carriage of resistant pathogens (although this rate does decrease over time) (Nasrin et al. 2002; Bryce et al. 2016). These resistant bacteria, although in usual circumstances causing no harm, can lead to invasive (resistant) disease – for example when a person's skin is cut or incised by a surgeon, or when bowel bacteria spread to other locations in a person's body, or when a person becomes immunosuppressed (Tischendorf et al. 2016; Safdar and Bradley 2008). Those who thus become 'carriers' of resistant bacteria can transmit such pathogens to others (whether the initial carrier is symptomatic or not) (Smith et al. 2004; Lerner et al. 2015; Jamrozik and Selgelid 2019).

Overuse of antibiotics in humans is thus a collective action problem – in some respects a classic 'tragedy of the commons' (Hardin 2009), but complicated, *inter alia*, by the transmission of resistance between pathogens and also the transmission of resistant pathogens between humans.[2] The (simplified) structure of the collective action problem is that each doctor or patient seeks individual benefit of the patient (minimising the risk of severe bacterial infection) by, respectively, prescribing and taking antibiotics even in cases where this may have only marginal expected benefits for the patient; but their decisions/actions collectively (in conjunction with other causal factors) bring about high levels of antibiotic resistance – which, in the long term, is a major threat to all.

Problematic treatment decisions (that contribute to resistance) are sometimes related to diagnostic uncertainty. When a patient has symptoms associated with respiratory illness, for example, there is often no sufficiently rapid and accurate test to determine whether it is caused by a bacterial pathogen. As a result of this uncertainty, combined with risk-aversion among doctors and patients, and a (mis)perception that a course of antibiotics 'does no harm' (or that the risks of side-effects and generating resistance are outweighed by potential benefits[3]), millions of antibiotics each year are taken when they are not required. Solutions that rely on individuals acting in accordance with the social optimum (especially if, in doing so, they take on more risk to themselves) are, at best, incomplete or, at worst, doomed.

The problems of both antimicrobial overuse and underuse are magnified in some low- and middle-income countries where many people lack access to basic diagnostic testing and antimicrobials—and/or where antimicrobials are commonly available without prescription (Holmes et al. 2016; Laxminarayan et al. 2016; Dar et al. 2016) (see Chap. 5). There is an inherent tension between 'access and excess', i.e. many die because they are unable to obtain diagnosis and/or antimicrobial treatment

[2] In standard commons tragedies, such as overfishing, individuals collectively deplete a common resource (e.g. by fishing), ultimately leading to its collapse. In the case of drug resistance, the resource (e.g. effective antimicrobials) can be depleted (in a way akin to standard depletion) through use of antimicrobial drugs, leading to resistance, but also, for example by the transmission of drug resistant strains from one person to another (regardless of whether either has recently used antimicrobials) – thus the relationships at play may be more complex than standard commons tragedies.

[3] The actual (as opposed to perceived) risks and benefits are rarely quantified 'at the bedside'.

when it is really needed while, at the same time, antibiotics are used when they are not required, leading to resistance. This, in turn, exacerbates problems of access – because the second line drugs required (after first line drugs have been rendered useless) are more expensive/less affordable (Laxminarayan et al. 2016; Dar et al. 2016). In parallel, the transmission of resistant pathogens is amplified by a lack of access to readily available clean water, sanitation, and well-resourced healthcare institutions. The burden of drug-resistant infections thus tracks poverty and social disadvantage both within countries and internationally (Llewelyn et al. 2017; Bryce et al. 2016; Guh et al. 2015) (See Chap. 16).

Transmission

Drug-resistant microbes are transmitted between human beings just like other non-resistant pathogens – via airborne or droplet transmission, skin contact, the faecal-oral route, sexual transmission, contact with infected bodily fluids, contaminated water and food, vector transmission (e.g. mosquitoes in the case of malaria), and so on. The epidemiological significance of transmission of some pathogens in some contexts is relatively well understood, whereas the transmission of the same pathogens in other settings may be different and/or less well-studied. In the case of drug-resistant bacteria, for example, in-hospital transmission is well-documented. Such transmission often occurs via contamination of the clinical environment and via healthcare workers – especially those who fail to adhere to basic hand hygiene practices (see Chap. 6), although controversy surrounds the optimum infection control policies to prevent transmission (Morgan et al. 2017). However, the transmission of resistant bacteria (and antibiotic resistance mechanisms) in the general community (i.e. outside healthcare facilities) is poorly understood, and much more evidence is needed to guide policy (Holmes et al. 2016; Dar et al. 2016). Transmission in the community is facilitated not only by direct human contact, but also general environmental contamination with resistant pathogens, the mobile genetic elements that confer resistance, and even antibiotics themselves – with polluted water systems being a key link in indirect transmission between human beings, and between animals and humans (Pruden et al. 2013; Martinez 2009). This problem is of greatest concern in low-income settings with poor access to clean water and sanitation, further exacerbating the inequitable distribution of harms from drug-resistant infection (Laxminarayan et al. 2016; Dar et al. 2016).

The global spread of drug resistance is greatly facilitated by modern air travel. Millions of people become colonised (usually without symptoms) with resistant pathogens or other (non-pathogenic) microbes containing genetic determinants of resistance every year in locations with high rates of resistance and then fly to regions where (whether or not those colonised are sick) resistant pathogens and/or resistance determinants are directly or indirectly transmitted to others (Kennedy and Collignon 2010; Östholm-Balkhed et al. 2013).

Antimicrobial Use in Animals and Agriculture

The widespread use of antibiotics in industrial agriculture and aquaculture, either as 'growth promoters' or in other mass prophylactic uses, has lead to pathogens developing resistance to the agents used. This has had consequences for both animal and human health. Consequences for humans occur when clinically significant pathogens (and/or resistance determinants) are transmitted from animals to humans (either directly via animal contact or consumption of animal products, or indirectly via environmental contamination with resistant pathogens and/or resistance determinants), when humans are themselves exposed to antibiotics used in the food chain (either in the products they consume, or because antibiotics and antibiotic residues are released into the environment), or when humans are exposed to pathogens (or other microbes) that become resistant (and/or carry resistance determinants) as a result of exposure to antibiotics in enviroments contaminated by agricultural use (Holmes et al. 2016; Schwaber et al. 2011; Birgand et al. 2016; Chang et al. 2015; Martinez 2009).[4] The links between animal and human health via our shared microbiome are complex, and the relative importance of different causal pathways in a particular setting is often difficult to quantify (Chang et al. 2015) (See Chap. 7). Likewise, although the agricultural industry uses more antibiotics in total tonnage than human healthcare, the relative contribution of agricultural antibiotic use to the epidemiology of resistant bacterial disease in humans is difficult to study, often unknown and likely varies widely in different settings (Holmes et al. 2016).

Consequences

Direct Harms to Human Beings

The true global burden of death and disease due to resistant infection is unknown, and from both ethical and scientific points of view there is an urgent need for more accurate estimates. One prominent appraisal published in 2015 suggested that at least 700,000 deaths occur each year due to drug-resistant infection worldwide, and that this annual death toll could rise to ten million by the year 2050 (Antimicrobial resistance: Tackling a crisis for the health and wealth of nations 2015). However, this analysis included only 6 pathogens and acknowledged that the true number is probably already far higher, especially given that more of the burden of disease falls on poor communities that often have incomplete disease surveillance systems and limited access to relevant diagnostic technology (Laxminarayan et al. 2016).

---

[4] In (1) microbes become resistant due to their exposure to antibiotics in animals' bodies; in (2) microbes become resistant due to their exposure to antibiotics in people's bodies (resulting from people's exposure to antibiotics in contaminated environments); in (3) microbes become resistant due to their exposure to antibiotics in contaminated environments.

The inequitable distribution of harms from resistant disease mirrors the inequitable distribution of infectious disease burden more generally. In both high- and low-income countries, the heavy burden disproportionately shouldered by impoverised people and communities is largely explained by 'social determinants of health' (e.g. lack of access to clean water, sanitation, wealth, education, access to a robust health system, etc). On many accounts of justice, wealthy individuals and societies have strong moral reasons to improve these basic determinants of public health for all (Selgelid 2008). Furthermore, since resistant pathogens (like other pathogens) spread across borders, the wealthy have increasingly strong self-interested reasons to provide assistance to others and to prevent others from developing resistant disease.

High rates of resistant pathogens (especially common bacterial species) undermine many of the advances of modern medicine – because the successes of surgery, transplantation, cancer treatment, immunosuppression, intensive care, and obstetric and neonatal care are very often contingent on being able to treat and cure infections. Increasing drug resistance thus has widespread implications for health and healthcare. Although patients who are unwell with other comorbidities are at the highest risk (both of carrying resistant pathogens – due to recurrent treatment and hospitalisation – and of invasive disease from these pathogens), even relatively healthy people are, and will increasingly be, harmed by resistant infectious disease.

Before the advent of antibiotics, a simple skin wound could lead to untreatable sepsis, amputation and/or death, and a 'post-antibiotic era' would entail a return to similarly grim prospects. Increasing drug resistance thus severely threatens the entire global population and, in addition, future generations.

Economic Consequences

Along with direct harms, drug resistance has severe economic consequences. Drug-resistant infections are more difficult (sometimes impossible) and more expensive to treat and cure, and they are more likely to result in incapacitation of the patient and significant economic losses for society. One estimate suggested that total global losses due to resistant infection between now and 2050 could total over $US 100 trillion (O'Neill 2015), meaning that there are powerful economic reasons to devise and implement effective measures to curb the problem (See Chap. 17).

As noted in several chapters in this book, the *availability of effective antimicrobials* has many features of a 'public good' in economic terms. Standard economic models predict (more or less accurately) that a free market in antimicrobials (i.e. with little or no regulation of access apart from price) leads to 'market failure' and the erosion of the good in question (i.e. availability of effective antimicrobials). In most societies, since access to antimicrobials occurs via healthcare practitioners, the 'market' is relatively controlled (as opposed to free). The incentive structures that lead to a collective action problem for doctors and patients (discussed above) nevertheless lead to a similar erosion of antimicrobial effectiveness – albeit at an attenuated rate, depending upon the degree to which regulations on prescriptions succeed. Private healthcare providers, in any case, can be difficult to regulate (see Chap. 5), especially where they are not part of a centralised and/or universal healthcare system.

Burdensome Public Health Interventions

The consequences of drug resistance for human beings are more than just matters of physical health and wealth. In many cases, public health surveillance and related public health practices have ethically salient implications for other aspects of well-being, including psychological well-being (e.g. due to experiences of stigma among carriers of resistant microbes – see below), as well as privacy and other freedoms (e.g. which are compromised by mandatory physical/social distancing measures such as isolation and quarantine). Well-designed public health surveillance and research should be conducted in order to clarify the health risks and costs of resistant infection and the risks, benefits, and burdens of potential public health interventions. High quality data would help policymakers determine whether imposing certain burdens on individuals would be justified as a means to improve public health (e.g. by reducing infectious disease due to resistant organisms) (Fairchild and Bayer 2004). Unfortunately, investment in surveillance for resistance has, globally, been very low and is only just starting to be improved, particularly in wealthy settings.

Those identified by surveillance as carriers of resistant pathogens while inpatients in healthcare settings sometimes experience stigma (Rump et al. 2017) as well as a wide range of effects on well-being, which some argue are best understood through a capabilities approach that explores the broader implications of public health policies for the flourishing of individual lives (see Chap. 13). Such an approach may also help to illustrate the broader aspects of human life that are jeopardised by the lack of access to effective antimicrobials, especially among children, for whom early severe infection may impair long term development (see Chap. 14).

Indeed, as more people become aware of resistance, and more community surveillance is conducted, apparently healthy individuals in the community may be increasingly identified as asymptomatic carriers of resistant organisms (See Chap. 12). Furthermore, such individuals might be monitored, offered or required to undergo treatment, and have other liberties (freedom of movement, free choice of occupation) curtailed by public health policy (Houston and Houston 2015). Those who have had recent contact with carriers might be tested and/or quarantined. There is thus frequently a tension between the aim to protect public health (by identifying infected individuals and reducing transmission of (resistant) disease) and the aim to avoid imposing significant burdens (in terms of compromised well-being, privacy and/or liberty) on individuals in order to prevent the spread of disease to others (Viens et al. 2009).

Responses1.

New Drugs

For many decades, even where the emergence of drug resistance was recognized, much of the response (or lack thereof) by individual clinicians as well as policymakers was grounded in (apparently unfounded) confidence that new antimicrobial drugs would be discovered and developed, meaning that resistance to older drugs was of limited significance. Despite early warnings of the consequences (Holmes et al. 2016; Honigsbaum 2016) – profligate use continued and indeed accelerated in humans, animals, and agriculture. Meanwhile, the restricted use of new antimicrobials as 'reserve' agents – although it may help to slow the emergence of resistance – means that there are disencentives to (profit-motivated) research and development of new antimicrobials. For this and other reasons, few new antibiotic classes or agents have been developed in recent decades (Norrby et al. 2005). Boosting more relevant research and development may thus require more public effort/funding and/or realignment of pharmaceutical companies' incentive structures (i.e. so that profit making becomes more compatible with developing products that are most important to global public health) (Banerjee et al. 2010).

New drugs (or other means of treatment/prevention) are arguably most urgently needed for infections that have become nearly pan-resistant (e.g. extensively drug-resistant TB, or multi-resistant gram negative bacteria). Vis-à-vis other responses that target particular causal pathways (e.g. restrictions on prescriptions practices or agricultural use) they would provide a cross-cutting solution to the problem of drug resistance – i.e. addressing the problem regardless of the specific mechanisms by which it was brought about.

It is clear, however, that policymakers (and, indeed, patients) cannot rely on new drugs to 'fix' the problem(s) of drug resistance, since (i) the development of new antimicrobial drugs has, in recent decades, been slow and/or relatively unsuccessful, (ii) the challenges underlying difficulties with drug development have thus far proven difficult to overcome, and (iii) without other interventions to curb the increase in drug resistance, we face a never-ending problem of finding new drugs. Thus, drug resistance requires a multi-faceted and global policy response – yet one that is also tailored to the specific problems and mechanisms of resistance in a given microbe and a given context.

Researchand Surveillance

Apart from finding new treatments, other kinds of research are urgently needed, including empirical research in diagnostics, microbiology, vaccines (and other non-drug interventions), as well as social science and public health systems research (Dar et al. 2016). As a starting point, there are large gaps in our knowledge of the epidemiology of most resistant pathogens. Improving local and international public health surveillance would help to determine the impact of various resistance mechanisms and evaluate the cost-effectiveness of interventions. Yet this, in turn, requires development of cost-effective and publically acceptable surveillance mechanisms that can be more widely implemented, including in LMICs, and political and scientific agreement on which data will be collected and shared (Tacconelli et al. 2017). It also requires careful attention to the ethical conduct of public health surveillance (World Health Organisation 2017b).

Reducing Use in Humans

There is an urgent need to reduce antibiotic use in human patients. The most ethically straightforward cases are those in which a person is prescribed (or purchases without prescription) an antibiotic (with a risk of side-effects and resistance) for a condition for which it will provide no benefit (e.g. a viral illness) or where a shorter course of antibiotics is as effective as a longer course but the latter confers an increased risk of resistance and/or side-effects. In such cases, antibiotic use constitutes a net harm to the individual and, through the risk of transmission of resistant organisms, to others.

One strategy to reduce use is to develop new diagnostics, so that patients and doctors can avoid using antibiotics where they are not required. But in the absence of perfect tests, changes in professional and public culture are also required. For example, doctors should address their own cognitive biases (see Chap. 8) as well as patient concerns about avoiding the complications of infection, and public awareness campaigns must emphasize that antibiotics are often not required and can themselves entail significant risk (to individuals and public health) (World Health Organisation 2015). International data suggest that some countries have made significant progress in reducing antibiotic use without a significant increase in severe infections (Bronzwaer et al. 2002).

Yet, as effective antibiotics become more and more scarce, there are more difficult ethical tradeoffs to be considered, involving greater uncertainty. For example, if antibiotics become reserved for severe and/or complicated infections – so that use is banned or dramatically reduced for patients with simple infections – many patients with a simple bacterial infection (e.g. mild pneumonia) may end up being more unwell for longer, or even at a small risk of severe outcomes (even though the vast majority will ultimately recover without specific curative treatment), because they do not have access to antibiotics.

Policy to reduce use in either the low risk or the higher risk cases cannot rely entirely on individuals, since the structure of the underlying collective action problem leads to strong incentives to 'free-ride' on others' reduction in use. Thus, some form of regulation is required – e.g. through antimicrobial stewardship (which has been a successful but resource intensive approach in healthcare institutions), and/or restrictions on physician prescribing. How best to design and enforce such regulation is an important matter for debate in public health ethics.

Reducing Use in Animals and Agriculture

As argued in later chapters of this volume (see Chaps. 7 and 18), antibiotic use and overuse in agriculture must also be reduced. First and foremost, many have argued that the widespread use in animals of agents that are critical to human health should be dramatically reduced and/or prohibited, especially when such agents are employed for non-therapeutic purposes (e.g. as 'growth promoters') (Marshall and Levy 2011; World Health Organisation 2017c). But even other drugs (and non-drug agents) may lead to the co-selection of resistance determinants for critical drugs among bacteria (and fungi) shared between animals and humans. The overuse of antibiotics in agriculture in part represents a palliative for the high rates of infection in crowded 'factory farms', suggesting that reforming farming practices would have the dual benefits of reducing animal cruelty and reducing drug resistant infections. Reducing or eliminating meat consumption would also obviate many of the dangers to humans of resistance in animals (although not all, since companion animals can also transmit drug-resistant infection (Guardabassi et al. 2004)). The fact that some wealthy countries have dramatically reduced or eliminated profligate antibiotic use in farm animals (in part by giving animals more space and improving infection control practices) often at little or no long term economic cost suggests that it is possible to minimise this driver of drug resistance (McEwen et al. 2018). Whether such practices will be successfully implemented in lower income countries remains to be seen (Dar et al. 2016).

Addressing Social Determinants of Health

Infectious diseases, in general, are more prevalent among poor people and communities in both high and low-income countries. Many aspects of social organization and the built environment (water and sanitation systems, health systems, etc.) alter the risk of acquiring infection, and the risk of transmission of resistance mechanisms. Historically, improvements in living conditions arguably contributed more to the decline in infectious diseases in developed/industrialised countries than discoveries of vaccines or antimicrobial treatments (McKeown 1976). One way of reducing the prevalence of drug resistant infection would be to reduce its incidence and transmission by addressing these (and other) such social determinants of health.

The rise of untreatable infections provides a new, and urgent, rationale to ensure universal access to the social conditions that enable healthy living. Even basic measures, especially if provided to all, could help minimize the transmission of resistance (e.g. by providing access to clean water and sanitation) and reduce the use of antimicrobial drugs (e.g. by providing access to high quality, and well-regulated, health systems). Since resistant infections routinely spread via international travel, wealthy nations have reasons not only to act locally but also to act globally by assisting others with less resources (see Chap. 21) – to reduce the incidence and international transmission of resistant infection (Selgelid 2008).

Infection Control

Infection control involves measures that aim to reduce the transmission of pathogens in an institution or community. In healthcare institutions, this typically involves screening of patients, monitoring of those carrying (and/or suffering disease from) resistant pathogens, use of personal protective equipment, and social distancing measures such as isolation and quarantine. In some cases, it also involves decolonization of patients. Methicillin-resistant *Staphylococcus aureus* (MRSA) decolonization, for example, involves the use of antibacterial solutions on the skin, hair, and nasal membranes. More dramatically, recent studies have reported successful use of faecal transplantation to decolonize those with highly resistant bowel organisms (Freedman and Eppes 2014; Crum-Cianflone et al. 2015). In many cases, screening for resistant pathogens in hospital does not involve/require informed consent of patients, on the grounds that screening and control measures are required in order to prevent harm to others. Such policies should nonetheless be based upon careful ethical justification as well as, where possible, evidence of cost-effectiveness (see Chap. 6), especially insofar as they infringe on the lives of individual carriers (who may or may not be symptomatic) in significant ways (see Chap. 13).

Infection control policies become more complex when they are applied in the general community. As more people in the community are identified as carriers of highly resistant pathogens, it remains to be seen what kinds of restrictions of individual liberty would or shoud be considered justifiable. When, if ever, for example, should travellers be screened on arrival from high-risk regions – and when should those who test positive for resistant organisms be offered (or required to have) decolonization – and/or be subject to monitoring and/or social distancing measures? Important questions such as these need to be considered (and re-evaluated) as more is learned about community and international transmission of drug-resistant organisms.

Vaccines

Vaccines are a cross-cutting intervention with the potential to obviate the need to prescribe antimicrobials for a range of pathogens. In some cases, furthermore, vaccines can prevent infections that would otherwise be untreatable/uncurable (e.g., due to high levels of drug resistance). Existing vaccines against tuberculosis and some bacterial infections (e.g. *Streptococcus pneumoniae, Haemophilus influenzae*) reduce the incidence of infections due to these pathogens and thereby reduce the use of relevant antimicrobials (Dar et al. 2016). Vaccines against specific resistant strains may also lead to their replacement (e.g. in a given ecological niche in the human body) by strains that are easier to treat (Dar et al. 2016), although longitudinal surveillance data regarding strain epidemiology and disease burden are needed to confirm whether such effects lead to a long-term net public health benefit.

Even effective vaccines against viral infections (e.g. influenza, common cold viruses) can lead to a marked reduction in antibiotic use since viral infections are often erroneously treated with antibiotics (Neuzil et al. 2000). New vaccines against malaria and typhoid may help to reduce antimicrobial use and resistance relevant to these pathogens. Because there is a great number of resistant pathogens for which we lack vaccines, however, this is an important area in need of further research and development.

Of course, discovering an effective vaccine may lead to the replacement of one collective action problem (antimicrobial overuse) with another (assuring high vaccination rates) – meaning that even this 'technical fix' would have limitations. Like the development of new drugs, in any case, new vaccines would form only one part of the multi-pronged approach needed to control the problem of drug resistance.

Conclusions

Drug-resistance is widely recognised to be one of the greatest threats to global public health in the coming decades. Its causes are complex, and more work is needed to determine the relative importance of different causes. The consequences for human health are already highly significant, and, if left unchecked, will be even more dramatic in the near future. These harms, taken together, represent a large, likely underestimated, and ethically salient burden of disease that disproportionately affects underprivileged people and communities worldwide. Yet the presence of untreatable and potentially fatal pathogens and the prospect of such infections becoming more common is a threat to all. Despite current uncertainties and urgent gaps in our knowledge regarding drug-resistant infection, there is a pressing need to develop and implement ethically informed policies to reduce rising levels of resistance and thereby mitigate or avert future harms and injustices. We hope that the subsequent chapters of this volume will make a significant contribution to this important area of public health ethics.

References

Banerjee, A., A. Hollis, and T. Pogge. 2010. The Health Impact Fund: Incentives for improving access to medicines. *The Lancet* 375 (9709): 166–169.

Birgand, G., L.S.P. Moore, C. Bourigault, V. Vella, D. Lepelletier, A.H. Holmes, et al. 2016. Measures to eradicate multidrug-resistant organism outbreaks: How much do they cost? *Clinical Microbiology and Infection* 22 (2): 162.e1–162.e9.

Bronzwaer, S.L.A.M., O. Cars, U. Buchholz, S. Mölstad, W. Goettsch, I.K. Veldhuijzen, et al. 2002. The relationship between antimicrobial use and antimicrobial resistance in Europe. *Emerging Infectious Diseases* 8 (3): 278.

Bryce, A., A.D. Hay, I.F. Lane, H.V. Thornton, M. Wootton, and C. Costelloe. 2016. Global prevalence of antibiotic resistance in paediatric urinary tract infections caused by Escherichia coli

and association with routine use of antibiotics in primary care: Systematic review and meta-analysis. *BMJ* 352: i939.
Carlet, J. 2012. The gut is the epicentre of antibiotic resistance. *Antimicrobial Resistance and Infection Control* 1 (1): 39.
Chang, Q., W. Wang, G. Regev-Yochay, M. Lipsitch, and W.P. Hanage. 2015. Antibiotics in agriculture and the risk to human health: How worried should we be? *Evolutionary Applications* 8 (3): 240–247.
Crum-Cianflone, N.F., E. Sullivan, and G. Ballon-Landa. 2015. Fecal microbiota transplantation and successful resolution of multidrug-resistant-organism colonization. *Journal of Clinical Microbiology* 53 (6): 1986–1989.
D'Costa, V.M., C.E. King, L. Kalan, M. Morar, W.W.L. Sung, C. Schwarz, et al. 2011. Antibiotic resistance is ancient. *Nature* 477 (7365): 457–461.
Dar, O.A., R. Hasan, J. Schlundt, S. Harbarth, G. Caleo, F.K. Dar, et al. 2016. Exploring the evidence base for national and regional policy interventions to combat resistance. *The Lancet* 387 (10015): 285–295.
Fairchild, A.L., and R. Bayer. 2004. Ethics and the conduct of public health surveillance. *Science* 303 (5658): 631–632.
Fleming A. 1945. *Penicillin. Nobel Prize lecture*.
Freedman, A., and S. Eppes. 2014. 1805 use of stool transplant to clear fecal colonization with Carbapenem-Resistant Enterobacteraciae (CRE): Proof of concept. *Open Forum Infectious Diseases* 1 (Suppl 1): S65. Oxford University Press.
Guardabassi, L., S. Schwarz, and D.H. Lloyd. 2004. Pet animals as reservoirs of antimicrobial-resistant bacteria Review. *Journal of Antimicrobial Chemotherapy* 54 (2): 321–332.
Guh, A.Y., S.N. Bulens, Y. Mu, J.T. Jacob, J. Reno, J. Scott, et al. 2015. Epidemiology of carbapenem-resistant enterobacteriaceae in 7 US communities, 2012–2013. *JAMA* 314 (14): 1479–1487.
Hardin, G. 2009. The tragedy of the commons. *Journal of Natural Resources Policy Research* 1 (3): 243–253.
Holmes, A.H., L.S.P. Moore, A. Sundsfjord, M. Steinbakk, S. Regmi, A. Karkey, et al. 2016. Understanding the mechanisms and drivers of antimicrobial resistance. *The Lancet* 387 (10014): 176–187.
Honigsbaum, M. 2016. Antibiotic antagonist: The curious career of René Dubos. *The Lancet* 387 (10014): 118–119.
Houston, S., and A. Houston. 2015. Screening and treating UN peacekeepers to prevent the introduction of Artemisinin-resistant malaria into Africa. *PLoS Medicine* 12 (5): e1001822.
Jamrozik, E, and M.J. Selgelid. 2019. Surveillance and control of asymptomatic carriers of drug-resistant bacteria. *Bioethics* 33 (7): 766–775.
Kennedy, K., and P. Collignon. 2010. Colonisation with Escherichia coli resistant to "critically important" antibiotics: A high risk for international travellers. *European Journal of Clinical Microbiology & Infectious diseases* 29 (12): 1501–1506.
Laxminarayan, R., P. Matsoso, S. Pant, C. Brower, J.-A. Røttingen, K. Klugman, et al. 2016. Access to effective antimicrobials: A worldwide challenge. *The Lancet* 387 (10014): 168–175.
Lerner, A., A. Adler, J. Abu-Hanna, S.C. Percia, M.K. Matalon, and Y. Carmeli. 2015. Spread of KPC-producing carbapenem-resistant Enterobacteriaceae: The importance of super-spreaders and rectal KPC concentration. *Clinical Microbiology and Infection* 21 (5): 470.e1–470.e7.
Llewelyn, M.J., J.M. Fitzpatrick, E. Darwin, C. Gorton, J. Paul, T.E.A. Peto, et al. 2017. The antibiotic course has had its day. *BMJ* 358: j3418.
Marshall, B.M., and S.B. Levy. 2011. Food animals and antimicrobials: Impacts on human health. *Clinical Microbiology Reviews* 24 (4): 718–733.
Martinez, J.L. 2009. Environmental pollution by antibiotics and by antibiotic resistance determinants. *Environmental Pollution* 157 (11): 2893–2902.
McEwen, S.A., F.J. Angulo, P.J. Collignon, and J.M. Conly. 2018. Unintended consequences associated with national-level restrictions on antimicrobial use in food-producing animals. *The Lancet Planetary Health* 2 (7): e279–ee82.

McKeown, T. 1976. *The role of medicine: Dream, mirage, or nemesis?* Princeton: Princeton University Press.

Morgan, D.J., R.P. Wenzel, and G. Bearman. 2017. Contact precautions for endemic MRSA and VRE: Time to retire legal mandates. *JAMA* 318 (4): 329–330.

Nasrin, D., P.J. Collignon, L. Roberts, E.J. Wilson, L.S. Pilotto, and R.M. Douglas. 2002. Effect of βlactam antibiotic use in children on pneumococcal resistance to penicillin: Prospective cohort study. *BMJ* 324 (7328): 28.

Neuzil, K.M., B.G. Mellen, P.F. Wright, E.F. Mitchel Jr., and M.R. Griffin. 2000. The effect of influenza on hospitalizations, outpatient visits, and courses of antibiotics in children. *New England Journal of Medicine* 342 (4): 225–231.

Norrby, S.R., C.E. Nord, and R. Finch. 2005. Lack of development of new antimicrobial drugs: A potential serious threat to public health. *The Lancet Infectious Diseases* 5 (2): 115–119.

O'Neill, J. 2015. Antimicrobial resistance: Tackling a crisis for the health and wealth of nations. In *The review on antimicrobial resistance*. Chaired by Jim O'Neill. December, 2014.

Östholm-Balkhed, Å., M. Tärnberg, M. Nilsson, L.E. Nilsson, H. Hanberger, A. Hällgren, et al. 2013. Travel-associated faecal colonization with ESBL-producing Enterobacteriaceae: Incidence and risk factors. *Journal of Antimicrobial Chemotherapy* 68 (9): 2144–2153.

Pruden, A., D.G.J. Larsson, A. Amézquita, P. Collignon, K.K. Brandt, D.W. Graham, et al. 2013. Management options for reducing the release of antibiotics and antibiotic resistance genes to the environment. *Environmental Health Perspectives* 121 (8): 878.

Rump, B., M. De Boer, R. Reis, M. Wassenberg, and J. Van Steenbergen. 2017. Signs of stigma and poor mental health among carriers of MRSA. *Journal of Hospital Infection* 95 (3): 268–274.

Safdar, N., and E.A. Bradley. 2008. The risk of infection after nasal colonization with Staphylococcus aureus. *The American Journal of Medicine* 121 (4): 310–315.

Schwaber, M.J., B. Lev, A. Israeli, E. Solter, G. Smollan, B. Rubinovitch, et al. 2011. Containment of a country-wide outbreak of carbapenem-resistant Klebsiella pneumoniae in Israeli hospitals via a nationally implemented intervention. *Clinical Infectious Diseases* 52 (7): 848–855.

Selgelid, M.J. 2008. Improving global health: Counting reasons why. *Developing World Bioethics* 8 (2): 115–125.

Smith, D.L., J. Dushoff, E.N. Perencevich, A.D. Harris, and S.A. Levin. 2004. Persistent colonization and the spread of antibiotic resistance in nosocomial pathogens: Resistance is a regional problem. *Proceedings of the National Academy of Sciences of the United States of America* 101 (10): 3709–3714.

Tacconelli, E., F. Sifakis, S. Harbarth, R. Schrijver, M. van Mourik, A. Voss, et al. 2017. Surveillance for control of antimicrobial resistance. *The Lancet Infectious Diseases*.

Tischendorf, J., R.A. de Avila, and N. Safdar. 2016. Risk of infection following colonization with carbapenem-resistant Enterobactericeae: A systematic review. *American Journal of Infection Control* 44 (5): 539–543.

Viens, A.M., C.M. Bensimon, and R.E.G. Upshur. 2009. Your liberty or your life: Reciprocity in the use of restrictive measures in contexts of contagion. *Journal of Bioethical Inquiry* 6 (2): 207–217.

White, N.J. 2017. Does antimalarial mass drug administration increase or decrease the risk of resistance? *The Lancet Infectious Diseases* 17 (1): e15–e20.

World Health Organisation. 2015. *Antibiotic resistance: Multi-country public awareness survey*. Geneva: WHO.

———. 2017a. *Ethics guidance for the implementation of the end TB strategy*. Geneva: WHO.

———. 2017b. *WHO guidelines on ethical issues in public health surveillance*. Geneva: WHO.

———. 2017c. *WHO guidelines on use of medically important antimicrobials in food-producing animals*. Geneva: WHO.

13

The Virtuous Physician and Antimicrobial Prescribing Policy and Practice

Justin Oakley

Abstract In this chapter, I outline some key patient-centred medical virtues and several community-centred medical virtues, and I consider what sorts of antimicrobial prescribing decisions such virtues would lead physicians to make. I argue that practically-intelligent virtuous physicians should also have an awareness of the sorts of cognitive biases that are especially likely to distort their antimicrobial prescribing decisions, and I urge physicians to develop ways of avoiding or counteracting such biases. Further, I argue that effectively addressing the impact of these biases and other countervailing factors that inhibit virtuous prescribing practices is the responsibility not only of individual physicians, but also of institutions and regulators. I outline some strategies that individual physicians, institutions, and healthcare policymakers could develop to help physicians hit the targets of those patient-centred and community-centred medical virtues, and to thereby play their part in redressing the problems of antimicrobial resistance.

Keywords Medical virtue · Practical intelligence · Justice · Antibiotic overprescribing · Cognitive bias

The detrimental health impact of antimicrobial resistance raises significant questions about physicians' antimicrobial prescribing decisions, so it is important to investigate what sorts of prescribing decisions about antimicrobials would be made by a virtuous physician in various contexts. Antimicrobial resistance has become a

---

An earlier version of this chapter was presented at the 2018 Effective Altruism Global Conference, Melbourne, where I received some helpful comments on this chapter. I also received some useful feedback on these ideas in medical ethics seminars at Monash University, and I thank students at these seminars for this. I am very grateful to Zeb Jamrozik for his resourcefulness and his excellent suggestions about relevant sources, and I wish to thank Michael Selgelid and Zeb for their invaluable advice with this chapter.

J. Oakley (✉)
Monash Bioethics Centre, Monash University, Melbourne, VIC, Australia
e-mail: justin.oakley@monash.edu

major global health concern, as the resistance of disease-causing microorganisms to antimicrobials can completely undermine the effectiveness of many antibiotics and other antimicrobials that are commonly used to treat a variety of diseases, and to lower the risks of post-surgical infections. The dwindling effectiveness of many antimicrobials has been implicated in a growing number of patient deaths worldwide, often from conditions such as respiratory and wound infections which had previously been responsive to antimicrobial treatments. Addressing what sorts of antimicrobial prescribing decisions a virtuous physician would make seems especially challenging for virtue ethics approaches to medical practice. For such approaches typically evaluate physician decision-making by reference to patient-centred role virtues like medical beneficence, medical courage, and trustworthiness, but tend to say little about broader medical virtues that help physicians act in the best health interests of the community, which is a crucial consideration in ethically justifiable clinician decision-making regarding antimicrobials.

In this chapter, I discuss some key patient-centred medical virtues and several candidate community-centred medical virtues, and I consider what sorts of antimicrobial prescribing decisions such virtues would lead physicians to make. I draw out the moral significance of these community-centred medical virtues by examining certain cases where prescribing an antimicrobial seems likely to be in the best interests of the patient in question, but seems unlikely to be in the best health interests of the community overall. In doing so, I consider some analogies with other sorts of cases involving seemingly divergent virtue directives, such as those involving psychiatrists breaching patient confidentiality to protect third parties from harm. Also, I argue that practically-intelligent virtuous physicians should have an awareness of the sorts of cognitive biases that are especially likely to distort their antimicrobial prescribing decisions, and I urge physicians to develop ways of avoiding or counteracting such biases. Further, effectively addressing the impact of these biases and other countervailing factors that inhibit virtuous prescribing practices is, I argue, the responsibility not only of individual physicians, but also of institutions and regulators. Therefore, I also consider the prospects of certain institutional and regulatory initiatives which aim to reduce antimicrobial over-prescribing by highlighting and undermining such biases in clinical practice.

Antimicrobial Resistance and Virtue Ethics

Rising global concerns about antimicrobial resistance has prompted many national and international agencies, professional medical associations, and policymakers to investigate what sorts of factors are contributing to this problem, and to the resulting significant increases in morbidity and mortality rates of certain diseases in many countries around the world. The accelerating resistance of microorganisms to antibiotics and other antimicrobial agents commonly used in medical treatment has substantially reduced – and at times entirely removed – effective microbial treatment options for some patients with serious conditions such as pneumonia, tuberculosis, or septicaemia, and a number of those patients have subsequently died. Further, antibiotic-resistant 'superbugs' like methicillin-resistant staphylococcus aureus (MRSA) have been found in significant quantities in some of the world's major hospitals, and many patients worldwide have died from hospital-acquired MRSA infections.[1] Antimicrobial resistance is a major problem in high-income countries and also in low- and middle-income countries. For example, China has the world's highest prevalence of MRSA, and this bacterium is associated with higher mortality rates for hospitalised patients there.[2] Also, the prevalence of multi-drug resistant tuberculosis is relatively high in countries such as India and Russia – it has recently been predicted that 12.4% of all cases of TB will soon be multi-drug resistant in India, and that 32.5% of all cases of TB will soon be multi-drug resistant in Russia.[3] It has also been reported that over 50% of microorganisms involved in hospital-acquired infections in Greece seem to be resistant to *all* available antibiotics.[4] Effective antimicrobial treatments have therefore become a somewhat scarce resource in clinical practice in a number of contexts, and many countries have now introduced new government regulations and clinical guidelines aimed at encouraging more responsible use and stewardship of antimicrobials. While antibiotics are one among several antimicrobial agents, I will focus here on the prescription of antibiotics, as inappropriate antibiotic prescribing appears to be a major contributor to antimicrobial resistance, which is why many of the efforts to improve antimicrobial prescribing practices are directed at antibiotic prescribing in particular.

This accelerating growth in antimicrobial resistance is due to a range of factors, including widespread farming practices, patient misuse of antimicrobials, and inappropriate antimicrobial prescribing practices by physicians. These contributing factors are now being targeted by a range of initiatives from government agencies, national and international medical and health care organisations, and at the level of hospital management. Thus, the WHO recently modified its longstanding *Essential Medicines List* by introducing recommendations that prioritise the use of some antibiotics over others in certain contexts – for example, the list recommends that amoxicillin be made widely available to treat common infections, such as pneumonia, but that other antibiotics should be reserved for use as a last resort when a life-threatening infection has failed to respond to other antibiotics.[5] And the clinical practice guidelines about antibiotic prescribing in Australia's *Therapeutic Guidelines: Antibiotic* also encourage the responsible use by clinicians of antibiotics in treating a wide variety of conditions, and thus discourage the over-prescribing of antibiotics.[6] However, questions have arisen about the effectiveness of clinical

---

[1] Staphylococcus aureus already exist in (e.g.) our respiratory tract, and some of those bacteria will already be antimicrobial-resistant, but antibiotic treatment allows those antimicrobial resistant S. aureus to potentially multiply.

[2] See Dan Cui et al. (2017), and Zhenjiang Yao et al. (2015).

[3] Aditya Sharma et al. (2017).

[4] Stavros Saripanidas (2016).

[5] See http://www.who.int/mediacentre/news/releases/2017/essential-medicines-list/en/.

[6] Antibiotic Expert Groups (2019).

guidelines aimed at improving antibiotic prescribing. For example, a recent Australian study concluded that "Antibiotics are prescribed for ARIs [acute respiratory infections] at rates 4–9 times as high as those recommended by clinical guidelines. The potential for reducing rates of antibiotic prescription and to thereby reduce rates of antibiotic-related harms, particularly bacterial resistance, is therefore substantial."[7] Physician decision-making in relation to antibiotics has thus been identified as a major contributor to the problem of antimicrobial resistance,[8] and so this remains a promising context on which to focus in developing effective ways of redressing this problem. In this chapter, therefore, I concentrate on the antimicrobial prescribing behaviour of physicians, and on what would plausibly be required of a virtuous physician in regard to antimicrobial prescribing.

The emphasis in virtue ethics on the character and moral psychology of virtuous agents have led some to regard this approach as excessively individualistic, and so it might be wondered whether virtue ethics is capable of providing useful guidance on addressing antimicrobial resistance, which is a complex multi-dimensional problem on an international scale. However, as noted above, physician prescribing behaviour is a major contributing factor to antimicrobial resistance, and so to this extent, focusing on what decisions a virtuous physician would make in relation to the prescription of antimicrobials would seem to offer a promising line of response to this problem. Further, recent empirically-informed accounts of the Aristotelian idea of practical intelligence (*phronesis*) emphasise the importance of agents being aware of, and having strategies to counteract, common decision-making biases that can divert their virtuous dispositions from hitting the target of the relevant virtue.[9] Physicians are evidently not immune from such biases,[10] and these biases may well contribute to physicians' inappropriate antimicrobial prescribing in certain sorts of cases.[11] So applying recent empirically-informed accounts of virtues and practical intelligence to physicians' roles and to their antimicrobial prescribing behaviour would seem to be a useful way of approaching the problems of antimicrobial resistance.

Generally speaking, virtue ethics evaluates actions by asking, 'what sort of person would do a thing like that?' For example, we can ask whether an action was generous or mean-spirited, courageous or cowardly, and we can examine whether this is the sort of thing which a kind person or a just person would do in the circumstances. Virtue ethics can therefore draw upon such considerations to provide the elements of a criterion of right action. A virtue ethics criterion of right action can be

---

[7] Amanda R. McCullough et al. (2017).

[8] See e.g. the US Centers for Disease Control and Prevention statement, 'About Antimicrobial Resistance': "The use of antibiotics is the single most important factor leading to antibiotic resistance around the world. Simply using antibiotics creates resistance. These drugs should only be used to manage infections." https://www.cdc.gov/drugresistance/about.html. [accessed 1 November 2018].

[9] See Justin Oakley (2018a, b).

[10] See Blumenthal-Barby and Krieger (2015) and Saposnik et al. (2016).

[11] See e.g. Jeffrey et al. (2014).

stated initially in broad terms as holding that: An action is right if, and only if, it is what an agent with a virtuous character would do in the circumstances.[12] Virtue ethicists have also applied such an appeal to exemplars in developing accounts of right action in the context of various professional roles, such as medical and legal practice. An influential version of these accounts highlights links between the proper goal/s of the profession in question – such as health and justice for medicine and law, respectively – and an Aristotelian conception of human flourishing, or *eudaimonia*. The proper goal/s of a profession can, in turn, provide the basis for an account of the role virtues for that profession. Thus in the case of medical practice, the role virtues for doctors can be understood as those character traits that enable doctors to serve the goal of health. These traits have been thought to include patient-centred dispositions such as medical beneficence, medical courage, and trustworthiness, along with community-centred dispositions such as justice.[13]

Medical Virtues and Antimicrobial Prescribing

We saw in the previous section that inappropriate prescribing decisions by physicians in relation to antibiotics is highlighted as one of the most important contributing factors to antimicrobial resistance and its resulting problems. Physicians in many countries are evidently over-prescribing antibiotics, and for a variety of conditions. For example, a recent study by Katherine Fleming-Dutra and colleagues found that during 2010–2011 physicians in US clinics prescribed antibiotics for acute respiratory infections at double the rates that were clinically appropriate for such infections – in other words, around half of those antibiotic prescriptions were clinically inappropriate.[14] Also, the 2018 national survey of antimicrobial prescribing practices in Australian hospitals found that 21.4% of antimicrobials prescribed during that year were classified as inappropriate prescriptions.[15] And a recent study using survey data from 2010–2015 on antibiotic prescribing rates in general practice found that Australian GPs are prescribing antibiotics for acute respiratory infections at rates up to nine times higher than those recommended by the national *Therapeutic Guidelines: Antibiotic*. These researchers found, for example, that "Despite the recommendation in these guidelines against prescribing antibiotics for bronchitis, general practitioners were estimated to have prescribed antibiotics for patients with bronchitis in 85% of cases during 2010–2015".[16] A subsequent interview with study co-author Chris Del Mar reported that he felt "doctors were acting out of a misplaced sense of caution, as many conditions requiring treatment with antibiotics

[12] Rosalind Hursthouse (1999).

[13] See e.g. Justin Oakley and Dean Cocking (2001).

[14] Katherine E. Fleming-Dutra et al. (2016).

[15] Australian Commission on Safety and Quality in Health Care (2020).

[16] McCullough et al. (2017), op. cit., p. 68.

share similar symptoms to those that do not.... doctors needed to stop considering a prescription for antibiotics as their first port of call. 'The idea that we have as GPs, that writing a prescription for antibiotics just in case, is probably not so effective..., That in fact not using antibiotics at all is actually safe, you don't end up with missed cases of meningitis and Lemierre's disease – all sorts of really nasty things.'"[17]

Given that patients frequently request antibiotics for acute respiratory infections, and are usually keen to get better sooner, it is perhaps not surprising that there is a tendency among physicians in many countries to over-prescribe antibiotics for such infections in responding to such requests. But while yielding to patient pressure results in physicians over-prescribing antibiotics, there is also evidence that antibiotics are prescribed inappropriately because physicians overestimate patients' expectations of receiving these drugs. Thus, in a 1997 study of antibiotic prescribing decisions by UK General Practitioners, Macfarlane and colleagues found that "Non-clinical factors influence the decision to prescribe antibiotics for nearly a half of those receiving one. Patient pressure was cited most frequently...and identified by the Audit Commission as an important reason for the excess use of antibiotics in the community. Pressure from patients to prescribe antibiotics, particularly for respiratory symptoms, has been identified as the commonest reason for doctors' discomfort with prescribing decisions. General practitioners can, however, overestimate patients' expectations. A quarter of our patients received antibiotics when they stated that before the consultation they had not wanted antibiotics".[18] A survey of 544 patients of inner London general practitioners found further evidence that physicians are overly influenced by their perceptions of patients' hopes and expectations of receiving a medication prescription, and those perceptions frequently seemed to be inaccurate: "A third [31%] of the prescriptions [which were sometimes for antibiotics] written in this study were either not indicated or not hoped for, with 3% being neither indicated nor hoped for.... The writing of nonindicated prescriptions was primarily associated with the doctor's sense of feeling pressurised [by the patient to write a prescription]".[19] This survey also found that "In a fifth [22%] of consultations in which a prescription was written, the prescription was not strictly indicated on purely medical grounds".[20] Overall, the strongest influence on a physician's decision to prescribe a medication was found in this study to be the physician's perceptions of their patients' hopes and expectations about receiving that medication.

---

[17] Angus Randall (2017).

[18] John Macfarlane et al. (1997), p. 1213. There is also evidence that UK General Practitioners have overestimated patients' expectations of receiving a prescription, not only in cases involving antibiotics, but also with other sorts of medication: see Nicky Britten (1995), p. 1084: "When general practitioners are surveyed they describe high levels of demand, but objective evidence consistently suggests that doctors overestimate patients' expectations. Reanalysis of published data shows that about a fifth of patients leave general practice consultations with prescriptions they did not expect."

[19] Nicky Britten and Obioha Ukoumunne (1997), p. 1509.

[20] Ibid, p. 1510.

In some of the above types of cases where physicians prescribe antibiotics inappropriately, they may well be acting from a beneficent motivation to serve the best interests of their patient in some way – particularly where, as mentioned above, physicians prescribe an antibiotic "just in case" the patient has a serious, albeit rare, type of infection where antibiotic treatment at that stage would likely benefit the patient in the longer-term. However, physicians are frequently in a position to accurately diagnose that a patient has the less serious condition of acute bronchitis, and to recognise that it is in the long-term best interests of such a patient not to be prescribed an antibiotic now.[21] Where physicians prescribing antibiotics are acting in misguided ways from motives of beneficence towards their patients, these cases can be usefully characterised as involving a failure of such motives to hit the target of the patient-centred virtue of medical beneficence.[22] Cognitive biases seem to be an important factor in explaining why physicians' beneficent motives can fail to hit the target of the virtue of medical beneficence in their prescribing decisions. An illuminating recent study of Australian GP trainees (registrars) describes their decision-making processes in deciding whether or not to prescribe an antibiotic for the patient. A number of these registrars explained that, while they realised prescribing an antibiotic was often not in the patient's best interests, and that it was important to avoid antibiotic over-prescribing, the registrars indicated how they rationalised prescribing an antibiotic in certain cases – for instance, telling themselves that it was in the patient's best interests to receive an antibiotic. The study found that: "Many registrars were concerned about patient safety and avoiding subsequent hospital presentations [for example, one registrar said]: *'I tend to probably cover things a bit more because…if something goes wrong I want to make sure that the patient is going to be safe.' (Registrar 9)*".[23] In certain cases this seems to be an overly cautious approach, which may indicate that a registrar is unduly influenced by the well-known 'framing effect', whereby possible losses loom larger to the agent than do possible gains.[24] The researchers also mentioned that: "Barriers to evidence-based prescribing included role-modelling outdated practices, or setting a precedent of

---

[21] See McCullough et al., op. cit. For a useful systematic review of studies on how individuals treated with an antibiotic for respiratory and urinary infections can subsequently develop a higher level of bacterial resistance to that antibiotic for several months, see Céire Costelloe et al. (2010).

[22] Christine Swanton emphasizes the importance of virtues 'hitting the target' of the contextually-relevant virtue, and she discusses various examples of candidate virtues that fail to hit their target (see Christine Swanton 2003). Similarly, Dean Cocking and I have argued that each virtue involves being guided by a 'regulative ideal': "To say that an agent has a regulative ideal is to say that they have internalised a certain conception of correctness or excellence, in such a way that they are able to adjust their motivation and conduct so that it conforms – or at least does not conflict – with that standard" (Oakley and Cocking 2001, op. cit., p. 25).

[23] Anthea Dallas et al. (2014), p. e564. While antibiotic over-prescribing seemed due in part to certain cognitive biases in the registrars, "many registrars described a dissonance between their attitudes to guidelines and their prescribing behaviours, producing dissatisfaction with their own prescribing…: *'There's probably been times where I've given them the script and kind of felt a bit disappointed in myself afterwards.'(Registrar 14)"* p. e563.

[24] See Amos Tversky and Daniel Kahneman (1981).

prescribing that created patient expectations and pressure on the registrar: *'I do know one supervisor in particular will give his patients antibiotics even for something that sounds very viral, and therefore when I see his patients, I feel I'm expected to do that as well, because his patients have been seeing him for many years. So they expect it too, so I'm definitely more likely to give his patients antibiotics even when I don't think it's justified.'"(Registrar 10)*[25] This sort of approach may manifest a form of 'authority bias', whereby the registrar shows undue deference towards the antibiotic prescribing practices of his or her clinical supervisor.[26]

According to some influential recent empirically-informed accounts of virtue and virtue ethics, acting virtuously requires (among other things) agents to employ certain deliberative strategies to counteract common decision-making biases and other countervailing factors which can impede virtuous actions. These accounts develop a comprehensive conception of virtuous character-traits, which include an awareness of situational factors that conduce to or inhibit virtuous behaviour.[27] The misguided beneficent efforts of those registrars who were (or could reasonably have been) aware that prescribing an antibiotic was not in their patient's best interests can be helpfully understood as failures to exercise the central Aristotelian virtue of *phronesis*, or practical intelligence, in this context.[28] Broadly speaking, *phronesis* is an overarching normative disposition that regulates the more specific dispositions involved in particular virtues, to enable their more context-sensitive expression. Developing such practical intelligence can help well-motivated agents to avoid two potential deficiencies that can undermine their attempts to hit the target of the relevant virtue – i.e. moral ineptitude, and failures of meticulousness. Moral ineptitude is shown by agents who are well-intentioned but lack sufficient practical know-how or emotional intelligence to succeed in bringing about the good which they intend to bring about. Unmeticulous agents have the relevant practical know-how and emotional intelligence, but their efforts fall short as they do not apply strategies to circumvent decision-making biases (and similar countervailing factors) that are prevalent in the context.[29] Thus, the registrars who prescribed antibiotics against their patients' longer-term best interests failed to exercise the virtue of practical intelligence here, because the registrars were not sufficiently meticulous in preventing cognitive biases and other countervailing factors from undermining their efforts to make prescribing decisions in their patients' best interests.[30]

---

[25] Dallas et al., p. e565.

[26] The phenomenon of 'authority bias' was famously observed in Stanley Milgram's experiments on obedience to authority. See Stanley Milgram (2010).

[27] See e.g. Daniel C. Russell (2009), e.g. p. 140; Nancy E. Snow (2009), p. 563; and Nancy E. Snow (2010), especially her pp. 34–7 discussion of how people can effectively confront and combat any prejudices they might hold. These conceptions of virtue and virtue ethics have been developed in response to 'situationist' critiques of earlier accounts of virtue ethics.

[28] Aristotle (1980); and Russell (2009), op. cit.

[29] For further details about these executive failings, and their relevance to practical intelligence and medical virtues, see Oakley (2018b), op. cit. See also Oakley (2018a), op. cit.

[30] See also Daniel Russell's helpful discussion of how agents may ascertain the specific ends of virtuous actions, in: Daniel C. Russell (2015).

Indeed, there is evidence of other cognitive biases diverting physicians' prescribing decisions from patients' best interests. For example, a recent US study found that as the number of prescribing decisions made by each primary care physician increased through the morning and into the afternoon, each physician became more likely to issue an antibiotic prescription that was not in the patient's best interests. This study suggests that good prescribing behaviour can be undermined by a form of 'decision fatigue' (a phenomenon seen in many other contexts), which seemed to lead the physicians to become less able to resist providing inappropriate antibiotic prescriptions.[31] So, developing ways of effectively addressing these (and potentially other) cognitive biases that appear to be contributing to physicians prescribing antibiotics in cases where this is likely to be contrary to the patient's long-term best interests, would seem a promising strategy supported by an empirically-informed virtue ethics approach (and perhaps also by certain other ethical approaches) to the problems of antimicrobial resistance.

Community-Centred Medical Virtues and Antimicrobial Prescribing Practice and Policy

Virtue ethics approaches to medical practice have tended to focus predominantly on patient-centred virtues, such as medical beneficence and medical courage, which help an individual doctor serve well the best interests of their patients. But while it is important that these virtues correct any physician tendencies to make unreflective assumptions about what prescribing decisions are best for their patients, patient-centred virtues are not the only role virtues which are relevant to ethically justifiable prescribing behaviour and the problem of antimicrobial resistance. For the antimicrobial prescribing decisions by physicians have also contributed to broader community harms, such as the diminishing effectiveness of antibiotic treatments for other patients, and the scarcity of more expensive, last resort, antibiotics due to their increasing use as first-line treatments (and which have become unaffordable to patients in some countries). So, ethically responsible antibiotic prescribing practices by physicians must also take into account the broader effects that their prescribing decisions are likely to have on the community. The virtuous antimicrobial prescriber thus needs to take account of a wider moral universe, beyond that of the best interests of their own patients. They would therefore be guided in their antimicrobial prescribing decisions by community-centred medical virtues, such as justice and a readiness to serve the broader community, along with patient-centred virtues such as medical beneficence. The virtue of justice requires physicians to allocate fairly the medical resources under their control.[32] In Aristotelian terms, allocating

[31] Linder et al. (2014), op. cit.

[32] For a useful discussion of how medical benevolence should be constrained by the virtue of justice, see Roger Crisp (2015).

medical resources fairly (particularly when medical resources are scarce) can be understood as making allocation decisions in such a way as to provide each person who is affected by the decision an equal chance of developing and exercising their capabilities to live a flourishing human life. These capabilities include those elaborated in the *Nicomachean Ethics*, such as being able to understand the world, to engage in practical reasoning about our lives, and to form personal relationships with others.[33] The readiness to serve others is another community-centred medical virtue, which requires physicians to make their services broadly available to the community, and so (for example) to avoid picking and choosing their patients according to the physician's personal preferences. This virtue is plausibly understood as applying to physicians *qua* professionals, who ought to provide this readiness to serve the community in return for being granted a monopoly of expertise over the provision of key goods – i.e. those that serve patients' health.[34]

In the context of antimicrobial prescribing, the virtue of justice requires physicians to consider whether prescribing antibiotics for patients in certain circumstances is likely to detrimentally affect the availability of effective antibiotics for other patients, even if there are grounds for believing that an antibiotic prescription is likely to be of some benefit to the former patients. While it is plausible to believe that physicians often serve the health of the community best by making antibiotic prescribing decisions that are in the best interests of their own patients, there will be cases where these two goals come into conflict – because the community's interest in constraining antimicrobial resistance can sometimes be served best by the physician refraining from providing an antibiotic which may be of some benefit to their patient. Where the likely benefit to the patient in such conflict cases is only marginal, the virtue of justice will require a physician not to prescribe antibiotic treatment to their own patient. Of course, it is possible that justice could also sometimes require withholding from a patient an antibiotic that is likely to be of greater than marginal benefit – for instance, where there is only a single last-resort antibiotic available, and one patient is likely to derive much greater benefit from receiving this antibiotic than is another patient, then justice could arguably require that the first patient be provided with this antibiotic. (This is analogous to situations where justice can plausibly require the allocation of the only available ICU bed to a patient who is likely to benefit more from this resource than will another patient, even if this second patient may suffer considerable harm as a consequence.) In what follows, I will concentrate on the first kind of conflict cases.

Suppose a child presents to their physician with acute otitis media. Prescribing an antibiotic in such cases would appear likely to confer marginal benefits for the child – but as Collignon explains, "with an absolute reduction in pain in only 5%. Most cases resolve spontaneously. Seventeen children must be treated to prevent

---

[33] See the capabilities approach developed by Martha C. Nussbaum (2006). Nussbaum draws on Aristotle's view that "the form of government is best in which every man, whoever he is, can act best and live happily" (*Politics* 1324a23–5). See also Justin Oakley (1994); and Millar, M. (2020).

[34] This community-centred virtue becomes especially relevant in discussions of ethically justifiable limits on conscientious objection by physicians.

one child having some pain after two days. Antibiotics have no effect on hearing problems or other complications".[35] In these sorts of cases, despite the possible minor benefits of the child receiving an antibiotic, the detrimental impact which such patterns of antibiotic prescribing have on antimicrobial resistance in the broader community suggests that the virtue of justice would require physicians not to prescribe antibiotics in such cases, and to provide the child with other medication, to relieve their symptoms. The dictates of justice in these sorts of cases can be compared with what justice would plausibly require of psychiatrists deliberating about whether to breach patient confidentiality to protect third parties from harm. Where a patient confides to his or her psychiatrist a credible threat to significantly harm a third party, and the psychiatrist is able to take steps to see that the third party is warned about this threat, the virtue of justice plausibly requires the psychiatrist to take such steps in the interests of this third party.[36] While maintaining absolute patient confidentiality might sometimes be in the best interests of the patient involved, and so might be thought consistent with the virtue of medical beneficence, the overarching virtue of justice requires that confidentiality be breached here. (Indeed, in many such cases this course of action will not be contrary to the *virtue* of medical beneficence – for instance, where confiding such a threat is actually a 'cry for help' from the patient – even if beneficence provides some grounds for maintaining confidentiality here).

But while the virtue of justice and its concerns for the broader interests of the community can in certain circumstances require physicians to refrain from providing a patient with an antibiotic that is likely to benefit that patient, there is evidence that physicians relegate these broader interests to the periphery of their antibiotic prescribing decision-making. A 2002 US survey of 400 generalist physicians and 429 infectious diseases specialists found that: "The risk of contributing to the problem of antibiotic resistance was ranked lowest, overall and by generalists, and second lowest by ID specialists"[37] The researchers concluded that "…neither generalists nor infectious disease specialists emphasize the relative societal risks of antimicrobial drug selection in their treatment decisions for patients with community-acquired pneumonia. Instead, they emphasize providing the newest and best treatments for each individual patient even though this approach may not be supported by current guidelines or public health policy".[38] One explanation of the insufficient weight given by these doctors to the risk of generating antimicrobial resistance was an overconfidence that their own antibiotic prescribing decisions were unlikely to negatively impact on antimicrobial resistance. This can be seen as an example of the cognitive bias known as 'the overconfidence effect', whereby agents have greater confidence in their judgements than is warranted by the evidence. There is much

---

[35] Peter J. Collignon (2002), p. 328.

[36] See, for example, the much-discussed 1969 case of Tatiana Tarasoff, as described in Marilyn McMahon (1992), pp. 12–16.

[37] Joshua P. Metlay et al. (2002), p. 90.

[38] Ibid., p. 93.

evidence that physician decision-making can be distorted by an overconfidence bias, which is one of the most frequently studied biases in medical decision-making.[39] Further evidence that cognitive biases can lead physicians to give insufficient weight to their own contributions to antimicrobial resistance is provided in an illuminating recent survey of 889 US physicians, which indicated that they often lacked insight into the broader harms of their own antibiotic prescribing decisions. Most of the respondents expressed concern about the problem of antimicrobial resistance. However, the researchers found that: "While 62% of respondents agreed that other doctors overprescribe antibiotics, only 13% agreed that they themselves overprescribe antibiotics".[40] The researchers concluded that "While most respondents agreed that other doctors overprescribe antibiotics, a much smaller proportion (especially of faculty) felt that they themselves overprescribe".[41] This significant underestimation by physicians of the contribution that their own antibiotic prescribing decisions are likely having on the broader problems of antimicrobial resistance can be characterised as an example of confirmation bias, where an agent interprets information in a way that confirms a view that they already hold, regardless of whether this information actually supports or undermines that view.

Thus, cognitive biases also seem to be diverting physicians' community-centred dispositions to act in accordance with the virtue of justice from hitting its target, in the context of their antibiotic prescribing decisions. A promising way of addressing this problem is for physicians to develop various 'debiasing' strategies, which can help them carry out what justice requires of them here in more practically intelligent ways. For example, Ian Scott and colleagues suggest that physicians' awareness of their cognitive biases, and their ability to counteract the detrimental effects such biases can have on medical decision-making, can be enhanced by providing them with powerful narratives of patients who have been harmed (e.g. by antimicrobial resistance), and by reflective practice and role modelling.[42] But while the prescribing decisions of individual physicians are clearly a significant contributor to the problem of antimicrobial resistance, effectively addressing this problem goes well beyond the responsibility of each individual physician to 'smarten up' their own decision-making about antibiotic prescribing by strengthening their medical virtues on their own initiative. For these individual efforts must be complemented by the responsibilities of governments, international organisations, policymakers, and healthcare institutions to create institutional and regulatory environments which are conducive to physicians hitting the targets of the role virtues of medical beneficence and justice. For it can sometimes be difficult for physicians in their antibiotic prescribing behaviour to succeed in hitting the targets of the virtues of medical beneficence and justice, when they are working in contexts where they are frequently

[39] See Saposnik et al. (2016), op. cit. Overconfidence and availability bias are the two most frequently researched biases in medical decision making, and they appear to be highly prevalent in this context (though their precise prevalence levels here have not been determined).

[40] Lilian Abbo et al. (2011), p. 715.

[41] Ibid., p. 716.

[42] Ian A Scott et al. (2017). See also Ateev Mehrotra and Jeffrey A. Linder (2017).

confronted with patients' requests for antibiotics, in circumstances where prescribing an antibiotic would be clinically inappropriate.

A good example of such government efforts is the Australian '*Choosing Wisely*' initiative, which aims to reduce antibiotic overprescribing (and other forms of poor clinical practice) by providing patients and physicians with guidelines and specific examples of when medications such as antibiotics would be inappropriate. For instance, one such guideline advises against prescribing antibiotics for patients with uncomplicated acute bronchitis.[43] These guidelines and examples on the *Choosing Wisely* website encourage discussions between physicians and patients about the appropriateness or otherwise of such medications in the circumstances, and make the boundaries of good medical practice more transparent to patients and doctors. Similarly, the UK Behavioural Insights Team successfully reduced the overprescription of antibiotics by sending letters to GPs in practices with relatively high rates of antibiotic prescription, stating that "80% of practices in your local area prescribe fewer antibiotics per head than yours".[44] Providing these doctors with such benchmarking information helped nudge them to recognise and counteract their biases towards prescribing antibiotics, and thereby helped enable these doctors' medical dispositions to hit their proper targets.[45]

Also, a worthwhile institutional initiative here could be to address authority bias through the creation of 'safe spaces' for junior doctors to be able to anonymously report established practices of poor antibiotic prescribing, without necessarily jeopardising their professional relationships with consultants and senior physicians.

Conclusion

The antibiotic prescribing decisions made by physicians have clearly played a significant role in increasing antimicrobial resistance. Due to their monopoly of expertise in their professional roles, physicians are especially well-placed to be aware of, and to combat, the broader problems which certain sorts of antimicrobial prescribing decisions can result in. Virtuous physicians owe the community a readiness to serve it by taking steps to reduce – and hopefully eliminate altogether – antibiotic prescribing decisions that are contrary to the virtues of medical beneficence and justice. In this chapter, I have outlined some strategies that individual physicians, institutions, and healthcare policymakers can develop to help physicians to hit the targets of those virtues, and to thereby play their part in redressing the problems of antimicrobial resistance.

---

[43] See *Choosing Wisely Australia*, *https://www.choosingwisely.org.au/*.

[44] Michael Hallsworth et al. (2016). See also David Halpern (2015).

[45] See also Kiran Iyer (2017), and Fay Niker (2018).

References

Abbo, Lilian, et al. 2011. Faculty and resident physicians' attitudes, perceptions, and knowledge about antimicrobial use and resistance. *Infection Control and Hospital Epidemiology* 32 (7): 714–718.

Antibiotic Expert Groups. 2019. *Therapeutic guidelines: Antibiotic, version 16*. Melbourne, Therapeutic Guidelines. https://tgldcdp.tg.org.au/guideLine?guidelinePage=Antibiotic&frompage=etgcomplete

Aristotle. 1980. *The Nicomachean Ethics*. Trans. W.D. Ross. Oxford: Oxford University Press.

Australian Commission on Safety and Quality in Health Care. 2020. *Antimicrobial prescribing practice in Australian hospitals: Results of the 2018 Hospital National Antimicrobial Prescribing Survey*, January 2020. https://www.ncas-australia.org/ncas-publications.

Blumenthal-Barby, J.S., and H. Krieger. 2015. Cognitive biases and heuristics in medical decision-making: A critical review. *Medical Decision Making* 35 (4): 539–557.

Britten, Nicky. 1995. Patients' demands for prescriptions in primary care. *British Medical Journal* 310 (29): 1084–1085.

Britten, Nicky, and Obioha Ukoumunne. 1997. The influence of patients' hopes of receiving a prescription on doctors' perceptions and the decision to prescribe: A questionnaire survey. *British Medical Journal* 315 (7121): 1506–1510.

Collignon, Peter J. 2002. Antibiotic resistance. *Medical Journal of Australia* 177 (6): 325–329.

Costelloe, Céire, et al. 2010. Effect of antibiotic prescribing in primary care on antimicrobial resistance in individual patients: Systematic review and meta-analysis. *British Medical Journal* 340 (18): c2096.

Crisp, Roger. 2015. The duty to do the best for one's patient. *Journal of Medical Ethics* 41: 220–223.

Cui, Dan, et al. 2017. Use of and microbial resistance to antibiotics in China: A path to reducing antimicrobial resistance. *Journal of International Medical Research* 45 (6): 1768–1778.

Dallas, Anthea, et al. 2014. Antibiotic prescribing for the future: Exploring the attitudes of trainees in general practice. *British Journal of General Practice* 64 (626): e561–e567.

Fleming-Dutra, Katherine E., et al. 2016. Prevalence of inappropriate antibiotic prescriptions among US ambulatory care visits, 2010–2011. *Journal of the American Medical Association* 315 (17): 1864–1873.

Hallsworth, Michael, et al. 2016. Provision of social norm feedback to high prescribers of antibiotics in general practice: A pragmatic national randomised controlled trial. *The Lancet* 387 (10029): 1743–1752.

Halpern, David. 2015. *Inside the nudge unit*. London: WH Allen.

Hursthouse, Rosalind. 1999. *On virtue ethics*, Oxford: Oxford University Press.

Iyer, Kiran. 2017. Nudging virtue. *Southern California Interdisciplinary Law Journal* 26: 469–492.

Linder, Jeffrey A., et al. 2014. Time of day and decision to prescribe antibiotics. *JAMA Internal Medicine* 174 (12): 2029–2031.

Macfarlane, John, et al. 1997. Influence of patients' expectations on antibiotic management of acute lower respiratory tract illness in general practice: Questionnaire study. *British Medical Journal* 315 (7117): 1211–1214.

McCullough, Amanda R., et al. 2017. Antibiotics for acute respiratory infections in general practice: Comparison of prescribing rates with guideline recommendations. *Medical Journal of Australia* 207 (2): 65–69.

McMahon, Marilyn. 1992. Dangerousness, confidentiality, and the duty to protect. *Australian Psychologist* 27 (1): 12–16.

Mehrotra, Ateev, and Jeffrey A. Linder. 2017. Tipping the balance towards fewer antibiotics. *JAMA Internal Medicine* 176 (11): 1649–1650.

Metlay, Joshua P., et al. 2002. Tensions in antibiotic prescribing: Pitting social concerns against the interests of individual patients. *Journal of General Internal Medicine* 17: 87–94.

Milgram, Stanley. 2010. *Obedience to authority: An experimental view*. London: Pinter and Martin.

Millar, M. 2020. A capability perspective on antibiotic resistance, inequality, and child development. In *Ethics and drug resistance: Collective responsibility for global public health*. Cham: Springer.

Niker, Fay. 2018. Policy-led virtue cultivation: Can we 'nudge' citizens towards developing virtues? In *The theory and practice of virtue education*, ed. T. Harrison and D. Walker, 153–168. London: Routledge.

Nussbaum, Martha C. 2006. *Frontiers of justice: Disability, nationality, species membership*. Cambridge, MA: Harvard University Press.

Oakley, Justin. 1994. Sketch of a virtue ethics approach to health care resource allocation. *Monash Bioethics Review* 13 (4): 27–33.

———. 2018a. Toward an empirically informed approach to medical virtues. In *The Oxford handbook of virtue*, ed. Nancy E. Snow, 571–590. Oxford: Oxford University Press.

———. 2018b. Creating regulatory environments for practical wisdom and role virtues in medical practice. In *Cultivating moral character and virtue in professional practice*, ed. David Carr, 83–95. London: Routledge.

Oakley, Justin, and Dean Cocking. 2001. *Virtue ethics and professional roles*, Cambridge: Cambridge University Press.

Angus Randall. 2017. Antibiotics: GPs prescribing to patients at up to nine times higher than current guidelines. ABC Radio, *The World Today*, 11 July 2017. http://www.abc.net.au/news/2017-07-10/australians-overloaded-with-antibiotics-research/8693600.

Russell, Daniel C. 2009. *Practical intelligence and the virtues*. New York: Oxford University Press.

———. 2015. What virtue ethics can learn from utilitarianism. In *The Cambridge companion to utilitarianism*, ed. Ben Eggleston and Dale E. Miller, 258–279. Cambridge: Cambridge University Press.

Saposnik, G., D. Redelmeier, C.C. Ruff, and P.N. Tobler. 2016. Cognitive biases associated with medical decisions: A systematic review. *BMC Medical Informatics and Decision Making* 16 (138): 1–14.

Saripanidas, Stavros. 2016. Antibiotic abuse in Greece. *British Medical Journal* 355: i6328.

Scott, Ian A., et al. 2017. Countering cognitive biases in minimising low value care. *Medical Journal of Australia* 206 (9): 407–411.

Sharma, Aditya, et al. 2017. Estimating the future burden of multidrug-resistant and extensively drug-resistant tuberculosis in India, the Philippines, Russia, and South Africa: A mathematical modelling study. *The Lancet: Infectious Diseases* 17 (7): 707–715.

Snow, Nancy E. 2009. How ethical theory can improve practice: Lessons from Abu Ghraib. *Ethical Theory and Moral Practice* 12 (5): 555–568.

———. 2010. *Virtue as social intelligence: An empirically grounded theory*. New York: Routledge.

Swanton, Christine. 2003. *Virtue ethics: A pluralistic view*. Oxford: Oxford University Press.

Tversky, Amos, and Daniel Kahneman. 1981. The framing of decisions and the psychology of choice. *Science* 211 (4481): 453–458.

Yao, Zhenjiang, et al. 2015. Healthcare associated infections of Methicillin-resistant *Staphylococcus aureus*: A case-control-control study. *PLoS One* 10 (10): e0140604.

Permissions

All chapters in this book were first published in EDRCRGPH, by Springer; hereby published with permission under the Creative Commons Attribution License or equivalent. Every chapter published in this book has been scrutinized by our experts. Their significance has been extensively debated. The topics covered herein carry significant findings which will fuel the growth of the discipline. They may even be implemented as practical applications or may be referred to as a beginning point for another development.

The contributors of this book come from diverse backgrounds, making this book a truly international effort. This book will bring forth new frontiers with its revolutionizing research information and detailed analysis of the nascent developments around the world.

We would like to thank all the contributing authors for lending their expertise to make the book truly unique. They have played a crucial role in the development of this book. Without their invaluable contributions this book wouldn't have been possible. They have made vital efforts to compile up to date information on the varied aspects of this subject to make this book a valuable addition to the collection of many professionals and students.

This book was conceptualized with the vision of imparting up-to-date information and advanced data in this field. To ensure the same, a matchless editorial board was set up. Every individual on the board went through rigorous rounds of assessment to prove their worth. After which they invested a large part of their time researching and compiling the most relevant data for our readers.

The editorial board has been involved in producing this book since its inception. They have spent rigorous hours researching and exploring the diverse topics which have resulted in the successful publishing of this book. They have passed on their knowledge of decades through this book. To expedite this challenging task, the publisher supported the team at every step. A small team of assistant editors was also appointed to further simplify the editing procedure and attain best results for the readers.

Apart from the editorial board, the designing team has also invested a significant amount of their time in understanding the subject and creating the most relevant covers. They scrutinized every image to scout for the most suitable representation of the subject and create an appropriate cover for the book.

The publishing team has been an ardent support to the editorial, designing and production team. Their endless efforts to recruit the best for this project, has resulted in the accomplishment of this book. They are a veteran in the field of academics and their pool of knowledge is as vast as their experience in printing. Their expertise and guidance has proved useful at every step. Their uncompromising quality standards have made this book an exceptional effort. Their encouragement from time to time has been an inspiration for everyone.

The publisher and the editorial board hope that this book will prove to be a valuable piece of knowledge for researchers, students, practitioners and scholars across the globe.

List of Contributors

Euzebiusz Jamrozik
Monash Bioethics Centre, Monash University, Clayton, VIC, Australia
Royal Melbourne Hospital Department of Medicine, University of Melbourne, Parkville, VIC, Australia
Wellcome Centre for Ethics and the Humanities and The Ethox Centre, Nuffield Department of Population Health, University of Oxford, Oxford, UK

Michael J. Selgelid
Monash Bioethics Centre, Monash University, Melbourne, VIC, Australia

Bridget Haire
Kirby Institute, University of NSW, Sydney, Australia

Gwendolyn L. Gilbert
Sydney Health Ethics, University of Sydney, Sydney, NSW, Australia
Marie Bashir Institute for Emerging Infections and Biosecurity, University of Sydney, Sydney, NSW, Australia

Ian Kerridge
Sydney Health Ethics, University of Sydney, Sydney, NSW, Australia
Department of Haematology, Royal North Shore Hospital, Sydney, NSW, Australia

Binh Nguyen
Woolcock Institute of Medical Research, University of Sydney, Sydney, NSW, Australia

Greg J. Fox
Woolcock Institute of Medical Research, University of Sydney, Sydney, NSW, Australia
Faculty of Medicine, University of Sydney, Sydney, NSW, Australia

Paul H. Mason
Woolcock Institute of Medical Research, University of Sydney, Sydney, NSW, Australia
School of Social Sciences, Monash University, Melbourne, VIC, Australia

Justin T. Denholm
Department of Microbiology and Immunology, University of Melbourne, Melbourne, VIC, Australia
Victorian Tuberculosis Program at the Doherty Institute, Melbourne, VIC, Australia

Phaik Yeong Cheah
Mahidol Oxford Tropical Medicine Research Unit (MORU), Faculty of Tropical Medicine, Mahidol University, Bangkok, Thailand
Centre for Tropical Medicine and Global Health, Nuffield Department of Clinical Medicine, University of Oxford, Oxford, UK
The Ethox Centre, Nuffield Department of Population Health, University of Oxford, Oxford, UK

Michael Parker
The Ethox Centre, Nuffield Department of Population Health, University of Oxford, Oxford, UK
Wellcome Centre for Ethics and Humanities, Nuffield Department of Population Health, University of Oxford, Oxford, UK

Nicholas P. J. Day
Mahidol Oxford Tropical Medicine Research Unit (MORU), Faculty of Tropical Medicine, Mahidol University, Bangkok, Thailand
Centre for Tropical Medicine and Global Health, Nuffield Department of Clinical Medicine, University of Oxford, Oxford, UK

Carl H. Coleman
School of Law, Seton Hall University, Newark, NJ, USA

Alberto Giubilini
Wellcome Centre for Ethics and Humanities, University of Oxford, Oxford, UK
Oxford Uehiro Centre for Practical Ethics, University of Oxford, Oxford, UK

J. Savulescu
Oxford Uehiro Centre for Practical Ethics, University of Oxford, Oxford, UK
Visiting Professorial Fellow in Biomedical Ethics, Murdoch Children's Research Institute, Melbourne, Australia
Distinguished Visiting Professor on Law, Melbourne Law School, University of Melbourne, Melbourne, Australia

Morten Fibieger Byskov and Marcel Verweij
Communication, Philosophy, and Technology, Wageningen University & Research, Wageningen, Netherlands

Babette Olga Rump
The Netherlands National Institute for Public Health and the Environment (RIVM), Bilthoven, Netherlands

Lisa Boden
Global Academy of Agriculture and Food Security, The Royal (Dick) School of Veterinary Studies and The Roslin Institute, University of Edinburgh, Edinburgh, UK

Dominic Mellor
School of Veterinary Medicine, College of Medical, Veterinary and Life Sciences, University of Glasgow, Glasgow, UK

Marco Liverani
Department of Global Health and Development, London School of Hygiene and Tropical Medicine, London, UK
Faculty of Public Health, Mahidol University, Bangkok, Thailand
School of Tropical Medicine and Global Health, Nagasaki University, Nagasaki, Japan

Lauren Oliveira Hashiguchi
Department of Global Health and Development, London School of Hygiene and Tropical Medicine, London, UK
School of Tropical Medicine and Global Health, Nagasaki University, Nagasaki, Japan

Mishal Khan and Richard Coker
Department of Global Health and Development, London School of Hygiene and Tropical Medicine, London, UK
Faculty of Public Health, Mahidol University, Bangkok, Thailand

Remmy Shawa
School of Public Health and Family Medicine, University of Cape Town, Cape Town, South Africa

Fons Coomans
Department of International and European Law, Maastricht University, Maastricht, The Netherlands

Helen Cox
Division of Medical Microbiology and Institute of Infectious Disease and Molecular Medicine, University of Cape Town, Cape Town, South Africa

Leslie London
Division of Public Health Medicine, University of Cape Town, Cape Town, South Africa

Michael J. Selgelid
Monash Bioethics Centre, Monash University, Melbourne, VIC, Australia

Justin Oakley
Monash Bioethics Centre, Monash University, Melbourne, VIC, Australia

Index

www.ingramcontent.com/pod-product-compliance
Lightning Source LLC
LaVergne TN
LVHW080607210926
848485LV00003B/111